A

THE NEW YORK ACADEMY OF MEDICINE: ITS FIRST HUNDRED YEARS

by Philip Van Ingen

. . . for review

Publication date . . .

July 1, 1949

Price . . . $10.00

Please do not release reviews before publication date

COLUMBIA UNIVERSITY PRESS

Morningside Heights, New York

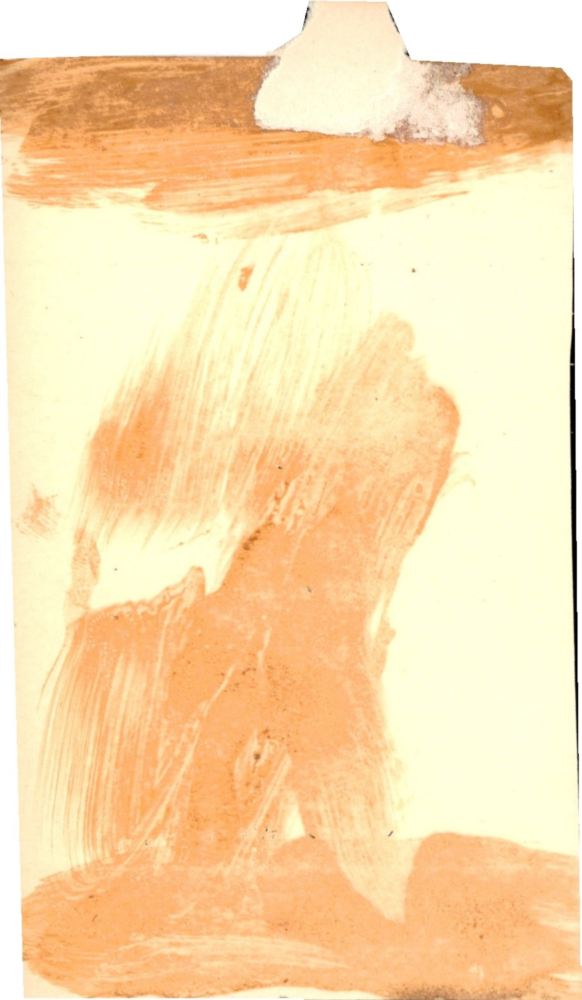

The New York Academy of Medicine

ITS FIRST HUNDRED YEARS

NUMBER VIII OF THE HISTORY OF MEDICINE SERIES
ISSUED UNDER THE AUSPICES OF
THE LIBRARY OF THE NEW YORK ACADEMY
OF MEDICINE

The New York Academy of Medicine

ITS FIRST HUNDRED YEARS

by Philip Van Ingen

New York: COLUMBIA UNIVERSITY PRESS

1949

PUBLISHED IN GREAT BRITAIN, CANADA, AND INDIA BY GEOFFREY CUMBERLEGE
OXFORD UNIVERSITY PRESS, LONDON, TORONTO, AND BOMBAY

MANUFACTURED IN THE UNITED STATES OF AMERICA

Preface

THE history of the New York Academy of Medicine is spread over some 6,000 pages of minutes of Stated Meetings, and meetings of the Trustees and the Council. There are as many or more pages of minutes of the Standing and Special Committees, of the Sections, and the Treasurer's records. To read through these volumes, and put related facts together in a readable form, was a time-consuming undertaking. Incidentally to decipher some of the old handwriting was a real task.

Every paper, essay, lecture, and report was supposed to be turned over to the Librarian to be filed and stored. But for thirty years the Librarian had no library in which to store them. Many reports were "read and ordered on file," their contents not being recorded. Diligent search has failed to uncover them. Some were ordered printed in the daily press. Photostats of some of these have been secured. Others were ordered printed in the medical journals and could be found, if the journal printed them, which was not always the case. All such material, either original or in photostat, is now in the Library of the Academy.

Long discussions of its own affairs, as well as controversial medical problems, took place with the Academy "sitting as a Committee of the Whole." Only the vote "to receive the report of the Committee of the Whole" is recorded. And occasionally it was voted that discussion of a matter be "stricken from the record." These discussions would undoubtedly have been illuminating.

Admission of the lay press was barred for many years, since the public was not considered capable of understanding medical matters. The lay press gained entrance, however, quite often and considerable information has been obtained from old newspaper files. Notwithstanding, the needle is often difficult to find in those haystacks.

The sixteen volumes of the *Transactions* and twenty-six volumes of the *Bulletin* are valuable source material. Between 1903 and 1925 the Academy published nothing, but the medical journals covered its proceedings very fully, and these have been carefully gone over. To the student of the history of the practice of medicine the early records are of the greatest interest.

The compilation of this history of the Academy was started in September, 1945. As work progressed, that Sword of Damocles—the year 1947—hung by a thread ever becoming thinner and thinner. The history, which was completed and turned over to the Council at the end of April, 1947, at the close of the Centennial ceremonies, attempts to describe the growth and work of the Academy during its first hundred years fully enough to be informative, and not long enough to be tiresome. Incomplete though it is, it is submitted for the information of the Fellows of the Academy and such of the general public as may be interested.

In compiling this material the author has been under deep obligation to the entire staff of the Academy and especially to that of the Library. He was free to wander where he pleased and had access to everything. By direction of the Librarian, Dr. Malloch, all limitations on the number of books he could take out and the length of time he could keep them were waived. The author was able to deal directly with the Photostat Division and, with the willing cooperation of Mr. Schumacher, was able to obtain immediate service, thus saving much valuable time. He is indebted to every member of the staff.

While it is difficult to pick out individuals, it is only proper he should express his special thanks to Dr. Malloch and Miss Doe, in charge of the Library, for constant advice, help, and encouragement; to Miss Helen Sayer of the Bibliographical Department for locating hundreds of references in the old journals; to Drs. Ashford and Galdston for detailed written information of the history of their Departments; to Mr. Eberle, the Comptroller, for his patience in giving and *explaining* details of financial activities; to Dr. Wilcox, the late Director, and to Dr. Craig, his successor, for special information and encouragement; to Dr. Baehr for his stimulating interest; and

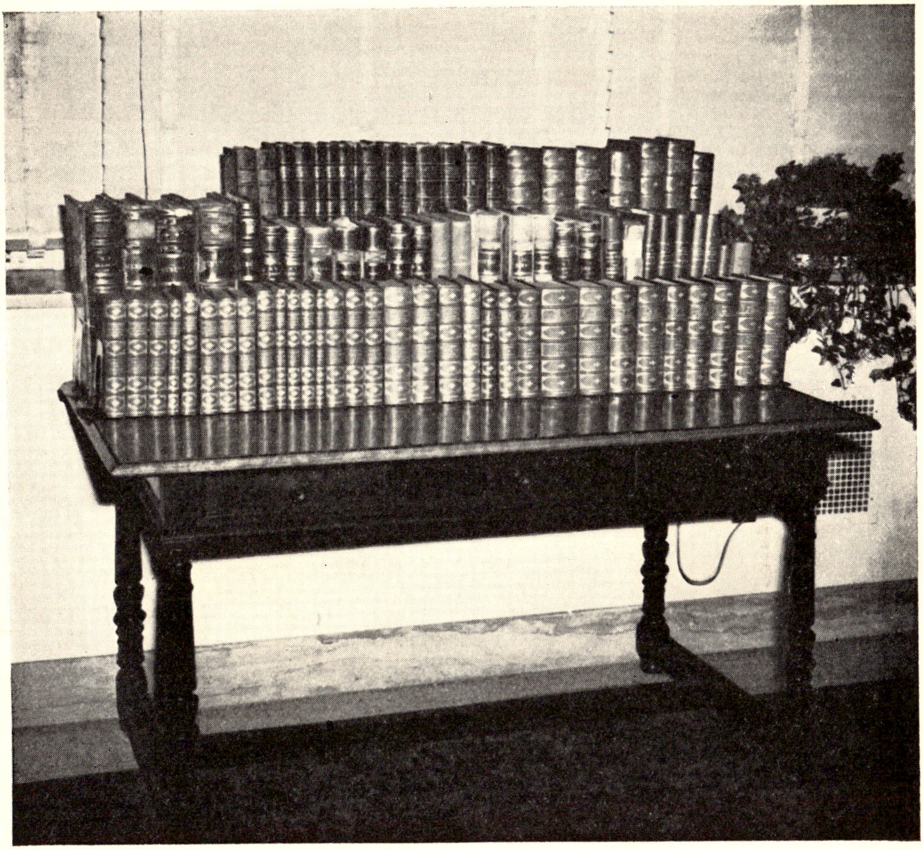

SOME SOURCE MATERIAL

to Mrs. Sproull, Secretary to the Director since 1925, for her help and patience in constant requests for information and inroads on her files of correspondence.

He is indebted to Dr. James Alexander Miller and Dr. Malcolm Goodridge for their help in matters occurring during their Presidencies.

And most especially is he indebted to Miss Gertrude Annan, in charge of the Rare Book Room. His work would have been more difficult without the help of her experience, constant and deep interest, helpful advice and criticism. In addition, beside her own time-consuming work, she volunteered to compile the very complete index for this volume. Too much appreciation cannot be expressed.

To those outside the Academy, he wishes to express his thanks to Miss Dorothy Barck, of the New York Historical Society, for help in locating and procuring photostats of old newspaper articles dealing with the Academy; to Mrs. Laura E. Smith, Library Consultant, for helpful information and especially in interesting Mrs. Joseph Devlin and Mrs. Frank Hennessy, to turn over to the Academy a priceless scrapbook of records compiled by their father, Mr. Brownne, who was the Academy's first Librarian and who filled that office for forty-five years.

To Mrs. John W. Brown and Mrs. Florence H. Watson de Muralt, granddaughters of Dr. John Watson, tenth President of the Academy, he expresses his thanks for donating Dr. Watson's autobiography written for Dr. John W. Francis, which threw much light on the founding of the Academy, and for other valuable source material.

To the Trustees and Council his thanks are due. They have been most generous in making the work as easy as possible, and have been very patient. His every request has been granted. Two offices have been provided, one for his secretary and one for himself. For a number of months two secretaries were really provided, the second being a two-machine "Soundscriber" outfit. It was thus possible to dictate while the previous day's dictation was being typed. This saved an enormous amount of time.

To his secretary Miss Mary Williams Lienau is due a debt of gratitude that cannot be adequately expressed. His personal secretary for thirty years, the niece of Dr. Linsly R. Williams, first Director of the Academy, she worked on this history with a personal pride and great patience. To meet the whimsies and demands of an historian working under "forced draught" was a long and hard grind. That the result contains no more mistakes or omissions, is largely thanks to her.

PHILIP VAN INGEN

New York
July, 1948

Table of Contents

Illustrations

The New York Academy of Medicine

ITS FIRST HUNDRED YEARS

Prologue

THE "EDITOR'S TABLE" of the *Annalist,* New York December 1, 1846, contains the following:

"The fourth anniversary of the Society for the Relief of Widows and Orphans of Medical Men was celebrated on Wednesday evening, 18th ult. About eighty gentlemen sat down to a beautiful entertainment prepared by M. Peteler at his saloon, No. 579 Broadway. The *Coup d'Oeil* of the supper table was extremely good, and the arrangements were highly creditable to the taste of the artist. Every delicacy of the season abounded upon the festive board, interspersed with many superb specimens of confectionery of the latest fashion; the creams, jellies and pastry, were of the finest description, and the sparkling wine circulated freely about the table. The room was brilliantly lighted, and the excellent arrangements made by the stewards who, regardless of self, exerted themselves indefatigably in behalf of their guests, contributed to make it, perhaps, the most agreeable and elegant entertainment ever offered to the medical profession in this city. At the cross-table, at the upper end of the room, sat the President, Dr. Delafield, having on his left Professor Mott, and on his right the Rev. Dr. Vermilyea, (who invoked the blessing upon the repast set before him, briefly, but expressively)."

After "ample justice" had been done to the "substantials and luxuries," the venerable President, Dr. Edward Delafield, spoke of the origin of the Society and the toasts began.

The third toast was "the Medical Colleges and Schools of our Country," to which "Dr. Mott pertinently replied, as the oldest medical teacher present, although modestly." He then gave the toast "The College of Physicians and Surgeons of the City of New York, which brought President Stevens on his legs. He said that speech making was an operation he was not well calculated to perform. . . . He congratulated the profession on the large assembly, upon an occasion of this kind; it was the initial step for an esprit de corps in the profession of the city, which was the *sine qua non*, without which it could not sustain its dignity and command respect. Instead of being anatomists of one another, the disjecta membra of the profession wanted to be brought together and become a body corporate. . . . He concluded a very appealing address by expressing the hope that the increasing unanimity in the corps would lead soon to the establishment of a medical hall, unconnected with hospitals or colleges, to contain meeting room, a library, etc., and be a place of general resort, both for ourselves and brethren from abroad. (Much applause.)"

After eight formal toasts had been offered and responded to, the article concludes; "Many volunteer toasts were given . . . and throughout the evening many excellent songs and stories were given. The entertainment passed off in the greatest harmony. . . . After the retirement of the President and the major part of the company, about forty gentlemen remained to prolong the festivities who voted Dr. Stevens into the chair. In consequence of the suggestion of this gentleman they organized themselves into a meeting, to discuss the propriety of establishing a local medical voluntary association, having for its objects the purification of the professional body, etc; the objects of which, will, when they shall have been matured by a committee appointed for the purpose, be made public, and promised the highest interest and advantage."

Thus was conceived the New York Academy of Medicine.

Founding of the Academy

Beginning on December 8, 1846, this notice appeared in several newspapers:

The subscribers request the regular practitioners of this city to meet on Saturday next, December 12th instant, at 1 P.M. at the Lyceum of Natural History, No. 561 Broadway.

The design of this call is to ask co-operation of our medical brethren in an undertaking intended to elevate the character of our profession and to advance its interests and increase its usefulness by furnishing facilities for medical intercourse, promoting harmony among its members, and offering means of mutual improvement therein.

In the prosecution of these objects it is proposed to establish an Academy of Medicine and Surgery and to provide a permanent place for its meetings.

Valentine Mott
Alex. H. Stevens
Isaac Wood

Dr. Valentine Mott was President and Professor of Surgery at the New York University Medical College, and sixty-one years old; Dr. Stevens, President of the College of Physicians and Surgeons, the older of the medical schools, fifty-eight; and Dr. Isaac Wood, President of the "Medical Society of the City and County of New York" as it was then called, fifty-four years old.

A "numerously attended meeting of the regular practitioners of medicine in this city" was held and Dr. John Stearns was made Chairman and Dr. Campbell Stewart, Secretary. These resolutions were offered:

First, Resolved that it is expedient to organize an Academy of Medicine in this city, which shall represent, if not embrace, the great mass of regular practitioners residing here.

Second, Resolved that it be expedient to procure a building to be devoted to the use of the Academy of Medicine and that shall also serve as a hall in which the regular members of the profession may meet on common ground.

Third, Resolved that a subscription be commenced for this purpose.

Fourth, Resolved that a Committee of (blank) be now appointed to prepare a Constitution and By Laws.

Many remarks were made upon the necessity of "changing the character of the profession," the "rampancy of quackery" which had deprived it of the confidence of the public; drawing a line between "science and roguery"; the exclusion of those who practiced Homeopathy even though graduates of a regular school, and so on.

Dr. Mott stated that any swerving from the path of professional rectitude meant exclusion, the least flavor or tincture of Homeopathy would not be recognized by those of the old school. "We must all alter our generation and be educated anew before we can believe in the doctrine of the infinitesimal."

Dr. Isaac Wood wished to exclude not only irregular practitioners, but also those who *met and consulted* with them. He desired membership to be considered as a guarantee to the public of the qualifications and respectability of the physician.

Thus were expressed the main motives for forming the Academy.

It was then voted unanimously that it was "expedient" to form such an Academy. The proposals to procure immediately a building and to commence a subscription for this purpose were laid on the table "for the present."

The appointment of a Committee to draw up a Constitution caused much discussion. It was finally decided that a committee of eleven be appointed; that the Chairman of the meeting be Chairman of the Committee and that he be empowered to appoint the other ten. Dr. Stearns promptly announced the Committee, which was no sooner done than objections were raised, it being noted that those who had called the meeting were not included in the list. Finally, after voting to reconsider, Dr. R. S. Kissam's motion prevailed—that "the gentlemen who had been named by the Chair should, together with those who had signed the call to the meeting, constitute the committee"—and the names of Drs. Mott, Stevens and

Isaac Wood were added to the list already announced, fourteen in all.

The meeting then adjourned to assemble at the same place on January 6 at one o'clock P.M., due public notice of the same to be given, through the press. Much valuable professional time must have been lost on that midwinter afternoon.

Under date of December 31, 1846, and after, there appeared, tucked away among various advertisements, the following notice. It is surprising that anybody saw it.

NOTICE—An Adjourned meeting of the regular Practitioners of Medicine of this city, will be held at the Lyceum of Natural History, No. 561 Broadway, on Wednesday, the 6th of January, 1847, at one o'clock P.M. to receive the report of the committee appointed on the 12th inst. to prepare a Constitution and By Laws for an "Academy of Medicine."

F. Campbell Stewart, M.D.
Secretary

At this meeting before the report was read, Dr. Stevens announced that the instrument about to be presented was the result of much care and pains on the part of the whole committee. It was not perfect, but changes could be made later and he hoped the Academy would adopt it as read. The Constitution and By Laws were then read.

"A friendly discussion ensued." After considerable discussion as to whether to act on each article, or adopt it as a whole, the Constitution and By Laws were adopted without a single adverse vote. This was a good start for the Academy.

The name selected was "The New York Academy of Medicine." The objects of the new organization were:

First. The separation of the regular from irregular practitioners.

Second. The association of the profession proper for purposes of mutual recognition and fellowship.

Third. The promotion of the character, interests, and honor of the fraternity, by maintaining the union and harmony of the regular profession of the city and its vicinity, and aiming to elevate the standard of medical education.

Fourth. The cultivation and advancement of the science, by our united exertions for mutual improvement, and our contributions to medical literature.

The Academy was to consist of Resident Fellows, "regular practitioners, resident for three years in the City, State, or vicinity," and Corresponding Fellows. "No proprietor or vendor of any patent or secret remedy or medicine, nor any empirical or irregular practitioner" could be admitted or retain his membership.

The Academy was to be administered by a President, four Vice Presidents, a Recording Secretary, two Corresponding Secretaries, designated for domestic and foreign correspondence, a Treasurer and a Librarian, all to be elected annually by ballot at the regular meeting in January. The President was to appoint, immediately after his election, five Standing Committees, each of which was to consist of five Resident Fellows,—Admissions, Finance, Medical Ethics, Publications, and a Council of Appeal.

The By Laws provided for regular meetings, the first Wednesday of each month, a quorum to consist of twenty-one. At each meeting all five Standing Committees, the Corresponding Secretaries, Librarian and Treasurer were to report—a long and tedious procedure for each meeting.

The Committee on Admissions was to guard the portals of the Academy and to see that no irregular or unqualified practitioner gained entrance.

The Committee on Finance was to recommend an "annual tax" not to exceed $3 per annum, prompt payment of which was to be considered a "point of honor." It was also required to provide quarters for the Library and Museum.

The Committee on Medical Ethics was to "hear and decide" all complaints of breach of etiquette or violations of medical ethics, and rule on all questions of medical ethics submitted to it.

The Committee on Publications was to superintend the printing of all orations, memoirs, or papers on uniform paper and page under title of *Transactions of the New York Academy of Medicine.*

The Council of Appeal was to decide all questions of violations of the provisions of the Constitution and could summon any Fellow to appear before it.

The unfortunate Librarian was given charge of "all books, pamphlets, manuscripts, anatomical or pathological specimens, apparatus, instruments, medals, coins or scientific property of whatever kind," and was to keep a catalogue and designate every article with the name of the donor. A copy of "every oration, memoir, or medical paper read before the Academy" was to be kept in his archives. Where he was to keep them was *his* problem.

The names of Resident Fellows were to be "published once each year in at least four of the newspapers of the city, certified by the President and Secretary."

These were the important items in the By Laws.

After much discussion it was decided that all present at the December meeting or at the present meeting should be enrolled as Founders, that the Chairman of the meeting should sign the Constitution first, then some of the elder members of the profession, the Committee on the Constitution, and finally the Secretary, to be followed by the others in alphabetical order.

After the presiding officer, three of the elder members of the profession were invited to sign—Drs. Gilbert Smith, seventy-five, Consulting Physician, Asylum for Lying-In Women and the New York Dispensary; James Manley, sixty-four; and Thomas Cock, sixty-three, Consulting Physician to the New York Hospital and Asylum for Lying-In Women, Vice President College of Physicians and Surgeons.

While the callers of the meeting, the Committee on Constitution, and the Secretary were signing, eleven other "elder members" were discovered and were invited individually to come forward and sign. They were Drs. J. P. Batchelder, sixty-two; F. E. Berger, fifty-six; Joseph M. Smith, fifty-seven, Attending Physician New York Hospital, Professor at the College of Physicians and Surgeons; W. W. Miner, sixty-six; John B. Beck, fifty-four, Professor at the College of Physicians and Surgeons; F. U. Johnston, fifty, Attending Physician, New York Hospital, and Consulting Physician, Asylum for Lying-In Women; Willard Parker, forty-six, Consulting Physician, New York

Dispensary, and Professor of Surgery, College of Physicians and Surgeons; C. R. Gilman, forty-five, Professor of Obstetrics and Diseases of Women and Children, College of Physicians and Surgeons; James L. Phelps, sixty-one; James Cameron, sixty-one; Thomas Van Beuren (age unknown; he died in 1848).

Dr. Hasbrouck, Sr., was invited to sign, but declined, not approving of the Constitution. In all, 132 signatures were affixed to the Constitution.

After electing a committee to nominate officers, they adjourned to meet a week later.

The *Annalist* of January 15, 1847, stated:

> The sixth of January last was a proud day for the profession of this city and one which is destined, we fondly believe, to be commemorated hereafter as the commencement of a new era in our science. It witnessed, we trust, the founding of the first great barrier between quackery and medical integrity; the first establishment of a stringent motive for ethical observance, the desire of standing well among one's fellows; and the first step toward a professional harmony of purpose and sentiment, the suppression of roguery and the elevation of the standard of professional qualifications.

The Editor of the *New York Medical and Surgical Reporter* intimates the intensity of feeling at this meeting. He tells us Dr. Mott, President of New York University School of Medicine, asked whether he could sign. He had used with great success Morton's patented anaesthetic "Letheon" (ether) having been assured by Dr. Warren, of Boston, that he knew the component parts. He was very anxious to sign, and said that "if he had done wrong, he would use it no more." Dr. Mott was probably the most important and influential person present. Dr. Stevens, President of the College of Physicians and Surgeons, immediately moved "that it is unbecoming for any member of this Academy to employ any secret nostrum." As it was admitted most of them used "McMunn's Elixir of Opium" and "Henry's Magnesia," it was voted to refer the matter to the Committee on Ethics, and Dr. Mott signed.

The Academy was thus founded January 6, 1847, for the next meeting is recorded as an "adjourned meeting of the New York Academy of Medicine."

On January 13, the Academy met at Lyceum Hall at 1 P.M. It was unanimously voted that as no officers had been elected the Academy was not yet organized, and therefore any person who desired to enroll, against whom nobody spoke, could sign as a Founder. Fifty-three did so, which, with 132 already signed, made the "Founders" 185 in number, and the list was closed.

The Committee on Nominations presented a list of thirty names, three for each of the ten offices, as directed. Drs. Mott, Stevens, and Isaac Wood, who were nominated for Vice Presidents, begged leave to decline "on account of their desire to promote the objects and interests of the Academy," which they thought they could do better from the floor.

Although officers were about to be elected, a Treasurer *pro tem* was appointed to collect at once the tax of one dollar, which had been imposed upon all who signed, to defray the "expenses of organization."

The vote for President was first cast. One hundred and twelve votes were counted and Dr. Stearns was declared President. He thanked the Academy for the honor and called for a divine blessing upon the new institution.

Dr. Stearns, the first President, was in his seventy-seventh year. He was well qualified to fill his difficult position. Graduating from Yale "with distinguished honor" in 1789, he attended lectures at the University of Pennsylvania, studying under Shippen, Wistar, and Rush. He did not wait to take an examination for a degree—a very common occurrence in those days—but began practice in Waterford, N.Y., in 1793. He proposed the formation of the State Society in 1806, and was its first Secretary in 1807 and for several years thereafter. In 1809, he was elected to the State Senate, and served till 1813, practicing in Albany from 1810 to 1819. He received the honorary degree of Doctor of Medicine from the Regents of the State of New York in 1812. He was President of the State Society in 1818, and was re-elected in 1819 and 1820. In 1819 he moved to New York, when he was forty-nine years old.

Dr. Isaac Wood, alert to enhance the ethical standards of the Academy, proposed two resolutions: that any member who consulted with a homeopath or other irregular practitioner be considered as having forfeited his membership, and that the Committee on Ethics be instructed to inquire into and report at the next meeting whether any improper members had already associated themselves with the Academy. Both these resolutions were referred to the Committee on Ethics.

Dr. Van Kleek had discovered that the order of business in the By Laws *omitted the reading of the minutes*, so he therefore offered an amendment to include that important item after roll call.

After this digression, and doubtless diversion, they voted for the other officers. While the Tellers were counting the votes, the President announced the various Standing Committees, as required by the Constitution.

The Tellers then announced the result of the election, and the first officers of the Academy were:

President: Dr. John Stearns

Vice Presidents: Drs. F. U. Johnston, Thomas Cock, John B. Beck, John W. Francis

Recording Secretary: Dr. F. Campbell Stewart

Domestic Corresponding Secretary: Dr. William C. Roberts

Foreign Corresponding Secretary: Dr. Benjamin Drake

Treasurer: Dr. Robert Watts, Jr.

Librarian: Dr. Thomas M. Markoe

Drs. Cock, Beck, Francis, Stewart, Roberts, and Drake had already been appointed on Standing Committees, so the direction and administration of the Academy was in the hands of twenty-nine men, all of the highest ethical and professional standing in the profession.

Dr. Isaac Wood then officially founded the Library by presenting a copy of "Paine's Commentaries" in three volumes. On this account, these volumes have stood in proud and undisturbed rest for many years in the Rare Book Room.

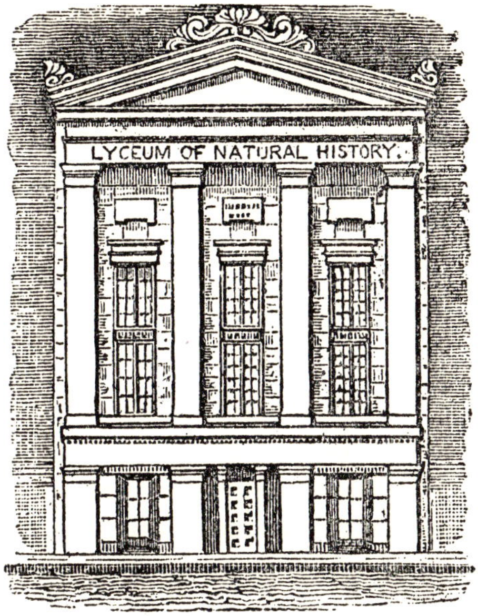

LYCEUM OF NATURAL HISTORY,
561 BROADWAY
Organization and First Stated Meetings Held Here

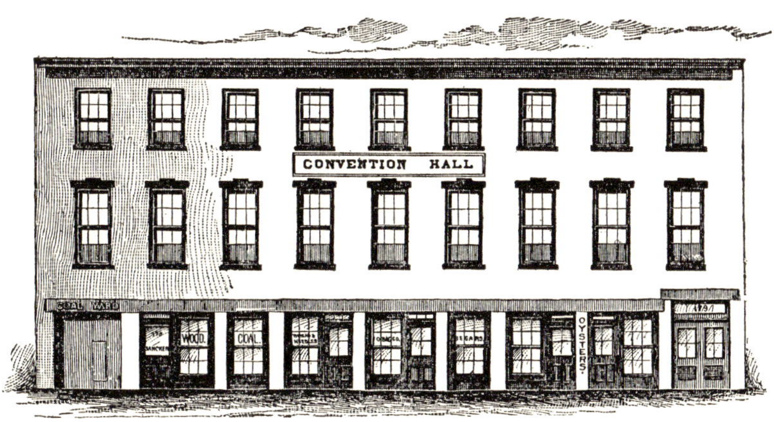

CONVENTION HALL, 175 WOOSTER STREET
Meetings Held Here from March 3, 1847, to July, 1850

The Academy met again on January 20, with 159 of its 185 enrolled members present. After considerable time was consumed by amendments offered to the two weeks' old Constitution and By Laws, it went into a Committee of the Whole. The Committee on Admissions had twenty-five names before it, and requested to be informed just what *did* constitute "regularity" and "irregularity." The discussion was long and "animated." After many definitions had been suggested, Dr. Manley's was accepted. It excluded "all homeopathic, hydropathic, chronothermal and botanic physicians, and also all mesmeric and clairvoyant pretenders to the healing art, and all others who at any time or on any pretext claimed peculiar merits for their mixed practices not founded on the best system of physiology and pathology, as taught in the best schools in Europe and America, and shall be deemed to exclude also all such persons as associate with them in consultation." This report was adopted without a dissenting vote.

The *Annalist* (New York) enthusiastically, and the *Boston Medical and Surgical Journal,* with dignified approval, commented at length on the founding of the Academy, and even from Berlin the *Allgemeine medicinische Central-Zeitung* noted: "AUSLAND . . . Zu New-York bildet sich eine Academy of Medicine and Surgery, welche alle legitimen Praktiker aufnimmt, Quacksalber verdrängen, die Ehre und Collegialitat der Aerzte heben will." (Foreign . . . In New York an Academy of Medicine and Surgery has been established, which receives all legitimate practitioners, rejects quacks, and will increase the honor and congeniality of physicians.)

1847

John Stearns

AFTER THESE FOUR long and argumentative meetings, the Academy held its first stated meeting, February 3, 1847, with eighty-seven Fellows present. The President read his inaugural address, which is chiefly notable for its brevity and the length of individual sentences. He closed by saying:

To elevate the standard of medical education, to exclude from our profession all ignorant pretenders, to enlighten the public mind on the subject of medicine and its collateral branches of science, and to take all necessary measures to promote the honor, the dignity, the respectability and the usefulness of the medical profession, appear to constitute the important topics for our future consideration.

After this, amendments already proposed were taken up. Dr. Calkins had strongly objected to the power of the Committee on Admissions to prevent any name from being voted on. He had moved that the Academy should vote on any name it desired, whether presented by the Committee or not. This was discussed and laid upon the table. The minutes state "Thereupon Dr. Calkins rose and stated that inasmuch as the Constitution, which he considered to be very imperfect, had been adopted without discussion, and as there appeared to be a disposition on the part of the Academy to prevent the introduction of amendments or alterations, which he thought important and necessary, he felt himself called upon to tender his resignation as a Fellow of the Academy."

Dr. Reese, none too pacific an individual, promptly moved that the Academy grant Dr. Calkins the privilege of withdrawing. Before the motion could be voted on, however, Dr. Calkins changed his mind and withdrew his offer of resignation. This amendment was later rejected by the Academy and Dr. Calkins resigned, the first Founder to do so.

The tenseness of the situation is illustrated in the election of Anniversary Orator, required to take place at the February meeting. Drs. Francis, Reese, and Manley had been nominated by a committee. After an attempt to suspend the By Laws and postpone the election until March had failed, it was put off for a week to an adjourned meeting. At that meeting, after another unsuccessful attempt to suspend the By Laws, it was voted to elect at another adjourned meeting a week later, at which 106 Fellows were present. It was then suggested that their past actions in the matter had been irregular, in which the President concurred. It was finally voted to expunge from the minutes the record of all actions considered irregular, which was done so thoroughly that we know nothing about what had been done.

While the Tellers were busy, the Secretary announced an acknowledgment in writing from Dr. J. R. Shearman that he had been guilty of violating one of the Academy's rules, by which he had forfeited his right to membership. His name was ordered erased from the list of Fellows of the Academy. His "offense against the rules" had been that he had consulted with a homeopath.

The Tellers then announced that Dr. Francis had been elected Orator, receiving 55 of 106 votes, and the election was promptly made unanimous.

The editor of the *Annalist* (incidentally Recording Secretary of the Academy) wrote at length about this meeting—"a very exciting one"—which "roused the fears of its warmest friends . . . for its stability." The Academy "had happily escaped the first dangers which threatened the shipwreck of her harmony," but he warned "the elements of tempest exist—a spirit slumbers easy to arouse and difficult to be again lulled."

The election for delegates to the National Convention in Philadelphia, which formed the American Medical Association, also caused much excitement. The Academy had voted it was "expedient" to send delegates, and discussed whether to send from five to thirty. Fifteen was decided as the number, and forty-one were nominated.

At the next meeting, the election was postponed to an adjourned meeting. It must have been a tedious affair. After a "ten minute recess," to "prepare ballots"—102 being present—as his name was read (184 on the roll call) each Fellow came forward and deposited his vote. The delegation elected attended the Convention and Dr. Stewart, the Chairman, reported to a later meeting by the new "magnetic telegram" that the Convention was organized.

During the first year, six meetings were held at the Lyceum of Natural History, 561 Broadway, and all at 1 P.M. In February the President, Secretary and Finance Committee were directed to procure a suitable room for meetings and to select a time for the same. They acted promptly and, on March 3, the Academy met at "Convention Hall," 175 Wooster Street, at 7 P.M. Except for special and anniversary meetings, all meetings were held here until July, 1850, and always in the evening. It was not a very attractive building, being built over a coalyard.

At first, almost everything was done through reference to committees, some for scientific reports, others for purely Academy affairs. The first of the latter was appointed to try to procure books for the Library. It sent out in April a circular asking if the recipients were willing to make a donation of medical books. The first page of this circular was a bookplate, which was to be signed by the donor and to be pasted in each book donated. It was too large to go in any octavo book.

Another committee was appointed to devise a seal for the Academy. It reported promptly that an "ancient medallion head of Hippocrates" had been selected. The motto suggested was HOMINES DEOS ACCEDUNT HOMINIBUS DANDO SALUTEM. It was immediately adopted, and "not more than $40" was appropriated for making the design. The seal shown is reproduced from the diploma issued to Dr. E. L. Beadle, dated January 6, 1847. As a model it leaves much to be desired. On the edge is the motto reading clockwise. Within, on either side of the head, is the divided word "Hippo-Krates" in Greek letters, which run counter-clockwise and which, read that way, shows the "Krates" upside down. This seal was in use until 1874.

Many other committees on minor subjects were also appointed. Six special scientific committees were appointed during the year.

The first was to investigate and report on "the use of Sulphuric Ether in mitigating pain in surgical operations" as extensively done in Europe. A committee of five was appointed, its report received and laid on the table. It was taken up again later, and an enlarged committee was appointed and instructed to make experiments on animals, otherwise investigate and report. That is the last heard of this committee.

In June, typhus fever was very prevalent and a committee was appointed to visit the hospitals, investigate the whole subject and report. They did so promptly, and the report was ordered printed in the daily press and medical journals. This was the first action of the Academy given to the press.

In August it was voted that a committee of eleven be appointed "to examine into the effects, proximate and remote, upon the general health of the City caused by the numerous distilleries, gas works, slaughter houses, milk establishments, lead manufacturies, tanneries and all other manufacturies and establishments which are, or may be styled nuisances, from their deleterious effects upon the health and particularly to report the effects upon the human economy of milk taken from kine tuberculously or otherwise diseased from improper food or confined situations in these milk establishments."

Dr. Gardner was appointed chairman. The Committee confined its work to the milk establishments, rendering a most detailed and creditable report thereon, which was published in the *Transactions* —eventually. The other "nuisances" were never taken up.

The Common Council of the City appointed a committee to study the subject of sewerage, and requested the Academy to investigate "in respect to the present and prospective sanitary condition of the city." A committee was appointed, but, apparently overwhelmed by the size of the undertaking, was discharged two years later without having made any report.

Another committee was appointed to cooperate with one from the College of Pharmacy on the subject of restriction of importation of adulterated and impure drugs. The reports of these committees caused long and animated discussions which occupied much of the Academy's time.

The five appointive Standing Committees had a large job. That on Ethics was very busy, but unfortunately its early minutes are not in existence. The first "charge against a Fellow" was presented March 3 and was referred to the Committee, which reported it had examined the charge, nothing was proven, and the charge had been withdrawn. Dr. W. W. Miner had been accused of consulting with a homeopath. Dr. Miner was elected Vice President the ensuing year.

The Committee recommended that hereafter charges should be presented to the Secretary in a sealed envelope, marked "Charge against a Fellow," that the Secretary should so announce it to the Academy, and that after being numbered it should be delivered unopened to the Committee. This recommendation was adopted. This, however, was the only charge presented during the year.

The Code of Ethics adopted by the American Medical Association was referred to the Academy's Committee on Ethics for their opinion. After study, they reported that, although the code was "not entirely in accordance with the views of the Committee," it was on the whole "well digested and suitable." On account of the advantages of one system of ethics for the whole profession, the Academy adopted it unanimously.

Dr. Gilman had previously made a motion that a committee be appointed to inquire whether any Fellows demanded and received a percentage on prescriptions sent to particular apothecaries. The Academy judged it "inexpedient" to investigate the matter.

The Committee on Finance had a hard time. The Treasurer was not one of its members, but he fairly frequently attended its meetings. One of its functions was to recommend the "tax" each year, and it explained at the start that owing to the many original expenses, it was forced to suggest the limit, three dollars, which the Academy approved.

But the Academy was not very far-seeing in financial matters. When Dr. Stout read a paper on "The Revelations of the Microscope," he concluded with a series of resolutions urging in substance that the first disposable funds of the Academy be devoted to the establishment of a laboratory—chemical, physiological, and pathological—with a Fellow in charge of each branch, and each

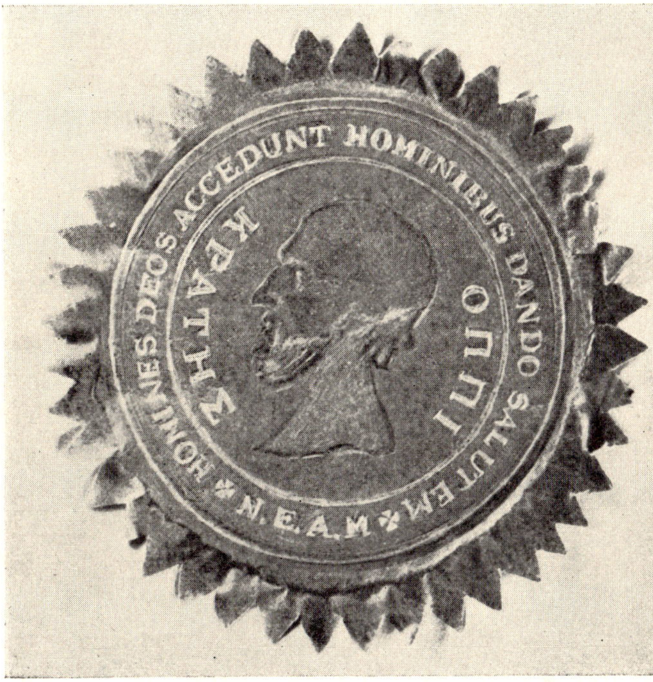
HOMINES DEOS ACCEDUNT HOMINIBUS DANDO SALUTEM
ΙΠΠΟ
ΚΡΑΤΗΣ
N.E.A.M.

THE ORIGINAL SEAL OF THE ACADEMY
USED UNTIL 1874

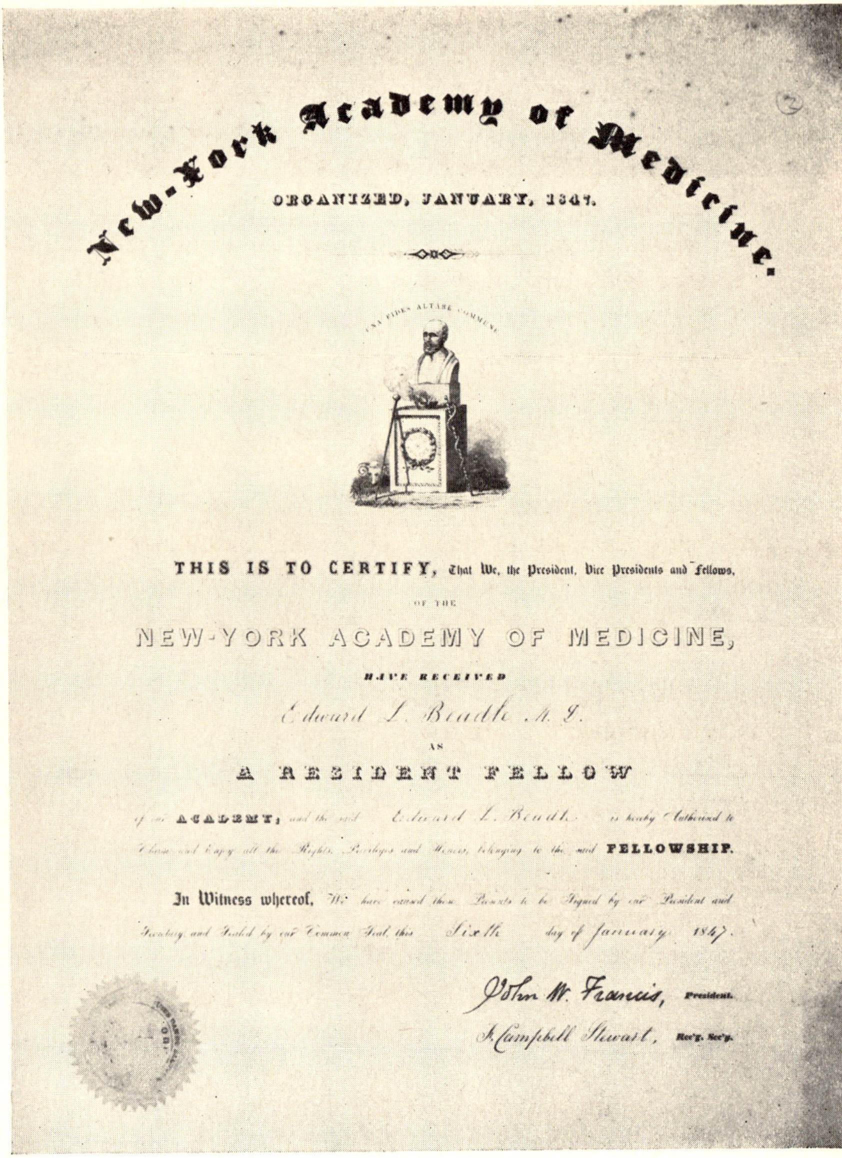

New-York Academy of Medicine.

ORGANIZED, JANUARY, 1847.

UNA FIDES ALTARE COMMUNE

THIS IS TO CERTIFY, That We, the President, Vice Presidents and Fellows,

OF THE

NEW-YORK ACADEMY OF MEDICINE,

HAVE RECEIVED

Edward L. Beadle M.D.

AS

A RESIDENT FELLOW

of our ACADEMY; and the said Edward L. Beadle is hereby Authorized to Claim and Enjoy all the Rights, Privileges and Honors, belonging to the said FELLOWSHIP.

In Witness whereof, We have caused these Presents to be Signed by our President and Secretary and Sealed by our Common Seal, this Sixth day of January 1847.

John W. Francis, President.

J. Campbell Stewart, Rec'g. Sec'y.

ORIGINAL CERTIFICATE OF FELLOWSHIP (REDUCED)

with an advisory council of three other Fellows. These branches were to examine pathological specimens submitted, test anatomical and physiological experiments reported, do original research, make medico-legal analyses, and test the purity of drugs of commerce. Nothing ever came of this.

Another example of this financial-dreaming is shown when, at a meeting in March, it was suggested that every member should be obliged to take one share or more of stock to pay for a building for the Academy, each share to cost $25, and to pay interest at not more than 6 percent. If each Fellow had bought two shares, the fund would have been about $11,250, and the interest would have amounted to $675, the total income of the Academy *if* dues were paid.

The Finance Committee had to warn the Academy that its function was to pay the bills authenticated by the officers. It had no other control, and it reported twice that the bills exceeded the income of the Academy. One reason was because the Fellows were strangely loath to pay their dues, and a collector had to be employed during the first year.

It may be mentioned that the Finance Committee paid out $66.38 for publishing the names of the Fellows of the Academy in the City Directory and in the newspapers, as required by the By Laws, and that the publication of Dr. Francis's Anniversary Address cost $141.

The members of the Committee on Admissions were the hardest worked of all. Nominations were referred directly to them by the Recording Secretary as received, often without the knowledge of the Academy itself. A rule was made that, after the Committee had made its first investigations, names should be reported to the Academy as "before the Committee." No name was ever refused recommendation on the first vote by the Committee; each candidate was always considered a second time after "seeking other information." The Committee had to remember always to try to "maintain the union and harmony" of the profession. One nomination caused much trouble. The credentials, medical standards, and moral character were entirely satisfactory, but it was felt "union and harmony" were threatened. The Chairman, Dr. Francis, called on the gentleman and explained their decision to delay action. He seemed satisfied, but insisted action be taken before the year was over. Wheels began to work within wheels. Dr. Mott, not a member of the Committee, moved that, as the Academy was not organized for the immediate profit or advancement of any individual member, and as the question might arise when the very discussion of membership *might* result in serious injury to the interests of the Academy without any advantage to the individual, when the Committee on Admissions unanimously believed that presenting a name might cause injury to the Academy, it should withhold it, with the consent of the President and Secretary, and consider it "as if not presented."

When in October the gentleman demanded action on his name, the Committee resolved to consider his name "as if not presented," and referred the matter to the President and Secretary, who upheld the Committee's action. His name was "not presented" to the Academy.

During this first year, 117 names came before the Committee and only 16 were not recommended to the Academy. Nine names were suggested for Corresponding Fellows, and five were recommended for election. The first to be elected a Corresponding member was Dr. Thomas T. Blatchford, of Troy. No name recommended by the Committee failed to be approved by the Academy, although there were usually a number of blackballs, sometimes five, six, or seven. The Council of Appeal held one meeting of organization. Nothing was ever referred to it throughout the year.

All told, twenty-three committees, including four of the Standing Committees, functioned during the year. The total membership of all committees was 145. They were filled by but 71 Fellows. Dr. Manley was a member of seven committees, Drs. Drake, Griscom, Isaac Wood, and Bulkley of five, and Drs. Buel, Buck, Carter, Stevens, Stewart, and J. R. Wood of four. The Academy was relying on its older and wiser (?) members.

The first paper on a scientific subject was read by Dr. Mott, March 3, 1847, on the treatment of ununited fractures. His method consisted in boring holes through the ends of the bone, passing

CODE OF MEDICAL ETHICS,

ADOPTED BY THE

AMERICAN MEDICAL ASSOCIATION

AT PHILADELPHIA, IN MAY, 1847

AND BY THE

NEW-YORK ACADEMY OF MEDICINE,

IN OCTOBER, 1847

NEW-YORK:

PRINTED FOR THE ACADEMY OF MEDICINE.

BY H. LUDWIG & CO., 70 VESEY ST

1848.

TITLE PAGE OF THE CODE OF ETHICS
ADOPTED IN 1847

ANNIVERSARY DISCOURSE

BEFORE THE

NEW-YORK

ACADEMY OF MEDICINE.

DELIVERED IN THE BROADWAY TABERNACLE,

November 10th, 1847.

BY JOHN W. FRANCIS, M.D.

[PUBLISHED BY ORDER OF THE ACADEMY.]

NEW-YORK

PRINTED BY HENRY LUDWIG, 70 VESEY-STREET.

1847.

TITLE PAGE OF THE FIRST ANNIVERSARY ADDRESS

silk setons through them, thus causing inflammation and eventual union. The setons were removed gradually, thread by thread, and union was usually obtained after "several months."

The second paper read was by Dr. Stout. He had moved that a scientific paper be read at the next meeting, and was promptly appointed to read it. It does not appear that this was either unexpected or undesired by Dr. Stout. His paper was "Revelations of the Microscope." The third paper, "by invitation," was read by Dr. Pliny Earle in July, "An Historical Sketch of the Institutions for the Insane in the United States of America." In September Dr. Batchelder read "Symptoms, Phenomena and Exciting Causes of Inflammation." The last paper of the year was Dr. Gilman's "Placenta Praevia."

The Academy was very anxious to publish papers read, in its own *Transactions*, and the papers of Drs. Mott and Earle and the report on milk were ordered printed. But apparently the Finance Committee called attention to the *cost*, and they did not appear until 1851, when the *Transactions* made their maiden bow.

While only five papers were read during the entire year, the reports on scientific subjects occupied considerable time, and the Academy was very busy with its own internal affairs. At the first Stated Meeting of the Academy Dr. Griscom presented a memorial to be sent to the State Legislature, endorsing a proposed law for registration of births, deaths, and marriages. It was voted to send the memorial, signed by the President, Officers, and Fellows of the Academy. It was also voted to endorse a memorandum to the Congress, urging legislation proposed by the College of Pharmacy to control the importation of impure drugs.

The third endorsement of legislation was a memorial to the Honorable the Legislature, urging State action for the care of youthful idiots. Thus the Academy early entered the field of public health.

The first Anniversary Meeting was held November 10. By arrangement, the Fellows assembled at the President's house and marched in a body to the Broadway Tabernacle two and one-half blocks away.

After an appropriate prayer, the President explained the objects for which the Academy had been organized, and introduced the orator, Dr. John W. Francis. The oration lasted two hours, after which a benediction was pronounced and the meeting adjourned. "Dodsworth's Cornet Band was in attendance and played appropriate music at intervals during the evening." The *Annalist*, after mentioning the distinguished occupants of the platform, said:

every other part of the room was filled, literally filled, to the very walls with well dressed persons of both sexes. Scarcely was standing room afforded either upon the floor or in the galleries. . . . Hundreds must have gone away disappointed being unable to obtain places. . . . The forceful manner in which, at the close of his discourse, the subject of legislative support of indigenous quackery, the bill of pains and penalties inflicted by its sects upon the community was adverted to, will not soon be forgotten.

In 1854, seven years later, the *Medical Times* referred to Dr. Francis's address "when 2500 were present." In a later number "Vindex" corrected the *Times*, stating the attendance was "upward of 4,000" and "nearly an equal number were turned away." At any rate, there was apparently a large attendance.

The months of December, 1847, and January, 1848, were very active ones. Six meetings were held. A committee had been formed to arrange the amendments already passed, and to consider those proposed and present a new Constitution and By Laws. It reported in December, with 104 members present. The report was ordered printed for an adjourned meeting to be held a week later. The Committee to nominate officers for the next year was also elected.

At the adjourned meeting, the Academy sat as a Committee of the Whole, discussed the amendments for three hours, and decided to sit again on the 15th. This time they sat for five hours, and another adjourned meeting was proposed but was voted down.

Two important matters therefore came up at the January Stated Meeting—the adoption of the new Constitution and the election of officers. One hundred and eight Fellows were present. Someone remembered that in March it had been voted to make a majority of *all* members necessary to change the Constitution, and there were 265 still in good standing. As there was not a majority of members present, an attempt was made to rescind the vote of March, which was declared out of order by the President, who was sustained by the Academy. Consideration was postponed to the following week; notices were to be sent earnestly requesting a full attendance.

Then the election of officers was taken up. It was decided that one Fellow who had not paid his dues for the year, but to whom the Academy owed more than $3, should be allowed to vote!

President and Vice Presidents were voted on first. The roll was called (265) and each Fellow cast his vote as his name was called. After the Tellers had counted the votes, watched by the Supervisors, it was announced no one of the three candidates for President, and only three of the four Vice Presidents, had received a majority.

When the vote for the other officers was counted, only a Domestic Corresponding Secretary, Treasurer, and a Librarian had been elected, but Dr. Watts had asked to be excused from running for Treasurer, and, being elected notwithstanding, he promptly resigned, so with President, Recording Secretary, Treasurer, and one Vice President still to be elected, they adjourned for another week.

On the 19th, it was announced that 56 Fellows who were "prevented from attending the last meeting" had sent in their votes for the new Constitution; this made 160 favorable votes and the Constitution was declared adopted. Seven hundred and fifty copies with the names of the officers (as yet unelected) and Fellows were ordered printed.

The election was then continued. New nominations had to be made. Eight were nominated for President and twelve for Vice President. The vote for each office was cast separately, with a roll call before each, and nobody was elected. Nominations were then made for all other officers and it was decided to vote for all on one ballot. There were four nominations for Assistant Secretary and Foreign Corresponding Secretary, two for Recording Secretary and Treasurer. This time things went better. Dr. Francis was elected President; Dr. W. W. Miner, Vice President; Dr. Stewart, Recording Secretary (reelected); and Dr. J. O. Pond, Treasurer. Corresponding Secretary was still undecided, so a fourth long roll call and vote occurred and Dr. Beck was declared elected.

After this long session, it was decided to postpone the election of the standing committees until the next stated meeting and, after expressing their thanks to Dr. Stearns, the Academy adjourned, and thus the first year terminated.

Twelve stated meetings were held, nine adjourned meetings, and the Anniversary, and there was also the organization meeting. The attendance varied; if an election of any kind was to be held, it was large. The only small meeting was in May, when all the officers were in Philadelphia to organize the A.M.A. At that meeting, they organized themselves into a "conversational meeting."

The "eventual" attendance was as high as 159 once, was over 100 five times, and over 90 twice.

1848

John Wakefield Francis

JUST WHY so much time was consumed amending the Constitution and By Laws is hard to understand, for the changes were few and relatively unimportant. The *first* object of the Academy was now "the cultivation and advancement of the science by united exertions for mutual improvement and contributions to medical literature"; this supplanted "the separation of regular from irregular practitioners," which became the third object.

The office of Assistant Secretary was established, an Executive Committee was substituted for the Council of Appeal, and the President was made ineligible for reelection. All Standing Committees were to be elected, and not appointed by the President, as previously.

The Constitution also provided for "reprimand, suspension, remission or expulsion" for violation of regulations on vote of four-fifths of the Fellows present. A member who had been expelled could not again be proposed for Fellowship, nor was he to be recognized by the Academy as a "regular practitioner." Amendments could now be made by a two-thirds vote of those in attendance, provided 100 were present, but only after due notice had been given.

The By Laws provided that the President and Secretary were ex-officio members of all Standing Committees.

The Committee on Admissions was to report such candidates "as may be worthy" within three months after nomination. If they failed to do so, the proposer could submit his candidate directly to the Academy, and if four-fifths voted affirmatively, knowing the candidate had not been recommended by the Committee on Admissions, he could be elected. Dr. Calkins, who had resigned over this question, won his point.

The Executive Committee was charged to "solicit and receive donations for the Academy; to recommend plans for promoting its objects; to provide a suitable room for meetings; to assist the several officers in protecting the property of the Academy and procure proper receptacles for the same; and in all things to superintend the general interests of the Academy." It is to be noted that a quorum for the Executive Committee consisted of all five members.

The annual tax was no longer limited to $3.00. Any Fellow indebted for one year's dues was excluded from voting at the election of officers. The order of business for each meeting still contained nineteen items.

A copy of the revised Constitution and By Laws was voted to be sent to "their Exellencies the Governor and Lieutenant Governor of the State, the Honorable Speaker of the Assembly, the Regents of the University, the Mayor and members of the Common Council of our city, the Clerks of the two Boards, the heads of departments in our city, officers of the State Medical Society, President of each medical society of the State, the editors of the several medical journals in the United States, and to the Commissioners of Emigration in our city." The legal authorities were to be informed of the organization of the Academy!

Dr. Francis, second President, emphasized that the Academy was now firmly established, had already received general and official recognition, and that its future was bright, but only if every Fellow contributed his best to the scientific discussions and to the application of modern scientific knowledge. Otherwise failure was ahead.

The election of the Standing Committees was carried out and a new setup was established, only one member of each of the former committees being reelected, except to the Committee on Publications, in which three former members held over. The elder members again predominated.

The vote for Orator was in striking contrast to that of the previous year. It was taken up promptly and only two ballots were necessary to elect Dr. Manley, although there were six candidates voted on.

The election of delegates to the A.M.A. was also a peaceful occasion. The Academy was entitled to twenty-six delegates. They agreed that the nominations should close when fifty names had been presented. Fifty nominations were promptly made. Of the twenty-six elected, nineteen were either officers of the Academy, or members of its Standing Committees.

Dr. John Stearns, the first President, died in March, 1848, and a special meeting was called to take suitable action. The Academy voted to attend his funeral in a body, to wear the usual badge of mourning for thirty days, to place the President's chair in mourning for six months and to invite all members of the regular profession and students of medicine to join with it at the funeral. The Assistant Secretary was requested to provide crepe bands for the Fellows when they met at the City Dispensary the next day.

Early in 1847 the Academy voted to issue certificates of Fellowship and instructed the "Committee on Books for the Library" to prepare a draft. This was done promptly, the form, in English, was adopted and 600 ordered printed, to be issued gratis to Fellows who had paid their dues. A form in Latin was also ordered prepared for Corresponding Fellows. In September, when finances were in difficulties, without rescinding the old resolution, it was voted to charge each Fellow 50 cents for his diploma. When the Secretary called attention to the conflict, the question was asked, where is the Latin diploma? A new committee was appointed to devise one in Latin for both Resident and Corresponding Fellows. It was not until April, 1848, that it decided to adopt the Latin form for Corresponding Fellows, and stick to the old English one for Resident Fellows.

Dr. Stearns had signed a few in blank before his death. In July, 1848, it was voted to issue those signed by Dr. Stearns to Fellows in the order in which they signed the Constitution. When these were exhausted, they were to be signed by Dr. Francis as President and all to be dated as of the date of election. In the Rare Book Room of the Academy is the diploma of Dr. E. L. Beadle, one of the Founders and No. 40 in the list of signers. It is signed by Dr. Francis as President and Dr. Stewart as Secretary. Perhaps some favoritism was shown. There is no diploma signed by Dr. Stearns in the Academy collections. This form was used, with many changes in the character of the type, until 1893, when a new certificate was adopted. There is no copy of the Latin Certificate at the Academy, but its form is on record.

In January a resolution was offered to appoint a committee of ten to be known as the Committee on Public Health to investigate the subject of cholera, "which seems to be approaching rapidly toward us, having already devastated the countries of Eastern Europe." The Committee was also to study all other epidemics as well as supervise sanitary conditions of the city. After being tabled until July, these resolutions were discussed and referred to the Executive Committee, who promptly reported that the objects of the resolution were "legitimately and properly one of the ends contemplated in the organization of the Academy," which should also study and record the relative values of various forms of treatment and other "philosophical measures" in abating and preventing epidemics. The public had a right to expect from the Academy that "no small share of their attention would be devoted to public hygiene." The long report ended with resolutions that "there shall be a permanent committee, consisting of seven Fellows appointed by the President, to be denominated the Committee on Public Health," whose duties were of a broad and extensive nature. This was unanimously adopted.

In December, when the report on cholera was expected, 134 Fellows attended. The report was so long that the first part, dealing with a history of cholera, was omitted for the present. In addition, Dr. Stewart read a long report of cholera as it appeared on a vessel recently arrived from England. After the Committee was instructed to report on the disease now at Quarantine, discussion was postponed a week to an adjourned meeting, at which 162 were present. The Academy sat as a Committee of the Whole for nearly three hours "without coming to any conclusion," and was permitted to continue a week later. Only fifty-three attended that meeting, but the Committee of the Whole discussed the subject for three more hours, and again were permitted to sit "at such time as the Academy might direct."

At this last meeting on the subject, Dr. Stewart proposed:

WHEREAS, The Academy of Medicine, embracing as it does nearly three hundred active practitioners, constitutes the highest medical tribunal of the city, it is incumbent upon it to watch over, guard and advise the citizens whose lives are committed to the care of its members in all matters pertaining to the public health, therefore

Resolved, That it is recommended to the Academy to appoint a committee to prepare an address to the public on the subject of Cholera, to be published officially in the daily papers of the city.

The preamble being stricken out, Dr. Stewart withdrew the resolution.

The Anniversary Meeting was held this year at the Church of the Crucifixion, and the address was delivered by Dr. Manley. This was a very different address from that of Dr. Francis the previous year. It was a very frank criticism of the medical profession and even franker and more critical of existing medical education as responsible for the low status of the profession. Dr. Manley started by saying, "I am not without apprehension, however, that some of the opinions which I may advance will not meet with the hearty concurrence of all whom I address, since interest is often found to conflict with duty so much as to warp the judgment even of those who aim to discharge it most conscientiously. . . . I shall speak of the abuses of medicine in connection with the education of physicians with a view to their correction."

He paid his compliments to the general public for their disregard of health rules and their acceptance of every form of quackery and sure-cures—adding that bounties awarded to medical men were mostly awarded "to those whose only wisdom is cunning and whose only moral is selfishness."

We are unwilling to believe that the practice of physic has with us been absolutely degraded to the condition of a *trade,* but we much fear it soon will be: the preliminary information of the pupil; the conduct of his medical education in some of our medical colleges; the measure of acquirement of the teachers themselves; their anxiety to profit by their situation to which accident, management, or the influence of political friends have promoted them; and the known fact that volubility of delivery, a fund of anecdote to amuse, rather than a store of scientific intelligence upon which to draw for the instruction of the students and a cultivated familiarity with them, which in effect defeats all proper discipline and destroys all the deferential respect which should attach to the character of instructors; and above all the indefinite multiplication of the schools contribute infinitely more to make it such than all other causes combined. Lecturing itself had become a trade, confessedly such, practiced more for its profits then for any other purpose.

He insisted the licensing power should be separated from that of conferring a degree. It was a fine and brave address, backed up by quotations from reports read at the American Medical Association meeting. When it came to voting for publishing the address, the motion was made to lay the matter on the table and narrowly escaped being adopted. It was finally voted to print the address. As to the number to be printed, Dr. Detmold moved to print 25 copies. (1,250 of Dr. Francis's address were printed.) Eventually 500 were ordered.

It is interesting that in March, 1849, Dr. Manley offered and the Academy adopted resolutions favoring the separation of the teaching and licensing power, which resolutions were sent to the American Medical Association. That Dr. Manley championed this cause, against intense opposition, and succeeded in having the Academy take such action, entitles him to a distinguished place on its honor roll.

The annual election was held in January. Ten names were presented for President, nineteen for the four Vice Presidents. The attendance was small, and when the question was raised, those in arrears of dues were allowed to come forward, pay and then vote. The President was voted for first and Dr. Mott was elected on the first ballot.

The election of the four Vice Presidents required three roll calls and three ballots, and two more (roll call omitted) for the other officers.

Resolutions were then passed thanking Dr. Francis for his "efficient, impartial and satisfactory" service as President, and the following on Dr. Stewart, the retiring Secretary:

Resolved, That the New York Academy of Medicine entertains a just appreciation and a proper sense of gratitude for many and efficient services which have been rendered by the late Secretary from the first organization of the Academy to the present time and at much personal sacrifice, with a far larger amount of labor than has fallen to the lot of many of the members, encountering many difficulties incident to organization without precedents or examples to guide him, and with a precision and punctuality almost unexampled, contributing essentially to the permanency of the Association, and adding greatly to its public reputation, in order that a formal record may be made of their sentiments, hereby tender their hearty thanks to F. Campbell Stewart, M.D.

Dr. Francis had been an excellent president. He gave much attention to its affairs, presided at all but one meeting, and as an ex-officio member of all Standing Committees, attended two-thirds of those of the Finance Committee, one-third of the Executive, and two of the Committee on Admissions.

Still more deserved was the action in regard to Dr. Stewart, the Recording Secretary. He served for two long years during this early formative period, and was only absent from one meeting each year, when he was perforce at the meeting of the A.M.A. In addition to his duties as Recording Secretary, he was also a member the first year of the Standing Committee on Medical Ethics. As ex-officio member he was present at all the meetings of the Finance Committee, all but two of the Executive, and over half of the Committee on Admissions.

On his retiring as Recording Secretary, he was elected chairman of the Committee on Admissions. In June he resigned, because he had been appointed by Governor Fish (whom he did not know personally) to the newly created position of physician to the Marine Hospital on Staten Island. He had long been active in public health matters. He moved to Staten Island and lived near the hospital. He did excellent work, but unfortunately he incurred the ill-will of the shipping industry, whose methods of running things he was forced to criticize. He finally resigned in 1851, remaining and practicing on Staten Island till 1855, when his father died and he returned to England never to reside here again. The original family name was Stewart Campbell, but Dr. Stewart's father, then professor of mathematics at William and Mary College, inherited the estates of "Stewart of Ascoy," became a British citizen, and changed his name to Campbell Stewart.

Dr. Stewart's later career with the Academy is interesting. He was elected Orator in 1851, but resigned because he had to go to England. There was no oration that year, but Dr. Stewart delivered it in 1852. He was Vice President 1853–1855, when, as already stated, he moved to England. In 1874 he was made a Corresponding Fellow. The Academy records show that he was made an Honorary Fellow in 1904, an honor he could not appreciate, for he had been in his grave since 1899.

Voting for Standing Committees occurred at this meeting. Each Committee was voted for separately. The effort to suspend the By Laws and omit the roll call each time, failed. Only one second ballot was necessary to elect the committees.

The Academy's second year was very much like its first, except perhaps the rivalry and jealousy were not quite so obvious.

The Standing Committees, elective now, did not work so well as the previous year. The Chairman of the Committee on Ethics reported early that important business could not be attended to on account of the "neglect of several of the members" to attend meetings. He asked the Academy to adopt some means to ensure attendance. A copy of his report was ordered sent to each of the delinquent members!

Although "important business had been referred to it," the Executive Committee never had a quorum (the entire committee) until September. The By Laws were by then amended, leaving the question of a quorum to the Committee, who set it at three. But the Committee did its work very satisfactorily.

The Committee on Admissions also had its troubles about attendance. It held eleven meetings, at which no quorum was present twice—once there was "no business." Nominations fell off very much during the year. The Committee only recommended twenty-two for Resident and two for Corresponding Fellows. It asked for instructions on what to do about applications for membership from practicing dentists who held medical degrees. The Academy decided that "the practice of dentistry is not sufficient to entitle a gentleman to membership in this body although he be a licensed

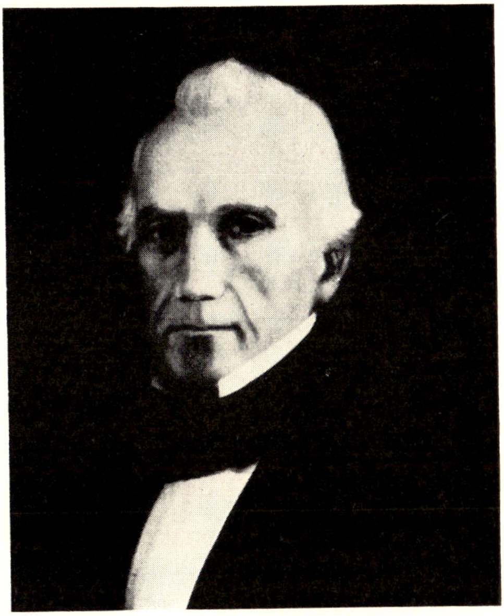

JOHN STEARNS, 1770–1848
First President, 1847

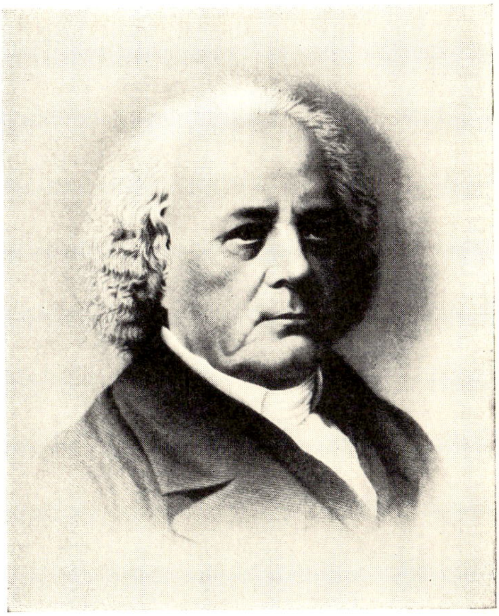

JOHN W. FRANCIS, 1789–1861
Second President, 1848
Reelected, 1855

physician, inasmuch as he is not a practitioner of medicine in the view of the Constitution of the Academy."

The Finance Committee held nine meetings, mostly well attended. It approved bills to the "Collector" of back dues for $17.92 (10 percent), and one for $44.82½ for publishing the list of Resident Fellows in "at least four newspapers." The Committee referred one bill to the Academy, incurred by the Public Health Committee, which had not been specifically approved. It was ordered paid but it was ruled that, hereafter, no bill should be paid except when officially authorized.

Dr. Stewart, the Recording Secretary, having that action in mind, reported he had prepared two letters of condolence and a number of documents ordered to be sent, but was holding them until the Academy authorized payment of postage. The Academy did so.

The Committee on Ethics only received one "charge," which turned out to be against two Fellows, for consulting with an irregular practitioner. The Committee decided the delinquents did not *know* the practitioner was "irregular" at the time, and dismissed the charges. This caused some protest, but their action stood.

Only six papers were read during the year, the first in July by Dr. Mark Stevenson on "Labor with Plurality of Births." Dr. Batchelder read one on "Proximate Causes, Indications and Methods of Cure of Inflammation," which occupied two meetings. Dr. Mott read two, which were ordered published in the *Transactions*. The Honorable Ashbel Smith, M.D., of Texas, was the first "outsider" to address the Academy. His paper, "Diagnosis between Yellow Fever and Bilious Fever," was, after some opposition, also ordered published in the *Transactions*. It was three years before any of them appeared in print. Dr. S. P. White read a long paper on "Acid Springs of Genessee County," which was *not* ordered published. But while the papers were few and far between, the discussion of cholera had occupied undivided attention for three meetings. The report on milk from cows fed on distillery waste was discussed at length at three meetings before it was finally referred to the Committee on Publications.

Other things which occupied much of their time were trusses, drugs, and apparatus referred to the Academy for an opinion. The giving of certificates of approval by individual Fellows was frowned on, although no definite action was taken on the subject. An apothecary submitted a sample of Sulphate of Bebeerine, "highly recommended by several eminent professional gentlemen of Scotland as a febrifuge and tonic"; another a specimen of fluid extract of Valerian with "certificates from several professional gentlemen." Three submitted samples of trusses and abdominal supporters. Hecker's "Farina of Wheat" was submitted by a physician, requesting an opinion as to its value as a food. ("Hecker's Farina" can be seen today on most grocery shelves.)

Each request resulted in a special committee of three to examine and report, and these reports called forth much discussion. There is no record of what most of them recommended.

1849

Valentine Mott

WITH THE ADVENT of Dr. Mott as President, we have for the first time a record of an inauguration with fitting ceremonies. The Chairman of the Executive Committee, flanked by the other members, presented the President-elect to Dr. Francis, who immediately gave an address of welcome, at the conclusion of which Dr. Mott was presented with a copy of the Constitution and By Laws and was conducted to the Chair. As soon as the other officers-elect had taken their respective seats, the President delivered his address.

The *Boston Medical and Surgical Journal* speaks in high terms of Dr. Mott's address:

"Its chief feature is a tone of hope and encouragement that the degraded condition of the profession may be changed and elevated to the position to which it is eminently entitled. Dr. Mott keeps the idea distinctly in view that New York is the city of American cities and it is easy enough to discover that he would like to have it considered the center of all that is grand and imposing in medicine and surgery." The report also called attention to Philadelphia's eminently successful medical institutions and stated that it was not to be expected in a country like this that one city—as London or Paris—could embrace all the genius and enterprise and learning of the country: "Medical schools spring up everywhere; hospitals are founded in the interior, and surgeons of widespread distinction reside thousands of miles from the old cities upon the seashore."

The Academy had spent much time and thought on preparing the diplomas for its Fellows. Now the question arose, what should be done about Fellows who moved out of town? It was finally decided to grant them "letters of dismission," which read:

We, the undersigned, Officers of the New York Academy of Medicine, by virtue of the authority in us vested, do hereby certify that A. B. is at this present date a Resident Fellow of this Academy in good standing and entitled to all the honor and consideration appertaining to said Fellowship.

Given at the City of New York this——day——

(To be signed by the President, four Vice Presidents, and Recording Secretary, with the seal.)

The Academy, however, reserved the right to withdraw such letters on sufficient cause.

The election of Orator was again a difficult matter. Dr. Manley's address had not been popular. An attempt to postpone action beyond the regular date failing, after two votes, Dr. J. B. Beck was elected, but declined. At a later meeting Dr. Stevens was elected, after two ballots, but he declined. It was not until August that Dr. Post was selected and accepted the office.

A strong contrast to this was the election of twenty-eight delegates to the American Medical Association. Only thirty names were put in nomination. It was voted that only a plurality vote should be necessary for election and, in case of a tie, the winner should be selected by the alphabetical position of his name! Two names were then withdrawn, and it was immediately voted the twenty-eight nominees be considered elected, and they were declared so.

Collection of dues or the "tax," as it was called, had been a difficult procedure from the very beginning of the Academy, although its payment had already been twice declared to be a "point of honor." It was decided that if the "tax" was not paid within twelve months, a collector should be employed and his 10 percent collection fee should be paid by the delinquent. This caused such protest that the latter clause was rescinded.

Later it was voted that at the next annual meeting those in arrears for *three years* (that is, from the organization of the Academy) should be stricken from the rolls, and that after another year, all delinquent for *two years* should be stricken from the rolls. It took several months of discussion before this was decided, and ten or more years before it was enforced.

In June a report was read from Dr. M. J. Bailey, Special Examiner, on the operation of the law regarding importation of adulterated and spurious drugs. In ten months some 90,000 lbs. had been condemned; including 3,353 lbs. of opium, 33,970 lbs. of "bark" (cinchona), and various amounts of rhubarb, jalap, gamboge, senna, myrrh, valerian root, croton oil, sarsaparilla, and iodine. The report was ordered given the widest circulation, and was reprinted —2,500 copies—from the *New York Journal of Medicine,* at a cost to the Academy of $61.30.

Five years later Dr. John Millington in his farewell address to the graduating class at Memphis Medical College, said, "The Medical Faculty of New York . . . obtained the establishment by Congress . . . of an inspection of drugs by appointed judges, in that port, and by a report of the New York Academy of Medicine in my possession, it appears that no less than 34,000 pounds of bark, etc." The report had been widely circulated.

But Doctor Bailey's activities were hurting unscrupulous importers, and he was subsequently removed from office by the Secretary of the Treasury. Thereupon the Academy sent very strong resolutions of protest to the President and Secretary of the Treasury. Apparently Dr. Bailey was reinstated, for we hear much of him later.

During this year the Academy took extraordinary action: at the suggestion of Dr. Samuel Pomeroy White, it was voted that the degree of M.D. should be bestowed by the Academy. Examinations were to be held by a board of examiners, standards of preliminary and medical education were established, a thesis was to be required, and even the fee to be charged—and divided among the examiners —was stated. But a month later sounder judgment doubted the constitutionality of establishing a new feature "uncontemplated in the Constitution." It was most desirable that the Academy's proceedings should be "unobjectionable from every point of view." The matter was reconsidered and action "deferred for the present" and that was the end of the idea.

The Anniversary Meeting was held at the Chapel of the University. Fifteen hundred cards of invitation and 100 circulars were printed (at an expense of $9.00). Every member received four cards and the Orator 100. Notices appeared in six daily newspapers —three insertions—which invited "the reverend clergy, members of the bar, the medical profession of the city and vicinity, and the general public." These notices appeared in pica type and occupied just seven-tenths of an inch in column.

The Committee secured the services of a clergyman and also of a policeman. Dr. Post's address was devoted to four general subjects: an enthusiastic comparison of medical knowledge of today as against the past; a defense of the regular profession during the recent cholera epidemic, claiming that the mortality was due to neglect of advice, delay in treatment, or a "depraved state"; an appeal for higher medical education; and finally a long castigation of quackery and especially Homeopathy. The address was ordered printed. It filled seventy pages and cost $55.98.

In January, when officers were to be elected, there were so few present when the meeting was called to order that the rules were suspended and the annual reports of committees and officers were heard first. When they came to the vote additional names were presented, although nominations had been closed at the last meeting. This was protested, but the Chair allowed them to be made.

It required three votes to elect Dr. Isaac Wood from the eleven candidates for President. After the officers were announced, the Secretary again stated the nominations had been closed at the last meeting, additional names had been nominated and that two of them had been elected. He moved that these elections be declared null and void. The motion was not sustained. Dr. Adams had ousted Dr. Vandervoort as Secretary.

Election of Standing Committees was deferred to a postponed meeting two weeks later. At that meeting a "retiring committee" was appointed to nominate. It presented the exact number of candidates to fill the offices and they were, naturally, all elected.

During the year the attendance was none too good, and in May for the first time there was no quorum. Dr. Mott presided at twelve of the sixteen sessions held, being absent only in the summer. The Committee on Admissions had little to do, and only six Resident and three Non-resident Fellows were presented for election. Very little was referred to the Committee on Ethics, and no charges were brought.

During the entire year only four papers were read, three of them by Dr. Batchelder. The other was, by invitation, by Professor Bureaud-Riofrey of Paris, on the Curability of Phthisis. Only a few cases were reported, Dr. Mott contributing two.

The year might be called the Academy's "Cholera Year," for little else was discussed in the months of February, March, and April. The Academy sat as a Committee of the Whole, each of these months. The report of the Public Health Committee on the subject was proposed for publication, but Dr. Stewart stated that in connection with the origin and mode of propagation of the disease and particularly with that form of it which recently prevailed at the Quarantine at Staten Island, at the City of New Orleans, and in the "Western Country," circumstances had occurred which were not yet fully and satisfactorily explained, and which were calculated to yield additional and important information in regard to the manner in which the disease was communicated. He therefore moved, and it was resolved, "that it is premature and inexpedient for this Academy to pronounce at the present time any positive opinion in regard to the contagious or non-contagious nature of Cholera."

The motion to publish the report was laid on the table, and the Committee on Public Health was instructed to prosecute their investigations and obtain all the available information on the subject, and report as occasion might present. As soon as these resolutions were passed, Dr. Batchelder read a paper on Cholera, discussing this very question of contagion and infection, upon the conclusion of which the resolutions submitted by the Committee of the Whole, which had been laid on the table, were again taken up and were adopted.

So, after many delays, the report got as far as the Committee on Publications but no further. In April a report (translation) of the disease as it occurred in Paris in 1832 (seventeen years before) was read, which resulted in another discussion in Committee of the Whole, and the whole subject was referred to a special committee of five.

The matter stayed with that special committee until October, when out of a clear sky Dr. Manley started things all over again, moving: "Resolved, as the deliberate opinion of this Academy, that Cholera is not a disease personally communicable." After considerable discussion, that matter was again referred to the Committee on Cholera.

In October the Trustees delegated two members to wait upon the Common Council, to ascertain what hygienic measures were proposed to be adopted in relation to the apprehended appearance of cholera. The members reported that the Academy would be informed when any matters were taken up!

Not so silent were the homeopaths, who issued this broadside: *

ADVICE TO THE PUBLIC IN RELATION TO CHOLERA

New York, June 2d, 1849

The undersigned, Physicians of the City of New York, believing that during the prevalence of Cholera, many lives are in danger of being sacrificed to improper modes of treatment, recommended in the newspapers, consider it their duty to warn the public of the danger of using the drugs generally recommended, and large doses of medicine of any kind. Since homeopathy has saved 91 out of 100 in thousands of cases of Cholera, we feel confident that it will cure almost every case, provided the physician is called immediately after the attack, and before any other treatment has been resorted to. But if any other medicines beside the appropriate homeopathic remedies are employed, or if several hours elapse, before the proper treatment is commenced, the cure will in many cases be impracticable by any treatment.

It is important that the community should be especially warned against the use of laudanum, and opium in any form, as well as calomel and all the advertised specifics.

During the prevalence of Cholera, every person should immediately consult his physician for the slightest diarrhoea, (whether with or without pain,) avoiding laudanum, and also cathartics even of the mildest kind. If medical advice cannot be obtained within an hour or two, the patient may take spirits of camphor a few times, in a dose of one drop.

Every person attacked with such diarrhoea, vomiting, cramps, colic or other symptoms, as give an apprehension that actual Cholera has com-

* Courtesy of the New York Historical Society, New York City.

menced, should take one drop of spirits of camphor in sugared water, every five minutes, and nothing else, until relief is obtained, or the physician arrives.

Twelve drops of the camphor, dropped in a table-spoonful of white sugar, may be dissolved in twelve table-spoonfuls of cold water, and one table-spoonful of this solution be given every five minutes. This, in most cases, will make an excellent foundation for the complete cure by the physician; but he should be immediately called, whatever may be the apparent amendment.

Spirits of camphor should not be used in large doses as a curative, nor by persons in health, in any dose, with the expectation of preventing the disease; but we believe that appropriate homeopathic medicines are efficacious as preventives.

We have not here given any advice for the use of other medicines beside camphor, believing it impracticable to point out the indications for each in a few words. Those who cannot consult a physician will find full directions in works written expressly on this subject.

[*Signed by twenty-seven homeopathic physicians.*]

1850

Isaac Wood

DR. MOTT made a very important valedictory address. After the usual flaying of irregulars in general, and homeopaths in particular, he discussed Academy affairs. He outlined what had been done to accomplish its original aims and frankly stated that he thought it had failed to advance medical science as much as might have been expected. This was due to a bulky "Order of Business." "Reports of Special Committees, the Reading of Papers and discussions thereon, and the Reception of Professional or Scientific Intelligence" stood 15th, 16th, and 17th on the Order of Business. This resulted in postponement of scientific papers, or these were "read to a beggarly account of empty benches." The result had been few papers and few discussions of scientific reports, except that on cholera. Too much time was wasted on arguments over administrative matters. The result had been poor attendance. All matters other than medical should be discussed as briefly as possible and the legitimate business, that of imparting information and discussion and observations thereon, should be promptly taken up.

When this should occur then, and then only, would the Academy rival European academies, its "transactions—(none as yet published)" would honor us. If the Academy should fail, "let quackery in its thousand forms and Homeopathy at the head flourish unmolested! You have given them the mastery of the field!"

Dr. Mott was also very insistent that the lay press should be excluded from meetings, as they were very prone to exaggerate "Doctors' differences of opinion," at the expense of the profession.

Dr. Wood, fourth President, in his Inaugural agreed with all Dr. Mott had said, and emphasized the need of a permanent home for the Library, which would ensure its increase. He thought trustees should be appointed and a charter obtained so that the Academy could hold property. He hoped this year would be known as the "working year" of the Academy.

Things started peacefully. The Anniversary Orator was promptly elected, and the President was authorized to accept "volunteers" for delegates to the forthcoming meeting of the A.M.A. in far off Cincinnati.

The question of securing a charter and the election of trustees had been suggested in 1849, and referred to a special committee. Its suggestion was that the trustees should consist of the officers of the Academy and that these trustees should supplant the Executive Committee. The plan was referred to the Executive Committee to consider. That Committee recommended that the Board of Trustees should consist of nine members, including the President, Recording Secretary, and Treasurer, and should supplant the Executive Committee. This of course caused lengthy discussion. The Executive Committee plan was finally adopted, and the Executive Committee immediately resigned. Two months later the first Trustees were elected—Drs. James Anderson, Galen Carter, E. L. Beadle, Willard Parker, J. Kearny Rodgers and J. H. Griscom. As the Legislature had adjourned, the matter of the charter of course lay dormant.

An important change in the Academy's organization was made this year. Dr. Batchelder had recommended in October, 1849, that nine scientific committees be appointed, to bring before the Academy "matters and things" pertaining to the several departments of medicine "as subjects for discussion, or such other action as shall be deemed best calculated to promote advance and diffuse professional knowledge and intelligence among its Fellows." These resolutions started on the usual long course. They were referred to a special committee of five, which reported favorably in December, and another long discussion followed. Not until April was the matter mentioned again, and then a committee of nine, plus the President and Recording Secretary, was appointed to nominate for the various committees, and another of three to propose the necessary alterations in the Constitution and By Laws.

But someone was suspicious that freedom of action and discussion might be curtailed, and it was therefore voted that every member should have the right to bring up any subject he desired, that the President could still call on any member for an expression of opinion, as could any Fellow through the President.

Finally in June seven scientific committees were elected:

Anatomy, Physiology and Pathology, five members

Surgery and Surgical Pathology, nine members

Theory and Practice of Medicine and Medical Pathology, seven members

Materia Medica, Botany and Therapeutics, five members

Obstetrics and Diseases of Women and Children, seven members

Chemistry and Pharmacy, six members

Public Health and Legal Medicine, nine members

Dr. Mott had certainly not exaggerated the time lost over minute details of organization. These first committees were strong ones, containing, with few exceptions, the most capable and active Fellows. It was the first effort to establish a *medical organization.*

The Trustees engaged the small Chapel of the University in Washington Square as a meeting place, at $7.00 per night, including fuel, light and ordinary janitor services. This was not only a distinct economy, for Convention Hall cost approximately $10.00 per night, but provided much more dignified surroundings for the Academy's meetings. The first stated meeting held there was on July 3, 1850.

On July 19, a special meeting was called that the Academy might express "as a public body" its sympathy with the nation at large, on the "afflicting intelligence" of the death of the President of the United States, Zachary Taylor. Resolutions were passed "that this Academy, uniting in deep and heartfelt regret, which at present overwhelms the entire American Republic, at the inscrutable dispensation which has removed from the sphere of his exalted station the Chief Magistrate of the Union, and desirous of uniting with the constituted authorities of this city in their public demonstration of sorrow at this most unexpected event, will as a body cooperate with the said public functionaries in such ceremonial as may be adopted on the occasion, etc."

It was voted to wear "the usual badge of mourning for sixty

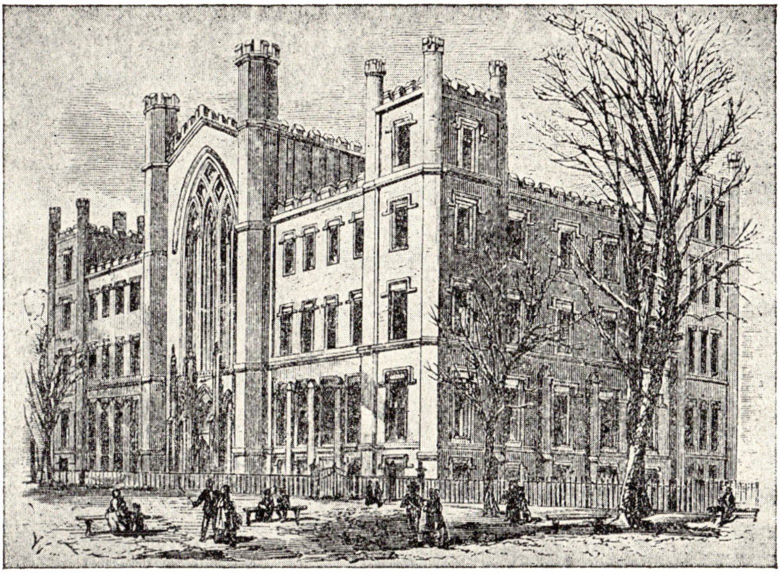

NEW YORK UNIVERSITY, WASHINGTON SQUARE
Meetings Held Here from 1850 to April, 1868

days," and to send a certified copy of these resolutions to the family, which the Secretary did.

The matter of cholera came up again, and it was voted that the report of the Committee on Public Health, submitted to the Academy in December, 1848, adopted, and ordered published, be referred back to the same committee for extension, "so that it may comprise the history, statistics, etc., of the late epidemic."

The fourth Anniversary was celebrated November 13, 1850.

The Fellows having assembled in the small Chapel of the University at one-quarter after seven o'clock P.M., the procession was formed at seven and a half o'clock, and entered the large Chapel. The Rev. Mr. Chambers, of the Dutch Reformed Church, made the opening prayer.

Dr. Wood, President, then after a few general remarks introduced the Orator, Dr. Joseph M. Smith, who delivered a discourse upon the Mental Phenomena of the Soldier.

There was a large audience who appeared interested.

The benediction by Rev. Mr. Chambers, concluded these exercises.

During the year, the subject of publishing transactions was often discussed. In May the Committee on Publications recommended that a "Bulletin" be published to appear monthly, or as material was at hand. Decision was wisely postponed until the Committee could get an estimate of probable expense. At the next meeting the Committee had changed its mind, and now favored issuing a volume of "Transactions" as "more conducive to its interests." The cost of a bulletin would have been $34.18 per issue of thirty-two pages in readable type. In July it was decided to publish the Transactions.

The scientific committees now began to recommend what should be published, although most of the papers had already been ordered published. This caused much discussion. Dr. Manley objected to the publication of *any* paper without its being read again, but the Academy did not agree with him.

Having decided on what to publish, it was suggested it would be wise to get an estimate of cost, which was later presented. A volume "similar in page, paper and binding to the *Transactions of the*

American Medical Association" would cost $456.00 for 500 copies. There would be some extra charges for table pages, or pages of rules and figures. Dr. Francis moved the matter be laid upon the table for future consideration—$456.00 was a lot of money. But later the Treasurer reported that he had $731.92 in the Treasury, with $301.00 awaiting collection, so the matter was taken up again, and the Committee instructed to proceed with the publication of the *Transactions* as soon as papers in their hands should amount to 350 printed octavo pages.

The annual election in January did not bring out the usual attendance, only sixty being present. The President was voted for first, after a roll call, and no one was elected. After a second roll call and vote, Dr. A. H. Stevens was elected by a large majority.

Election of four Vice Presidents required three ballotings, the roll call being omitted after the second ballot. Other officers were elected without much difficulty, there being more than one candidate for only two positions. All were elected on the first ballot.

This really was the Academy's most successful year. It had taken three years to get started. Much time was still spent in unproductive discussion, but things were definitely better. Thirteen meetings were held and the average attendance was sixty-six. Dr. Mott's hope for prompt attendance was not fulfilled, for the meetings opened with an average attendance of only twenty-eight.

The enrolled membership was announced as 250. During the first four years 304 had signed the Constitution, of whom nineteen had died, eight being victims of typhus or cholera.

Only one charge was brought against a Fellow. The Committee on Ethics decided it was clearly a case of malpractice with no question of medical ethics involved, so it asked the charge be dropped. After vigorous discussion it was eventually voted to drop the matter.

The Finance Committee had recommended the Annual Tax be only $1.00, but the Academy made it $2.00, "in order to build up the Library."

The Committee on Admissions presented only ten candidates for Resident, and five for Corresponding Fellowship. It asked for in-

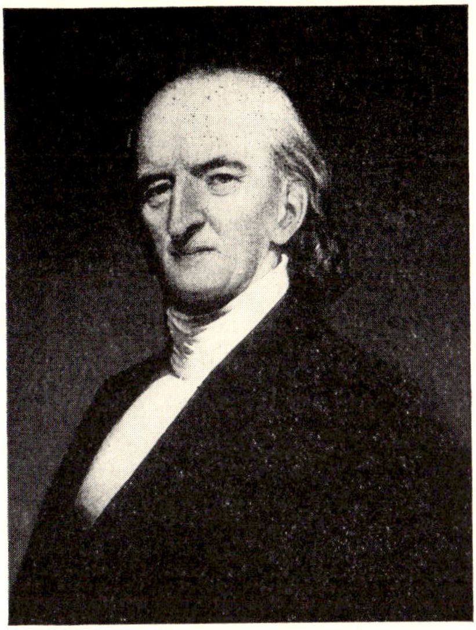

JAMES R. MANLEY, 1782–1851
Orator, 1848

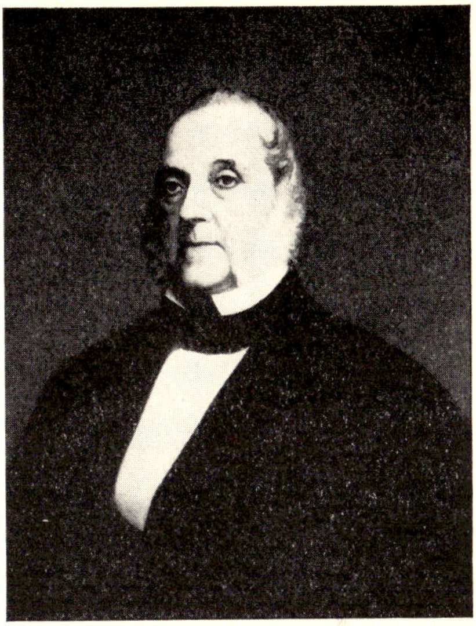

VALENTINE MOTT, 1785–1865
Third President, 1849
Reelected, 1857

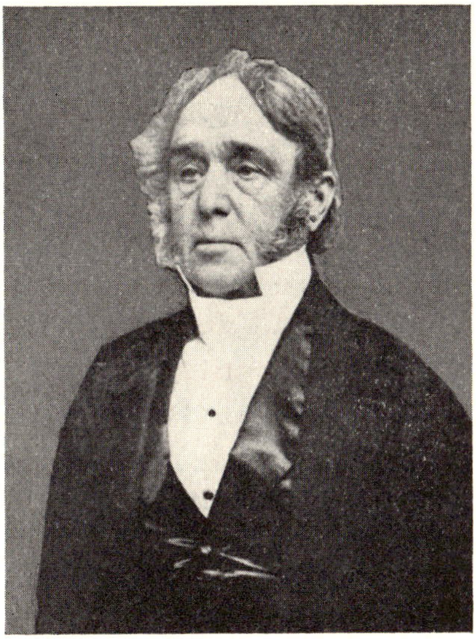

ISAAC WOOD, 1793–1868
Fourth President, 1850
Reelected, 1853

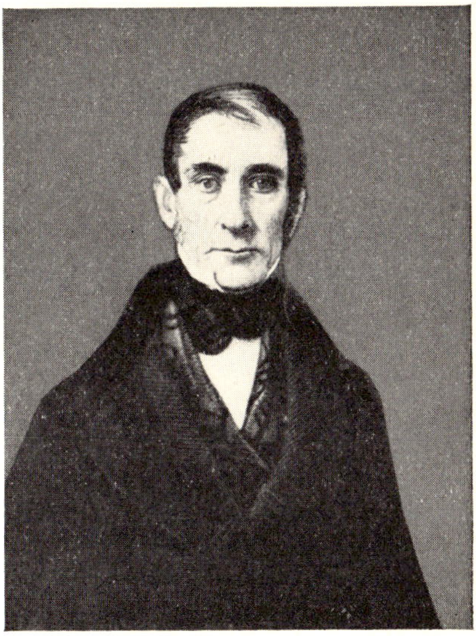

ALEXANDER H. STEVENS
1789–1869
Fifth President, 1851

structions in the case of Dr. C. E. Isaacs, who had been in the Army for five years and had lost his diploma. He had submitted a certificate from the University of Maryland, however. The Academy decided his credentials were satisfactory.

The Treasurer had handled $1,073 and had spent $314, of which $167 went for printing. He announced twenty-two delinquents for one year's dues, thirty-one for two years' dues, and nineteen for three. The Academy did nothing about it.

The scientific committees were working well and recommended several subjects for discussion at later meetings. Eight papers were read and six of them were important. Dr. Buck's two on "Tracheotomy," and on "Oedema of the Glottis"; Dr. Van Buren's two on "Tracheotomy," emphasizing the value of chloroform in such cases, and on "Amputation at the Hip" with presentation of the results, and Dr. Metcalfe's on "Chloroform as an Anesthetic," were really excellent papers. The latter caused discussion which occupied most of the time during three meetings. At the second one, the attendance was 100. The points emphasized were: the necessity of the recumbent position; no contraindication in operations about the nose and throat; that in children it might be used to great advantage; in valvular diseases of the heart it might be cautiously administered, but not in fatty degeneration of the heart; that much depended upon the purity of the article used, and that when pure, it might be continued for an indefinite period without danger, but that in certain conditions chloroform would prove fatal.

Dr. J. R. Wood read a valuable paper on "Morbus Coxarius."

Numerous cases were reported at various times. Several of post-pharyngeal abscess caused much discussion.

Dr. Metcalfe, who was a noted humorist, in reply to whether anyone had seen "any cases of an infectious nature similar to epidemic disease," stated that he had seen one, which if it had occurred last year would have been called *Asiatic* cholera. He came into the hospital with colic, vomiting, purging, and cramps—coming on after eating abundance of cabbage and drinking freely of beer. "He recovered promptly with Tincture Opii internally, and ice to the soles of his feet."

Dr. Reese, in his *New York Medical Gazette*, stated: "Every meeting since the presidency of Dr. Wood has been rendered interesting and profitable by a large attendance of the Fellows of the Academy, by the reading of papers, and by the exhibition of medical and surgical cases, some of which have been of very great interest."

Dr. Wood's hope that it might be a "year of action" was evidently fulfilled.

1851–1855

Alexander H. Stevens · Thomas Cock
Isaac Wood · Joseph M. Smith
John W. Francis

AND NOW BEGAN five rather discouraging years. Attendance was small; and lack of harmony and even open friction were painfully evident.

Dr. Stevens, the last of the "Callers" of the original meeting to be elected, became the fifth President. He was sixty-two years old. Graduating from P. and S. in 1811, he sailed for France to pursue his studies. He carried dispatches to our Minister, and was captured by an English warship. Soon released, he studied under Sir Astley Cooper and Abernethy and later in Paris. Returning to America, he was again taken prisoner by the English but on his release he returned and served as a surgeon in the Army till 1814.

In 1817, when only twenty-eight, he was appointed Attending Surgeon at New York Hospital, where he served for twenty-three years. When the Faculty of P. and S. resigned in a body in 1826, he became Professor of Surgery, resigning in 1837 because of ill health. In 1843 he was elected President of P. and S. and occupied that position when elected President of the Academy. He had virtually retired from practice.

On assuming the Chair he was addressed by Dr. Wood and presented with a copy of the Constitution. In his inaugural he hoped that the meetings would be considered "one great consultation, with the *older members* bringing forth papers for the benefit of the *younger.*"

Things seemed to start off very well. The Trustees, Standing, and Scientific Committees were elected with remarkable ease, reelections being the rule. The Academy was apparently well satisfied with work done the previous year.

Similarly, the following month, Dr. F. Campbell Stewart was promptly elected Orator, the roll call being dispensed with. When the twenty-fifth delegate to the A.M.A. meeting at Charleston (the number allowed) had been nominated, the President declared the nominations closed, and the list was elected. Not much "valuable time" was wasted in these elections.

Dr. Mott, determined to promote scientific discussion, reported during March and April on his "observations" during his recent trip to Europe. He spoke on "Vesico-Vaginal Fistula" (results discouraging, in which the Academy concurred), on the "radical cure" of hernia, by invagination of the sac and causing suppuration to destroy it, and at two meetings on "Vaccination" and its history. He mentioned the method (French) of inoculating at twenty or thirty different sites, to obtain "more constitutional effect"! In May he read his classical paper on "Ligation of the Subclavian Artery for Aneurism," which was published in the *Transactions*.

June 23, 1851, the Academy was incorporated by act of the Legislature. The Trustees had been active in pushing the matter; the necessary notices had been published in two papers and efforts had been made "to see" some of the city members and obtain their interest. Dr. Adams, the Recording Secretary, had been in Albany and presented a draft of the desired charter, which had been prepared in advance. There had been some opposition. Dr. Reese tells us in his *Medical Gazette*,

> The incorporation of this body, it seems, is resisted by two petitions from the city, very appropriately committed to Senator Brandreth. The opposition is said to be from physicians in this city, but there must be some mistake in this, for a friend in Albany who has seen one of the petitions having over two hundred signatures, finds but four who call themselves physicians, and neither of them can be found in the Directory, nor have they ever been heard of before. . . . The incorporation of the Academy is a matter of so little importance to anybody except its own members that it is difficult to imagine any motive to oppose it. We learn that the ground is that it will be a monopoly.

When the news was reported in July, it was voted that "in consideration of important services rendered the Academy" a copy of the *Transactions* should be presented to Dr. C. D. Robinson of the Senate, and Drs. Perry and Tuthill of the Assembly. Drs. Denison of Onandaga and Bottom of Wayne County, were also included for services rendered. The presentation of the *Transactions* to the State Library and Smithsonian Institution, voted at this same meeting, was perhaps a thank offering.

It was not until seven months later that it was remembered to offer thanks to Augustus Schelt, Esq., of New York City, for gratuitously drawing up the draft of the charter and using his influence to secure its passage.

At the suggestion of the State Medical Society, Dr. Adams had added to the charter the right to appoint one delegate to the State Medical Society.

As the summer came on, Dr. Mott got into trouble. Of just how it started, we have no official record. From a communication to the *Boston Medical Journal,* quoted by the *Medical and Surgical Journal,* and with the help of marginal notes therein by Dr. Purple, we learn the facts.

There was in New York at this time a physician known as Edward H. Dixon, who was a thorn in the side of the Academy. He owned and published a magazine called *The Scalpel.* Clever, an able practitioner, but utterly devoid of accepted ethical principles, he devoted much of his attention—to put it mildly—to ridiculing the Academy. He had been a student of Dr. Mott's in the "old Rutgers School." Dr. Mott was always very sympathetic toward his old students and in some way Dixon persuaded Dr. Mott, *ex-President of the Academy*, to give him some kind of a "certificate"; this he published in the *Boston Medical and Surgical Journal* and in one other periodical.

This caused a storm in the Academy. It was felt that the certificate brought "disgrace" upon the regular profession. Two letters were read from Dr. Mott, the first to Dr. Dixon upbraiding him for publishing the certificate when he had given his word he would *not,* and the other apologizing to the Academy, expressing regret and sorrow and appealing to its forbearance, because the certificate was given with a "solemn pledge" that it would not be made public.

Dr. Mott was very important to the Academy and apparently his excuses were accepted, but at the August meeting, Dr. Galen Carter being in the Chair, the minutes state "Dr. Mott occupied the floor for some time in support of his motion that all that part of the minutes of a previous meeting, under the head of New Business, be stricken out."

Dr. Reese, in his *Medical Gazette*, records,

After a spirited discussion, in which many members took part, the presiding officer, Dr. Carter, decided that all the action taken at the previous meeting on the subject of the Ex-President was irregular and directed the record to be stricken out, which was done by a nearly unanimous vote, after an appeal taken from the decision of the chairman, in which that officer was sustained. The Committee, and that report to which we alluded in our last, were of course annihilated. Dr. Batchelder gave notice that he would bring forward the subject in a constitutional way, at a subsequent meeting. This is undoubtedly desirable, as we hope thorough work will be made in rebuking and prohibiting all endorsement of quacks and quackery on the part of any Fellow of the Academy, including the Professors of each of our Colleges, if they should be found in the same category, hypothecated in this instance.

Dr. Batchelder was true to his word, and the next month the Academy went into a Committee of the Whole on the state of the Academy. After a session of two hours, the Committee rose and the Chairman reported that the Committee had under consideration a question of ethics and that after considerable discussion the subject had been indefinitely postponed.

In October the subject of certificates was again brought up and after much discussion, in which Dr. Detmold stated that, in view of recent occurrences, he was in favor of abolishing all laws on ethics, the President was authorized to appoint a committee of five to revise the Constitution. That ended the matter for the present.

Since July, 1850, the Committee on Publications had been waiting to print the *Transactions* until, as ordered by the Academy, the volume should consist of 350 pages. Nothing having happened by

THE

TRANSACTIONS

OF THE

NEW YORK

ACADEMY OF MEDICINE.

INSTITUTED 1847

VOL. I.—PART I.

PRINTED FOR THE ACADEMY.

NEW YORK:
PUBLISHED BY S. S. & W. WOOD, 261 PEARL STREET.

1851.

TITLE PAGE OF THE INITIAL PORTION
OF THE TRANSACTIONS

April, and many Fellows becoming impatient, it was voted that all material now in hand be published at once, as "Part I, Volume I. of the *Transactions* of the Academy."

After much discussion it was voted to print 750 copies; $200 was appropriated to pay for them. By June, Part I was reported printed, with lithographs illustrating Dr. Mott's paper. Dr. Beadle wanted it distributed at cost, Dr. Vandervoort, *gratis*, to those who had paid their dues. When it was decided not to issue it gratis, the Secretary called the Academy's attention to the fact it had voted in April, 1849, to issue all publications gratis, and it was then voted, to meet the situation, that "Transactions" did not come under that rule.

As a final chapter the Committee reported that the total costs amounted to $341.33 (as against the $200 appropriated), that Messrs. Wood were acting as publishers (33⅓ percent commission), and that 16 copies had been sold to Fellows at 75 cents. In spite of this marked increase in the expected cost, the Academy reconsidered its previous decision, and voted to give each Resident and Corresponding Fellow one copy gratis, and six copies to the author of each paper published, extra copies to be sold to Fellows at cost, and free copies to be sent to such medical journals as the Committee decided upon. Dr. Beadle proposed that the annual tax be raised to $3.00 to meet this expense, but his motion was tabled.

The *Boston Medical and Surgical Journal* wrote at some length about its copy. It had "rarely examined a series of medical and surgical papers with more satisfaction." Those of Dr. Mott were particularly commended, and the review closed by saying the Academy was "conferring peculiar favors upon the whole brotherhood of practitioners when it sends forth a publication like this."

The meetings in the fall were largely dominated by Dr. Batchelder. He offered a series of preambles and resolutions in regard to quacks, unprincipled and unmoral physicians. The first one called upon "all colleges, schools and institutions authorized to confer degrees" to withhold them from those unqualified by skill or morality and to claim their right to reclaim diplomas from unworthy and unethical holders.

The second proposal was that a committee of five be formed to call upon the profession and laity to petition state legislatures to alter the charters of institutions giving medical degrees so as to require of all applicants evidence of moral character, and reminding the institutions of their duty to revoke degrees in cases of conduct "unworthy the honor which should ever accompany the degree of Doctor of Medicine."

The third proposal called attention to a suggested plan that hospitals should organize medical schools, when approved by chartered medical societies, which would liberalize the "business of instruction and republicanize our medical schools." The Academy was urged to approve the plan and appoint a committee to memorialize the Legislature to grant to such hospitals, "supported wholly or in part by the bounty of the public" and having 100 beds or more, the right to organize as such and also to force existing medical institutions to establish connection with such hospitals.

The Academy went into a Committee of the Whole to discuss the last, with the result of the appointment of a special committee to report at a later meeting. This committee heartily approved of the object "as second to none which have ever engaged the attention of the Academy," and urged a committee to memorialize the Legislature for a general law on the subject, and to report at the next meeting. This was strongly advocated by some and as strongly opposed by others, who claimed that the resolution was indefinite, that the hospitals should be first consulted, that it should be referred to the State Society, and so on. But the motion was carried by a large majority, the memorial was presented and adopted, and another committee of three was appointed to circulate it throughout the state.

Dr. Batchelder, having accomplished this, now turned upon the New York Medical College as having "assumed an attitude and policy hostile to the honor, dignity and welfare of the medical profession," in having issued a degree to a person named Elliott. He called upon the Academy to withhold from the College "their countenance and support until it shall have changed its policy and come to be wholly on the side of the profession and the public." He also proposed that the conduct of several distinguished Fellows who were present "at what purported to be an examination" be censured, and that they be admonished "to be more circumspect in the future with regard to the professional company they keep and the certificates they give, and to abstain most religiously from encouraging and countenancing quacks of every kind and quackeries of every sort."

The Academy adjourned without taking action, but Dr. Batchelder brought the matter up at the next meeting again. Dr. Horace Green, President of the College, was present this time and read the certificate of the Censors of the Examination. The New York Medical College was the only one in the city which had carried out the recommendations of the State Society that degrees should be recommended by censors not connected with the teaching staff. He inquired why the New York Medical College had been selected for censure. Dr. Batchelder retorted because in his judgment "this was the most flagrant outrage upon the rights of the profession which had ever occurred and far transcended all other acts of the kind."

The discussion became quite intense. Dr. Anderson, always a calming influence, questioned the jurisdiction of the Academy. Drs. Beadle and Detmold were in favor of indefinite postponement. Dr. Batchelder then withdrew his motion.

When the minutes were read at the next meeting and a motion to strike out all that related to the moral character of the gentleman under discussion had been lost, the difficulty was solved by the adoption of Dr. Beadle's motion that "Dr. Batchelder's remarks were inquiries and not charges"!

In November two special meetings were called on account of the deaths of two important Fellows. The first was Dr. J. Kearny Rodgers, a very distinguished and able surgeon, one of the Staff of the New York Hospital. He had been a Founder of the Academy, its Vice President three times, and a Trustee twice. Very strong and appreciative resolutions were passed and fifty-eight members attended his funeral in a body.

The second meeting was called on the death of Dr. James Manley, who had been the second Orator of the Academy and made a most excellent address. He also was a Founder and had served on many committees of the Academy. He was always a calming influence in troubled waters. "Many disagreed with him—none ever questioned his honesty or sincerity."

The election for officers was a very peaceful one, and there was little competition. Dr. Cock was elected President on the first ballot, the four Vice Presidents on two ballots. All the other offices were filled on one ballot except the Assistant Secretary, which required two.

During the year only fourteen Resident and two Corresponding Fellows were elected, membership amounted to 222 Resident and 17 Corresponding. What the scientific committees did, if anything, is unrecorded.

Financially the Academy was doing very well, the Treasurer reporting $611.27 in hand, with $222 of the tax still unpaid. The collector had turned in $330 in back dues. Advertising the list of Fellows cost $30.41.

Dr. Stevens only attended seven meetings.

The Anniversary Address was omitted, because of Dr. Stewart's unexpected trip to Europe.

1852

Dr. Thomas Cock, the sixth President, was sixty-nine. He had studied medicine under the celebrated Dr. Valentine Seaman, and later became his partner. He had been a Trustee of the College of Physicians and Surgeons and was its Vice President. After fifteen years' service as Attending Physician to New York Hospital, he had become "Emeritus." He was one of the "elder statesmen" to sign the original Constitution, and is fourth on the roll. He had been Vice President of the Academy 1847–1849, serving on the old Council of Appeals, and he had been fairly active in its affairs.

At the first Stated Meeting Dr. Cock was ill and could not be present to be inaugurated. It was a particularly unproductive year for the Academy. Only three papers were read, two by Dr. Gardner—one on the meat supply of New York, the other on rupture of the perineum. Dr. Gilman described the anatomy of the Taenia, and showed many interesting drawings. He said it used to be thought they reproduced spontaneously, but now it was known they were abundantly supplied with reproductive organs.

A discussion on "Diphtheria and Croup" lasted through two meetings and brought a good attendance. Those diseases were a mystery to the profession at that time. Cases starting in a mild way, with sore throat, ended with dyspnoea, cyanosis, and death, with or without tracheotomy. Others with severe initial symptoms, and with membrane in the throat, all recovered. And still others, with severe sudden dyspnoea, yielded promptly to emesis and other treatment. Particularly baffling were those beginning with a membrane and high fever, which developed into scarlet fever. It was still a mystery when the discussion was concluded.

Another stated discussion was on "Cholera Infantum," a disease occurring among the poor and in hot weather, and more prevalent in Philadelphia and in the South than in New York. Dr. Reese remarked that 100 children had died from it in one week in the city. The remissions in the morning and exacerbations at night suggested a relation to intermittent fever. He considered it a malarial disease. When cholera infantum prevailed in the summer, intermittent and remittent fever prevailed in the autumn. He thought quinine a reliable remedy. Practically everyone disagreed with Dr. Reese. The discussion was postponed to a later meeting, but was not taken up again.

A third discussion was on "Tracheotomy in Croup." Dr. Batchelder monopolized most of the evening, without contributing much.

Among the very few other case histories reported, Dr. Detmold presented three and demonstrated a "speculum" for examination of the interior of the eye.

The Academy was active in matters of public health. Through its committee in this field, resolutions were passed stressing the importance of vital statistics and Congress was memorialized through the Honorable David T. Jones, urging publication of mortality tables in the forthcoming Census Report. They were published, showing deaths by cause, age, sex, nationality, season of the year, duration of illness, occupation, color, and by status as freemen or slaves. This was the first attempt to compile vital statistics by the Federal Government.

Dr. McNulty called the attention of the Academy to the inadequate rate of remuneration for medical services rendered the city on call of the police, its dangerous character and the difficulties of collection of fees, and urged that the Common Council be requested to inform the police when to call a physician, and to authorize the payment of bills on voucher signed by the Captain of Police; also to establish a more "just and liberal standard" of compensation. The unfairness of the situation was generally admitted, but Dr. Detmold hoped the Academy would not appear before the public in the matter. It was proposed to adopt a scale of prices and send it to the Common Council, and also to refer the matter to the Finance Committee. The resolutions were finally laid at rest on the table.

The Committee on Public Health and Legal Medicine presented an elaborate report, setting forth the insufficiency of the present dispensary system to meet the necessities of the sick poor and noting the inadequate remuneration of the physicians in attendance, which rendered it impossible for them to do their duty faithfully. It recommended that one or more physicians and apothecaries be appointed for each city Ward, to be paid adequate sums for their services and to be required to live in their respective districts, and as these District Physicians, in their daily attendance on the sick and poor in the cellars and garrets, necessarily came in contact with the filth and improper ventilation which were frequently the cause of the very diseases they were called upon to treat, they would form the most competent sanitary police, and they should be empowered to report upon and remove such nuisances as in their opinion were injurious to the health of the district. The report was received with great favor by the Academy, and after discussion was referred back to the Committee jointly with the Committee on Publications, with power of revision and publication.

In August, Dr. Griscom reported that it had been printed in full in the New York *Times*, from which it had been copied in all the daily press. (Photostat copy in the Academy.) In September, he reported that two thousand copies had been printed (at a cost of $53.00), which the Committee proposed to distribute, five to each Fellow of the Academy and the balance to the heads of departments, the Common Council, and all other public bodies. It was voted to memorialize the Common Council and Trustees of the several dispensaries, and appoint a conference committee, with power. Of what that committee did, if anything, we have no knowledge.

By April, Dr. Cock had regained his health, and was able to assume his presidential duties. He addressed the Academy, recounting his experiences and difficulties in obtaining a medical education and telling about the small private societies which had existed in the city at that time. He closed by hoping that the Academy's time would be spent in discussion of medical subjects rather than on legislation. He also hoped that the obituaries of many former members, long undelivered, would be presented promptly.

Dr. Shanks promptly started trouble by calling the Academy's attention to the fact "apparent to every reflecting physician that the gratuitous medical college cliniques in connection with indiscriminate elemosinary medical services of dispensaries degraded the practice of medicine by leading the public to the false and pernicious view" of undervaluing and scorning the services of "regular educated and legally practicing physicians" and by encouraging them to trust and *pay* the "boasting medical humbug or empiric or the advertising quack nostrum vendor." He therefore moved that "gratuitous medical, surgical, obstetrical, or pharmaceutical services" by physicians at medical cliniques, college or otherwise, "savour of quackery and as such meet with the decided disapprobation of this Academy." His resolution also included a call to "every high-minded and legal practitioner throughout the land who has the welfare of the public and the honor and dignity of the profession at heart" to discountenance such clinics and do all in his power to cause their "total abolition, or a sweeping reform." These resolutions caused much discussion, and were laid over to an adjourned meeting, the printing of notices thereof being ordered.

At the adjourned meeting Dr. Reese took over and proposed two resolutions which were both adopted. The first was:

> WHEREAS, The duty of rendering medical and surgical services to the poor and destitute without fee or reward, is one of the universal and perpetual obligations upon every member of our liberal profession; therefore
>
> *Resolved,* That no Fellow of this Academy shall be countenanced in making exclusive pretentions to benevolence by public advertisements or private cards, circulars, or other device, publicly offering advice, medicines or operations to the poor gratis, either in his individual capacity or in virtue of any office or position he may hold in any clinique, school, college, or other public institution.

It was also resolved that these resolutions be published in the medical journals of the city.

Encouraged by this success, Dr. Reese then presented his second resolution:

> WHEREAS, The cliniques now held at the medical colleges as at present conducted, are or may be made tributary to the private interests of the professors at the expense of other and younger members of the profession, depriving them by an odious monopoly of practice and operation and often to fees to which they are justly entitled, therefore resolved, as the sense of this Academy, that to prescribe for or operate upon the legitimate patients of any other physician, knowing them to be such, although done gratuitously at a clinique, is equally unwarrantable and unprofessional, with similar interference with the patients of another in private practice, and in either case is a violation of the code of medical ethics adopted by this body.
>
> *Resolved,* That the possible perversion of these cliniques to the private emolument of those conducting them by transferring patients to their private offices and thus exacting fees from those found able to pay, divests the cliniques of all pretext for professing to be public charities and should be scrupulously guarded against in all our colleges by stringent rules.
>
> *Resolved,* That a copy of these resolutions be sent to the authorities of the several medical colleges in this city.

The resolutions were carried. Dr. Griscom then desired that his name should be recorded as voting against sending the resolutions to the colleges. It had also been voted to send them to the American Medical Association.

This was bound to cause trouble and Dr. Reese was never loath to cause it. It came promptly. At the next meeting in May a letter was read from Dr. J. W. Draper, on behalf of the Faculty of New York University, acknowledging the receipt of the resolution and stating, "The University does not recognize the authority of the Academy of Medicine." The note was laid upon the table. Dr. Mott had been conducting free clinics, notices of which had appeared in the papers. He promptly wrote the Academy tendering his resignation. This was also laid upon the table.

Then the Secretary announced that he had received a "charge against a Fellow," which was handed over to the Committee on Ethics as Charge No. 2. It proved to be a charge against Dr. Mott. Who presented it we do not know. It was always referred to as Charge No. 2.

Matters lay dormant—outwardly—until January, 1853, when the Committee on Medical Ethics reported that they had had Charge No. 2 under consideration and, in view of all the circumstances of the case, they had arrived at the conclusion that no further action was demanded. Nothing more is recorded. The report was accepted and adopted.

Dr. Detmold then moved that the resignation of Dr. Mott be taken from the table, where it had lain since May. On motion of Dr. Anderson, it was resolved that Dr. Mott be allowed to withdraw his resignation. In the meantime Dr. Mott had discontinued his advertisements in the papers.

A committee to revise the Constitution and By Laws had been appointed the previous year, and in April made its report through Dr. Batchelder, the Chairman. The report was brought up at an adjourned meeting two weeks later. Sixty-four attended and discussed the amended Constitution. At another adjourned meeting the By Laws were discussed, and both were finally adopted and ordered printed.

The new Constitution established four classes of members, Resident, Non-Resident (and Fellow permanently removing from the city and not resigning, automatically became one), Corresponding (increased to 200), and Honorary. The purposes of the Academy were now three terse, simple ones: first, the cultivation and advancement of the science of medicine; second, the promotion of the character and honor of the profession; third, the elevation of the standards of medical education. No mention is made of separation of the sheep from the goats, or the outlawing of any "proprietor or vendor of any patent medicine, or secret remedy or medicine." Care was taken, however, to cover the difficulties caused by Dr. Mott's indiscretions. The By Laws stated that "no Fellow shall countenance, encourage or patronize by advertising, giving certificates, or in any other way whatever, an irregular practitioner, proprietor or vendor of any nostrum, patent, or quack medicine," and made the further sweeping statement that "any act which unfavorably affects the character of the medical profession shall be deemed a chargeable offense." The Committee on Medical Ethics was required, when charges were presented, to endeavor to "reclaim" offenders before proceeding against them "in manner and form." If that clause had been in effect when Dr. Mott's case came up, he would have escaped action on the charges, for in both instances he had been "reclaimed."

The President and Corresponding Secretary were made ex-officio members of all Standing Committees. The list of Fellows was no longer to be published "in at least four of the daily newspapers," but "an official catalogue of Fellows" was to be published when ordered by the Academy.

The new By Laws now required that business should only be transacted at the meetings of January, May, and September, except that nominations for officers and Orator were to occur in December. The Committee on Admissions was to report every month on candidates for fellowship. The three business meetings kept the same order of business, with its nineteen items.

In an editorial, the *New York Medical Times* stated,

> We congratulate our brethren of the profession upon the change at last effected in the Constitution of that body, which restricts the transaction

of ordinary business to only four meetings in the year especially set apart for that purpose leaving the remaining meetings entirely free for the discussion of scientific and practical subjects; indeed furnishing no other occupation for such evenings. The Academy therefore is now thrown upon its resources, which are abundant and will doubtless develop themselves as occasion may demand.

In November, the sixth Anniversary Meeting was held in the large Chapel of the University. After the usual prayer, Dr. Stewart spoke on "The Standing of the Medical Profession and its Claims upon the Public." The meeting closed with a "blessing." The Trustees' Minutes state that "the attendance was good as to numbers and respectability." The address was a straightforward statement of facts, in excellent English, and free from many of the absurdities and exaggerations of previous addresses. It is an interesting document today.

Financially it had been a good year for the Academy. Fellows were still delinquent in paying dues, and $50.80 of the income went to the collector for securing $508 of dues.

Publications cost only $105.20. After paying all bills, including one for $4.50 for "loan of candelabra and candles" for the Anniversary Meeting, the Treasurer had $682.39 in the Treasury.

Otherwise it was a discouraging year.

1853

The Annual Meeting in January, 1853, devoted to official business, was poorly attended, only forty being present. The last two years had been progressively unsatisfactory. Discord was rampant, and the selfish, sordid element in the Academy was more active and vociferous.

Dr. Isaac Wood was called back to again serve as President. His first term had been an excellent "working year." Perhaps he was called back to pull the chestnuts out of the fire. An entirely new set of officers was elected, except Treasurer and Librarian. Drs.

Galen Carter and James Anderson, always to be trusted, were reelected Trustees; most of the members of the Scientific Committees were reelected.

The year proved to be the most unsatisfactory of any in its history. The Fellows seemed to be losing interest. The attendance was for the most part poor. Only four papers were read during the year; the first, by Brown-Séquard of Paris, on various aspects of fracture of the spine, brought out the largest attendance of the year—sixty.

Dr. Griscom's paper on hospital hygiene caused a long and animated discussion. It was considered so important that it was printed at once, all by itself (no other papers being on hand) as Part 2, Volume I of the *Transactions*. The other two papers were trivial.

There were three formal discussions. The first, on hiccough, was monopolized by Dr. Batchelder who considered it due to spinal irritation, to be treated by cupping, leeching, and blisters to the spine. The second discussion was supposed to have been on croup, but the suggested treatment by quinine caused a diversion, and the discussion ended up on the treatment of rheumatism by quinine. The third was on lead poisoning. The majority believed that absorption was through the air passages but might be through the alimentary tract.

Dr. Buck reported a case of dislocation of the humerus beneath the pectoral muscles, reduced under ether with difficulty. Dr. Detmold thought dislocations reduced under ether were more likely to recur! Dr. Detmold exhibited a thumb, torn off by machinery. The discussion was chiefly on what must have been the condition of the muscles when the accident happened.

The President exhibited a pair of "Perkins Metallic Tractors" and Dr. Francis explained that Dr. Perkins came to New York to cure yellow fever with the tractors, died of the disease himself, and was buried in "Washington Parade Ground" (Washington Square), then called Potter's Field. In 1894 Dr. Wood's son presented these tractors to the Academy, where they still are.

In February a committee of nine, previously appointed to prepare a table of fees for professional services to be adopted by the Academy, reported. This was a subject many other societies had attempted to "standardize," and the committee's efforts met with the usual fate. It was voted to print 300 copies of the report and submit it to the Fellows for discussion at the next meeting. The discussion took place in March, but the *Medical Gazette* tells us, "The general sentiment appeared to be adverse to any action on that subject by the Academy, but as the hour was late, the report was deferred."

Nothing more was done until September, when discussion was resumed, and taken up again in October. This time the members voted that "it is expedient for the Academy to adopt a fee bill." Finally the Academy, sitting as a Committee of the Whole, voted to postpone the whole matter indefinitely. Most of five meetings were devoted to this topic. This is typical of many matters discussed at length by the Academy.

Dr. E. H. ("Scalpel") Dixon had his fling at the Academy on this subject in the *Scalpel:*

> The last effort of our academic friends was of a financial and literary character, and reflects high credit upon their imitative faculty. They published a list of prices for the various surgical operations, with consultations, etc., precisely after the manner of a bill of fare, or the prices of a trade's union!

Nominations were made at the December meeting, and after candidates were proposed for the various officers, it was voted that the President, with the other officers of the Academy, when elected, be a committee to appoint the various committees of the Academy for the ensuing year, as well as the delegates to the American Medical Association and the State Medical Society.

The Trustees now in office were renominated for the ensuing year.

When the Academy voted in January, only forty Fellows were present. Dr. J. M. Smith was elected President on the second ballot.

The Anniversary Oration was not given this year. Dr. Swett had been elected Orator, but he resigned on account of poor health. Dr. James Stewart was elected to fill his place, but he declined the honor. It was then decided to omit the oration.

The State Medical Society had expressed a wish that the Academy should be legally permitted to have a larger representation than one member. The State Charter was therefore amended, and the Academy became entitled to five delegates.

The Scientific Committees did not work well, and their chairmen complained. Attendance was frequently too small to establish a quorum. The Academy instructed the Secretaries of the Committees to inform all members that they were expected to attend and, if they could not do so regularly, they were requested to resign. No resignations were reported.

The Committee on Admissions presented candidates for twelve Resident and three Corresponding Fellows, who were all elected.

It was voted to employ a stenographer to record the proceedings of the Academy, if one could be obtained for $75 a year! The Secretary reported failure to do so at that price, and the matter was laid on the table.

1854

"Dr. Wood made some interesting remarks" upon retiring, and Dr. Joseph M. Smith, having been officially conducted to the Chair, made his address, which pointed out the manner in which the Society might continue to be useful and, in an increasing degree, exert a beneficial influence upon the profession both in this city and throughout the United States.

Dr. Joseph M. Smith, seventh President, was sixty-five when he assumed the office. He attended medical lectures at Columbia and was licensed to practice by the Medical Society of Westchester County in 1811. In 1815, he graduated from the College of Physicians and Surgeons. A tremendous student, he was a professor at P. and S. from 1826 and in medical practice did only consulting work. His reputation was based on his work and writings during an epidemic of typhus fever and as a member of the Consulting Committee of the Board of Health during the cholera epidemic in 1849. In Europe he was recognized as an authority on epidemics. It was said of him he was never known to have shown temper, remaining placid under all conditions.

For the first time the Academy showed little interest in the election of the Standing and Scientific Committees. Their selection had been left to the "officers-elect." Sixteen of the twenty on the Standing Committee, and over half the members of the Scientific Committees were reappointed.

At the first meeting Dr. Stewart, the efficient and enthusiastic first Recording Secretary of the Academy, announced that a large sum of money had been collected in 1853 to entertain the American Medical Association, meeting in New York. Although lavishly entertained, there was a considerable surplus, which a meeting of the subscribers voted unanimously to turn over to the Academy as the beginning of a building fund. Every contributor was allowed to withdraw his share, if he desired, but few did, and 166 medical men presented $1,736.22 to the Academy. Of them 51 were not members. The donation was accepted, ordered deposited with the Treasurer, and the Academy directed the Treasurer to pay $2,500 to the Trustees, "to be invested by them as an accumulating fund for the purpose of purchasing a site and erecting a building for the use of the Academy, said fund to be invested in bonds, mortgages, or Government or New York State stock, at not less than 7 percent interest."

During the year Dr. Gardner reported he had noticed a "new form of quackery" exhibited on Broadway—"Pulvermacher's Magnetic Machine." The newspapers, lay and medical, had carried extensive notices, and a pamphlet had been published stating that the machine had the approval of the Academy, "thus placing the Academy and some of its members in a false position." The instrument had been shown to the Academy by Dr. Detmold the previous December, and the Committee on Pharmacy had reported it an instrument of requisite efficiency, with the advantage, for medical purposes, of being more portable, more readily available, and more economical.

Dr. Taylor said that his name had been quoted without authority, and Dr. Metcalfe said that he had allowed it to be used at

Bellevue and refused a certificate, but had given his written opinion which, italicized and perverted in meaning, had been published contrary to agreement.

Dr. Reese, in his *Medical Gazette*, notes, "An interchange of opinion took place, which indicated a disposition to be more guarded in future individually and collectively, in recommending any patent article, which is a wise resolution if adhered to."

In April the "Anatomical Bill" was passed by the Legislature and the Academy voted its thanks "to the several gentlemen, professional and others, through whose agency the stigma hitherto attached by law in our State to the study of Anatomy and the dissection of dead bodies has been removed."

During the summer it was proposed that the Academy organize a vaccine bureau for gratuitous vaccination of the poor of the city and for furnishing pure matter for the use of its members. The Trustees were to apply to the Common Council for the use of a room for the purpose, funds to cover the expense of an attendant, light, fuel and stationery, because of the steady increase of small-pox in the previous winter, when it was believed 600 cases occurred in the city. The matter was laid on the table.

In October Dr. Corson announced that twenty Fellows had subscribed a total of $100 to allow the Academy to offer a prize of that amount for the best practical essay on cholera infantum "the most destructive of the many diseases which in our large American cities are so fatal to infant life." The offer was accepted, the contributors thanked, and a committee of five appointed to take charge of the matter.

At the November meeting, the President announced that this should have been the Anniversary Meeting, at which the Oration was to be delivered. The President of the Board of Trustees explained that no room could be secured for this evening which suited Dr. Griscom, the Orator, and they had engaged "Clinton Hall" on Astor Place for the next evening. Rather short notice. No mention is made of this meeting in the records of the Academy, but the *New York Medical Times* tells us:

"There was a very large attendance, both citizens and Fellows, the room being filled, and more interest apparently exhibited, than at any celebration since the address of Dr. Francis at the Tabernacle in 1847, when 2,500 persons were present." The editor criticized the place where the meeting was held, which was "subterranean" and was not susceptible of proper ventilation. Dr. Griscom replied the room *was* ventilated and that was why it had been chosen. "It does not follow because a room is 'subterranean,' it is not susceptible of ventilation, as anyone knows who knows anything of pneumatic philosophy." The editor retorted that it *was* installed with ventilators, but the air was so bad because it was also *damp*.

Dr. Reese, rather critical of the Academy, stated in his *Medical Gazette*,

> Dr. John H. Griscom delivered the late Oration of the New York Academy of Medicine, on the "Geological Formations of the State of New York," as we learn by one of the daily papers, which must have been misled by its reporter, for by extracts since published, it seems to have been an omnium gatherum on matters and things in general and ventilation in particular. The selection of orators of late years in this and some other scientific bodies would imply that the qualifications for the post is "to know a little of everything and nothing profoundly."

In November, the Academy took a very important step. At Dr. Batchelder's suggestion, a committee had been appointed to consider the propriety of dividing the Academy into sections. The Scientific Committees had been unsatisfactory. The plan was adopted, and in January the Academy was officially divided into Sections, and the By Laws were amended accordingly. The system of Sections has therefore been in existence for 92 years.

From its inception the Academy had had much difficulty in collecting its annual dues. In December the Finance Committee recommended that all Fellows who had refused to pay their dues by January, 1854, should be reported at the Annual Meeting, and that this should be printed in the announcement of the meeting. The Trustees were already authorized to drop anyone in arrears for two or three years, but they had been very loath to do so, and alone had the power to do it.

The first paper was read in August. It was on cholera, by Dr. Dupierris, of Havana. He could not speak English well enough to read it, so Dr. Adams did it for him. He claimed cholera was not contagious, but was due to an unknown gas in the atmosphere, which, if a predisposition existed, would cause the disease.

This paper, and the general discussion of cholera, occupied two meetings. Dr. White disagreed with Dr. Dupierris, being convinced that the disease was infectious, or communicable—in a bad atmosphere. Dr. Detmold, always a practical person, said Dr. Dupierris' theory of a peculiar gas was only a theory, and did not advance our knowledge of the disease, especially as to its contagiousness; his belief that the disease was an involvement of the vital ganglionic system, was another theory, unsupported by facts; theories got us nowhere. All agreed pretty well that there was a prodromal period of diarrhoea, always painless, and if this was properly and promptly treated, few would succumb to the advanced stages of the disease, unless their habits were bad.

It was not until December that any Fellow presented a paper, and then two were read, one by Dr. Gardner on uterine hemorrhage, and the other by Dr. Horace Green on the treatment of diseases of the larynx and trachea by the topical use of nitrate of silver, and the catheterization of the bronchi with a view to injecting remedies into them, and also into tuberculous cavities. We shall hear more about the latter paper.

Though there were few papers, the Academy was busy. A report on "Solid Milk" from the Committee on Public Health caused long discussion and it was later published in the *Transactions.* Four other subjects were discussed; poisoning by lead (adjourned from the previous year), operative midwifery, fistula lacchrymalis, and dysentery.

A remark of Dr. Stevens during the discussion of lead poisoning is of interest. He stated that in those countries where goitre prevailed, the rain water contained not a particle of iodine, which was not the case in other countries.

"Operative Midwifery" was chiefly concerned with the best methods of destroying the child in difficult labors; Dr. Henschel exhibited a cephalotribe and described the cases in which he had used it.

The discussion of fistula lacchrymalis was short, "owing to the lateness of the hour." That on dysentery was chiefly concerned with the best way of stopping diarrhoeal discharges.

An unofficial discussion occurred between Drs. Detmold and Isaac Wood who exchanged discouraging experiences on the result of treating hydrocephalus by puncture.

Dr. Buck's excision of the knee joint for ankylosis was the only case reported during the year.

The elections for 1855 were very peaceful. Dr. John W. Francis was for a second time elected President. All the Trustees and Standing Committees were reelected.

1855

At the first meeting it was announced that Dr. Francis had declined the election, but the matter was laid on the table. At the next meeting he wrote definitely refusing the office on account of the recent death of his son, which disinclined him to do anything of a public nature. This also was laid on the table. Influence was evidently brought to bear, and eventually Dr. Francis turned up in May and presided thereafter.

The Academy shortened its order of business. At Dr. Stewart's suggestion the roll call was abolished, and the Assistant Secretary was instructed to keep a register in which all Fellows should enter their names, on arrival, and as soon as a quorum was thus established the business of the evening was to commence. After April, 1855, therefore, there is no record in the minutes of attendance.

Considerable time was again wasted over what should be done with Fellows delinquent in their dues. The Treasurer had been ordered to report at the annual meeting in January all Fellows delinquent for several years, which he attempted to do. Much discussion and vigorous objections ensued, and action was postponed till February, the announcement of the subject to be inserted in the notices for that meeting. When the Treasurer offered his report again, its reception was objected to. The Chair decided it was out of order, containing "matter not contemplated in the resolution." His decision was appealed from, but he was sustained by the Academy.

Dr. Bolton moved to strike from the rolls all who were in arrears for three years or more, but Dr. Stewart proposed, as a substitute, that the names of all Fellows in arrears for three years or more be inserted in the notices until May and, after that date, all still in arrears be considered to have forfeited their membership. This was carried unanimously.

But in spite of that action, the next month it was voted that delinquent Fellows be referred to the Trustees and the Treasurer for investigation and report on the causes of nonpayment of dues. In April the Trustees and Treasurer offered an amendment to the By Laws as follows:

> First, those Fellows who are in arrears for three or more years for nonpayment of dues, having been notified of such indebtedness and neglecting to pay the same, shall be considered to have forfeited membership.
>
> Second, the Board of Trustees are hereby empowered to remit a part or the whole of the dues of any Fellow who is unable to pay.

The proposed amendments appeared in the May notices and, after objections to their adoption, it was finally voted to refer the whole matter back to the Trustees and the Treasurer, with instructions to report a "classified list" of delinquents, setting forth the causes of nonpayment, as they had been directed to do in March.

That was the end of the matter for the year. One pities the Treasurer! It was not until the latter sixties that anything was really done. Five meetings had been largely given over to this subject, with no decision.

At the meeting of the previous December, Dr. Horace Green had read a paper on "Catheterism" of the trachea and bronchi. Dr. Green, who had long claimed he could make direct applications of a solution of silver nitrate to the interior of the larynx, recapitulated his experiences. This subject had caused much angry discussion for many years. But Dr. Green's main purpose now was to convince the Academy that he had passed a catheter through the vocal cords into the trachea, injected strong solutions of nitrate of silver into it, and also into either main bronchus, at will; that this had never been done before; that these injections greatly benefited the patients; and that similar treatment *might* be done with tuberculous cavities, with relief; and, finally, that it could be done with ease by the "dextrous surgeon."

A number of those who heard him were his avowed enemies, notably Dr. J. G. Adams, Foreign Corresponding Secretary. A committee of seven was ordered to "inquire into and investigate the treatment proposed." This committee, consisting of Drs. Parker, chairman, Stevens, Isaac Wood, J. O. Stone, James Anderson, Fordyce Barker, and J. T. Metcalfe, reported in June. It had held eight meetings, the first to organize and outline its plans, which were:

1) to ascertain whether direct medication of the lungs by means of catheterism of the air tracts had been before accomplished;
2) to ascertain whether the operation could be performed by the dextrous surgeon with ease and facility and with perfect safety to the patients;
3) to ascertain as far as possible the therapeutic results of this method of treatment.

The committee decided that the passage of the catheter into the trachea could be best determined by "rational signs." Two meetings were held at Dr. Green's office and three at Bellevue Hospital; there was an interim meeting to discuss progress, and the final one to adopt the report. Three entire meetings of the Academy were devoted to this matter. The report was prefaced by the detailed minutes of all the eight meetings of the committee, and the findings were recorded under twenty headings. The first question was answered by the statement that catheterism of the trachea had been performed since the time of Hippocrates. The whole committee was satisfied that the tube could be passed into the trachea. As to the value of the treatment, the report frankly stated time alone would tell.

These three statements were definite answers to the expressed purposes of the investigation, and the report should have ended there, but it went on to make statements about the use of the probang, the proper curve of the instrument, the value of the "rational signs," and how to tell the difference when the tube was in the trachea or in the esophagus; also how much the patient's sensations could be relied on, and whether any "dextrous surgeon" could perform the operation, which was doubted.

Dr. Barker, one of the committee, spoke in dissent of the report. Asked if his remarks were "a minority report" he said the committee report had only been submitted twenty-four hours before and he had not had time to write a proper minority report, but would at a later meeting. After much dispute the matter was laid on the table, and it was agreed to meet again in two weeks.

This time Dr. Barker was ready, and he read a most impressive report. Dr. Barker was an able speaker. His conclusions were:

1. Direct medication of the lungs by means of catheterism of the air passages was first proposed and carried out by our associate member, Dr. Horace Green (not "since the time of Hippocrates" as in the committee report).

2. The process could be performed by the dextrous surgeon with ease and facility and with perfect safety to the patient.

3. The results of this method of treatment, whether it had been employed in bronchial affections or in the commencement of tuberculosis, had already afforded the most gratifying indications that practical medicine would be greatly advanced by the discovery.

After long and rather acrimonious discussion, the reports, both majority and minority, and the paper also, were ordered published as part of the *Transactions* and were ordered circulated before the next meeting.

When they met next month, many had not received the report, but the Academy went into a Committee of the Whole and discussed the matter. It was brought out that only four members of the Committee had signed the majority report. Dr. Stevens sent a letter explaining he had only been at the meetings at Dr. Green's office and so sent in his own memorandum, which considered the passage of the catheter as claimed absolutely proven without doubt. Dr. Anderson wrote that he had only voted that the passage of the tube was possible, and had refused to sign the rest of the report. Dr. Green spoke very well in defense of his paper and practice, and was patient in answering many pointed and unfriendly questions.

It wound up by the Academy adopting the verdict of the Committee of the Whole, "that having considered and discussed the subject referred to it, it recommended to the Academy to lay the subject on the table."

"The Academy then adjourned, after midnight, with the thermometer about 90 degrees."

Thus were three meetings wasted.

During the first half of the year, the newly formed Sections did not run very smoothly.

In March, all the Sections had been organized except that of Chemistry, Dr. Henschel, the chairman, announcing that he had been unable to obtain a meeting, no member appearing at the time appointed. He tendered his resignation as Chairman and member of the Section, which was accepted, and Dr. Bulkley was appointed in his place. Dr. Bulkley subsequently withdrew also.

In April, being called upon for reports, the Sections on Anatomy, Surgery, and Chemistry made none. The others presented written reports which were ordered on file. This caused some discussion in regard to the duties of the Sections, but no definite action was taken.

No provision was made for the meeting places for the Sections, some of which were quite large—Theory and Practice, 36; Obstetrics and Diseases of Women and Children, 34—a goodly number for the chairmen to receive at their offices. The Trustees were asked to make inquiries as to rooms for the Section meetings, but there is no record of their having taken any action.

In August each Section was again called upon and none presented any report. Dr. Batchelder then read a paper upon the duties and rights of the Sections. After considerable discussion, the matter was referred to a special committee, composed of the chairmen of the several Sections, to prepare instructions for the guidance of each Section, and to report to the Academy at the earliest moment possible. Dr. Batchelder, the father of the idea, was later added to the committee and became its chairman.

Next month the committee presented its report, which was adopted, as follows:

1. All papers and subjects referred by the Academy to the respective sections shall be considered and discussed by the sections and a report thereon made to the Academy.

2. Each section shall recommend a subject for discussion before the Academy at least once every six months, and appoint a member to open the discussion.

3. All original papers shall be first read before the Academy.

4. Each section shall appoint, annually, two or more of its members to read an original paper before the Academy.

5. A brief abstract of the cases regularly reported in the sections may be made to the Academy.

On November 6, the Anniversary Meeting was held in the large Chapel of the University. "Prayer was offered by the Rev. Mr. Hutton." After a brief address by the President, Dr. Watson delivered his discourse upon "The State of Medicine among the Ancients." "The lateness of the hour at which it was commenced preventing the Orator from completing his address," the Academy voted its thanks to Dr. Watson for "his able and interesting discourse" and requested him to deliver the remaining portion at his convenience and also to furnish a copy for publication.

In December the Academy suspended the order of business to hear the "remainder" of the Anniversary Address, which was read by Dr. Watson "in part." The next February he was asked to conclude his address, but Dr. Watson declined to occupy more time. It was a prodigious discourse, and as published occupied 222 printed octavo pages, and cost $287.27 to print. Dr. Watson, however, later contributed $152 toward the expense; the Academy voted its thanks.

It had been a troubled year for the Academy, and little was accomplished. It could not make up its mind what to do about delinquent members. It struggled during three meetings to decide what stand to take about Dr. Green and his paper, and nothing was decided. Having reorganized on a Section basis, the Sections were not working well.

Only three medical papers were read. Of these, one by Dr. Buck on badly united fractures, treated by refracture and traction, was valuable and was published in the *Transactions*, Volume I. Dr. Stone, of New Orleans, read a paper by invitation, on yellow fever, which caused much discussion and was published in full in the *New York Daily Times*, of October 8, 1855. Dr. Stone felt that yellow fever was a specific disease, the same in all areas, unmodified by topographical causes or different climates. He was sure one attack protected against other attacks. Almost everyone was likely to have it. Everyone was susceptible until "acclimated," by which he meant "had the fever." It was caused by deterioration of the vital powers, due to some unknown cause. As to contagion, it was "incapable of generating its own poison." Those who were apprehensive contracted the disease. Those who were not, did not. It was a self-limited disease and did not need to be treated, only managed—this meant, to secure perfect rest.

The third paper, on puerperal convulsions, read by Dr. Barker, caused considerable discussion and was published in the *Transactions*, Volume I.

There were no "stated discussions" and no case of interest was reported. A "self-adjusting hygrometric regulator," an apparatus to introduce fumes of chloroform into the vagina and uterus, and a new uterine sound were demonstrated and discussed. Two specimens of cod liver oil, thought to be "very fine" by their sponsors, were shown, and were "referred to the Section on Chemistry to report on their quality and to the Section on Materia Medica to report a mode of disguising the taste."

The Trustees reported the Building Fund amounted now to $2,762.50, which the Academy voted to increase to $3,000 "as soon as the state of the Treasury would permit." The Treasurer then reported he had a balance of $340.37 in the Treasury. The appropriation to the Building Fund was not made.

Only sixteen Resident, and four Corresponding, candidates were recommended for election by the Committee on Admissions.

Another year had passed with little enthusiasm or initiative shown and things were definitely on the down grade. Dr. Francis, as a recalled President, had not helped much, if at all.

1856–1858

Willard Parker · Valentine Mott
John P. Batchelder

1856

THE RETIRING President made a brief valedictory address. Dr. Kissam, Chairman of the Trustees, introduced Dr. Parker to Dr. Francis, who extended him a warm welcome and presented him with a copy of the Constitution.

Dr. Parker, the eighth President, was only fifty-six years old. Receiving his medical education at Harvard, he had been Professor of Surgery at Vermont Medical College (Woodstock, Vt.), Berkshire Medical Institution (Pittsfield, Mass.) and Ohio Medical College (Cincinnati), and was called from there to become Professor of Surgery at the College of Physicians and Surgeons in 1839. A splendid teacher and very popular with his students, he was also one of the most successful and well-known surgeons in New York.

In a brief address he emphasized the needs of a permanent home for the Academy and recommended consideration of the immediate purchase of a site.

Both Dr. Francis and Dr. Parker were asked for copies of their addresses for publication, but both declined on the ground that it would be wiser to reserve the funds of the Academy for other purposes.

A committee of five, including the President and Secretary, were immediately appointed to take steps to secure a site for the Academy. In May the Committee reported that it was "feasible" to do so "under certain conditions" and suggested the appointment of another committee to carry out the purpose. It was moved to make the present committee a committee "with power." The words "with power" caused long discussion, and it was finally decided that the committee report just what powers should be given to it. In September the report was presented and occupied most of one meeting. It was finally adopted.

The committee was to consist of the President and Chairman of the Board of Trustees, ex officio, and five permanent members, who could not be removed until the expiration of their trust. Vacancies were to be filled by the committee itself, which was further empowered to collect subscriptions, make loans, and conduct any other necessary financial arrangements. After completion of the building, the committee was to have authority to lease any portions of it in order to pay expenses and interest and was to continue to do so until all debt was extinguished, unless relieved of individual responsibility by the Academy. When requested to do so, the Trustees were to hand over the Building Fund to the committee, which was not to be held accountable for its acts until the conclusion of its work, or until it should resign. It was given authority to apply to the Legislature for any further powers needed. The Committee certainly had broad powers!

Election of the committee was postponed until the next meeting, when Drs. Anderson, J. M. Smith, and the Treasurer, Dr. Pond, were appointed to nominate the sixteen candidates for five positions as permanent members. In the interval, the Finance Committee probably had been heard from, and in November the election was "indefinitely postponed"—for ten years.

In May, 1855, the Committee on Prize Essay on Cholera Infantum had succeeded in collecting the prize money from its subscribers and advertised the competition in the *Medical Gazette* and *Medical Times*. In March, 1856, the sealed envelope containing the name was opened before the Academy, and Dr. James Stewart was announced the winner. The essay was referred to the Committee on Publications, and when printed it was to be discussed, the President to appoint four members to open the discussion, one for each part, Etiology, Pathology, Symptoms, and Treatment. The essay was printed in full in the *Transactions*, occupying sixty-four pages, but there is no record of its ever having been discussed.

Dr. McNulty reported a message of the Mayor regarding the

new City Charter, and presented resolutions that all medical places be filled by regular physicians and that they be suitably paid. The resolution was "cordially received," and a committee of three was appointed to draw up a memorial to the Legislature. The memorial was sent, and the committee also drafted a law to cover the matter. A year later the Chairman asked that the Committee be discharged, as its efforts had "proved unavailing."

In June, Dr. Watson referred to the "honor due Dr. William W. Reid, of Rochester, for his improvements in the method of reduction in dislocations" and moved that the thanks of the Academy and a gold medal costing "not less than $100" be sent him by the Academy. Dr. Stevens was strongly in favor of this, but Dr. Barker thought the subject ought to be investigated first. A special committee was appointed to report. Nothing more is heard of the medal, and quite properly, for in July the Finance Committee reported that because of the remissness of members in paying dues, the funds in the Treasury were very low. The Committee did not feel authorized to recommend an extra assessment unless the Academy decided to do that, or to use the interest on the Building Fund, or to ask for voluntary contributions. The Treasurer's books showed that only forty-five Fellows had paid their dues for 1856 by July 1. The total funds received from all sources had been only $240. There is no record that the Academy took any action.

During the year, on recommendation of the Trustees, the By Laws were finally amended to read: "Any member who neglects to pay his annual dues for two or more years shall forfeit his membership, provided that he shall have received one month's notice thereof from the Trustees."

Professionally it was a much more active year. Eleven papers were read, but only four of them by Fellows. Dr. C. E. Isaacs presented two very valuable reports of original work on the "Intimate Structure of the Kidney," with numerous illustrations. Dr. S. Conant Foster read an excellent paper on "Atelectasis of the Lungs." All these were ordered published in the *Transactions*.

"Outsiders" read the other papers. Dr. Simpson of Edinburgh, a Corresponding Fellow, sent one on "Carbonic Acid Gas as an

Anaesthetic in Uterine Disease," claiming that it produced better results than chloroform when injected into the uterus. Dr. Fair of South Carolina spoke on yellow fever.

A Mr. J. B. Richards discussed the causes of imbecility and idiocy, and mentioned as causes: (1) abuse of the procreative power; (2) intemperance of the father; (3) intermarriage of relatives; (4) low physique of the father from overwork; and as less important, (5) poor diet; (6) sudden fright of the mother early in pregnancy.

Dr. M'Elheran, M.R.C.S., Edinburgh, discussed "Comparative Anatomy of the Human Crania," which the *New York Journal of Medicine* tells us "fixed the attention of the Academy for two hours."

Dr. Brown-Séquard described his investigations on the physiology of the nervous system, and Dr. Barton of New Orleans, at a special meeting, spoke on yellow fever, emphasizing the influence of high temperature and a moist atmosphere in producing it.

For the first time we learn something of the Section activities—but not from the minutes. The *New York Journal of Medicine* reported in detail nine meetings held by the Sections on Surgery, Obstetrics, and Materia Medica. The discussions were very like those of small private medical societies. Anybody talked about what interested him. And the older and more impressive Fellows took a very active part. In the Surgical Section they discussed everything from the propriety of killing the nerve of a tooth and then filling it, the treatment of moles and phymosis, to the removal of tumors of the uterus and ovariotomy.

The Section on Public Health were much impressed by the food value of preparations of the "Marine Algae" and recommended that the manufacturers be given permission to publish its report; but the Academy was learning the dangers of such action and decided, instead, on publication in the *Transactions,* where it appeared as "Report on Alga Chocolate and Biscuits."

In July Dr. Detmold resigned as Anniversary Orator, so no Anniversary Address was delivered in 1856.

Financially the year had been difficult. At its close, the Treasurer reported a balance of $70.34½, with outstanding bills of $27.31.

The Academy then voted to raise the annual tax from $2.00 to $3.00.

When the Committee on Admissions asked for a decision as to whether a resident of Newark was eligible for Resident Membership, being outside the state, it was finally voted "that while the doors of the Academy are always open to all respectable physicians, yet no practitioner residing beyond the limits of the State of New York can be considered eligible for Resident Fellowship."

The Committee recommended a candidate for election, but the Academy sent the name back because it was said he owned a drugstore selling patent medicines. The doctor denied any connection with any drugstore, so his name was put up again and he was elected.

Much less time was given to discussion of administrative matters and more to the main purposes of the Academy. Dr. Parker was a much better President, attending eleven of its thirteen meetings, and surrendering the chair occasionally to take part in discussions. Except in finances, it may be said to have been the first encouraging year in some time.

When the Academy voted for a new president, Dr. Valentine Mott was elected, the third to be called back in five years.

1857

In his Valedictory Address, Dr. Parker congratulated the Academy upon its general prosperity and harmony and expressed his satisfaction that the discussion of scientific subjects had occupied so large a portion of its time. Dr. Kissam, Chairman of the Board of Trustees, introduced the President-elect to Dr. Parker and the Academy.

"Dr. Parker addressed Dr. Mott, handed him a copy of the Constitution and By Laws, and conducted him to the Presidential Chair, from which Dr. Parker retired, escorted by the Trustees. The Vice Presidents were invited to take seats upon the platform and the Secretaries-elect commenced their duties."

So began the official year of 1857.

His election was really a triumph for Dr. Mott. He had been

in troubled waters many times. Even his right to sign the original Constitution as a Founder had been questioned, but he had signed it. He had been before the Academy for giving a "certificate" to a "notorious quack," and had had considerable trouble clearing himself. His cards offering free advice and treatment to the poor at his college clinic caused charges to be brought against him. He had offered his resignation in 1851 and a year later was "allowed to withdraw it," which he must have done in 1853 for he paid his "annual tax" in November of that year, but did not pay it in 1852. His name does not appear as taking part in the Academy's proceedings after 1851 until his election. He was seventy-two years old when he assumed the presidency for the second time.

It was essentially a scientific year. Dr. Isaacs opened, in February, with a paper on the functions of the malpighian tufts and the elimination of solid matter from the kidneys, based on experiments on animals. In April he read another paper, "The Extent of the Pleura above the Clavicle," also based on original experiments, which "was listened to with much interest." Both of the papers were real contributions to medicine. In 1858 permission was granted to have the illustrations of the first paper electrotyped, to be sent to Dr. Brown-Séquard in Paris for republication in the *Journal d'anatomie et physiologie.*

The chief subject of discussion was puerperal fever. This occupied most of the year, at intervals, was continued into the following year, and developed into a battle-royal between Dr. Alonzo Clark, Professor of Pathology and Practice of Medicine at P. and S., and Dr. Fordyce Barker, Professor of Obstetrics and Diseases of Women and Children at New York Medical College.

Dr. Francis opened with a long paper summarizing the literature to the present day. He felt sure the disease was contagious and cited cases of apparent transmission by the hands and clothing of physicians. In treatment depletion must be used with great caution. Dr. J. M. Smith continued with a paper aiming to prove the "identity" of Erysipelas, Typhus and Puerperal Fever "to a certain extent." Puerperal Fever was not a disease *sui generis*, but an idiopathic fever, one of a group, arising from similar conditions whose essential pathological element was a poisoned state of the blood. The forms of disease associated with it were typhus and its modification typhoid fever, erysipelas and hospital gangrene. It was caused by a subtle poison, the "ochletic miasm of Gregory," gaining entrance to the blood and producing symptoms according to "certain morbid predispositions of the system existing at the time of its reception in the circulating blood."

After endless details, Dr. Smith concluded that puerperal fever arose from: noxious air from foul discharges of puerperal women in crowded, ill-ventilated lying-in hospitals; absorption of putrecent matter lodged in the post-partum vagina or uterus; exhalations of typhus fever, erysipelas, and gangrenous diseases; emanations from the human body after death; and that the miasm may attach itself to the persons or clothing of midwives and physicians and thus be conveyed to the lying-in chamber. Finally, he emphasized the necessity of preserving and maintaining the purity of person, clothing, bedding, floors, furniture, and atmosphere, and warned physicians to be always mindful of the danger of their being the agents of disseminating the disease, "in epidemic puerperal fever seasons."

Dr. Clark then took over. He saw no relation whatever between typhus and puerperal fever. The lesions were entirely different. Erysipelas and puerperal fever, however, did go hand in hand. He was convinced it was transmitted by the hands, clothes, and breath of physicians. At autopsy he had always found inflammation of the peritoneum, veins of the broad ligaments, lymphatics without any inflammation in the veins or the inner surface of the uterus ("endometritis").

At two subsequent meetings Dr. Barker monopolized the stage. He believed it was a "zymotic disease," altogether distinct from inflammation. The original cause was "vital depression," and the lesions were all secondary to that. He criticized Dr. Clark for reliance on findings in the dead house. Dr. Smith had regarded it as an idiopathic fever, Dr. Clark as a local phlegmasia. If that was so, the theory of contagion was untenable. If the cause was a poisoning of the blood, with secondary manifestations in the generative organs, everything was reconcilable.

Dr. Clark in replying stated Dr. Barker's "zymotic disease" was an indefinite and objectionable term. Typhus, smallpox, measles, cholera infantum, croup, whooping cough, syphilis, and many others were usually classified as such. Pathological studies had revolutionized our ideas of medicine. This ended the discussion for the year.

Rheumatism was another subject discussed. The general opinion was that the alkalis were the best treatment and that they tended to prevent cardiac complications. Dr. J. M. Smith quoted Dr. Rush that a fractured leg might be the exciting cause of yellow fever, and thought that after an injury a person well charged with lactic acid might develop articular symptoms. Dr. Hubbard said alkalis had failed to relieve pain in his own case, but colchicum had!

Dr. Horace Green's paper on "Lesions and Functions of the Epiglottis" took one hour to read. He emphasized the importance of topical treatment, as positively arresting cases which would otherwise terminate fatally.

"Dr. Squibb of the Navy" read a paper on chloroform. It was his first appearance at the Academy, in whose activities he later, as a Fellow, took a very active part.

Several other papers of little importance were read, making a total for the year of ten, not including those in the puerperal fever discussion.

Dr. Griscom read a long report on yellow fever from the Section on Public Health and Legal Medicine. Dr. Watson criticized the report as illogical, because the fact that a disease was sometimes imported did not prove it could never originate in a place. The Committee was authorized to publish the paper as read before the Academy, but no printed record of it has been found.

A very creditable report on Borden's concentrated milk was submitted by the Section on Materia Medica. Specimens had been examined as to purity and quality, and were found to be perfectly satisfactory. The whole actual process, from milking the cow to the final concentration of the milk, had been carefully investigated by the Section. The extent of vacuum used, the amount of evaporation, and the temperature to which the product was submitted, and all other details were studied. The Section was convinced it was a safe and valuable substitute for fresh, country milk, and that it would last in an hermetically sealed can for months. It was recommended to the Academy very strongly. The report was referred to the Librarian for filing, and leave was given to publish it as read before the Academy. There is a copy on file at the New-York Historical Society.

The Anniversary Address was delivered at the New-York Historical Society's rooms by Dr. J. Marion Sims, on "The Use of Silver Sutures in Surgery." It was illustrated by many drawings explaining the details of operations in which silver sutures had been used, including everything from gynecological operations to simple skin repair. (A lady sitting by Dr. Barker asked, "What is this silver suture?" Dr. Barker replied, "A new-fashioned backstitch.") Dr. Sims was an enthusiast on the technique. His address was rather self-congratulatory, and it is not strange that there were repercussions. The *North American Chirurgical Review* of July, 1858, published a very critical twenty-page article.

In January, at the elections, Dr. Batchelder was elected ninth President by a large majority, and the vote was made unanimous.

It required four ballots to elect the four Vice Presidents.

While ballots were being prepared for Orator, Dr. Clark withdrew his name as a candidate. It would appear that he was perhaps a little irritated over Dr. Barker's criticism of his remarks on puerperal fever, for he also had declined to run for President. The Academy was disposed not to accept Dr. Clark's withdrawal as candidate for Orator, and showed it by unanimously electing him. He again declined the honor. The resignation was accepted, and the election of Orator was deferred to April.

As in the previous year, a committee had been appointed to nominate members for the Standing Committees. On the former occasion that Committee had renominated all but four of the twenty members for reelection. This year the committee went even further in the opposite direction, and presented a completely new slate, not one former member being renominated.

The report was accepted, but when it came to adopting it there was trouble. In spite of the Secretary's remarks that to accept and then refuse to adopt was not "considerate to the Committee," they did not adopt it, and it was laid on the table, and, as the hour was late, the Academy adjourned.

The Constitution provided that Standing Committees were to be elected annually "by ballot or otherwise," and should serve "until others are chosen to perform such duties as may be assigned to them." The records of the Committees on Admissions and Finance show the same members serving in 1858 as in 1857. It seems probable therefore that the report never left the table and the Committees continued automatically.

Later, "Dr. McNulty begged leave to speak to a question of privilege, and did speak." He had been Chairman of the Nominating Committee. That is all that is said in the minutes, but Dr. Reese announced in the *Medical Gazette* that Dr. McNulty "repelled sundry personal attacks made by Fellows, both in and out of the Academy, imputing to him a conspiracy to revolutionize the officers at the late election and rescue the Academy from the rule of certain cliques. He at the same time avowed himself to be zealously in favor of reform and proposed to favor young physic in lieu of old fogyism, etc." Earlier in the year Dr. McNulty had inquired by whose permission an apothecary's advertisement was suffered to appear on the cover of one of the publications. The Committee on Publications was asked to explain, but never did.

During the year Dr. F. U. Johnston died and a special meeting was called. Long and appreciative resolutions were adopted, after which the meeting adjourned to attend the funeral wearing "the usual badge of mourning." Dr. Johnston was a very distinguished man. The grandson of the celebrated Dr. Samuel Bard, he started studying under him, and then was in the office of Dr. Hosack. He served as "Walker and Resident" at New York Hospital, and for eighteen years was Attending Physician there. He was an active opponent of the then theories of treatment, "drawing out, driving out, and sweating off." While he detested quackery, he was rather sympathetic to Homeopathy, but "so far only as it was limited to doing nothing when nothing was required to be done." He had been a Vice President of the Academy, and was sixty-two years old when he died.

It had been a very active year for the Academy and comparatively peaceful. Except for some irritated feelings in the intensity of the discussion on puerperal fever and the nominations for Standing Committees, there were no encounters.

But financially it had been a very bad year. In May the Treasurer announced a deficiency in the funds, and the Academy promptly instructed the Finance Committee "to raise at once the necessary funds for the Treasury"! A loan of $50 each was secured from Drs. Beadle and Watson. In September the Treasurer reported that the Academy was in debt $95.54 over and above this loan. The Academy really did try to cut down expenses. The publication of Dr. Isaacs' paper on the kidney had been very expensive, $360 for the plates alone. The possibility of publishing the *Transactions* regularly in the medical journals was considered. It was poverty that caused the Academy to allow the publication of papers "read before the Academy" elsewhere than in its *Transactions.* Dr. Isaacs' two papers were the only ones read in 1857 that were published by the Academy.

It also considered substituting the columns of the daily press for official notice of its meetings, but that was given up. Cooper Union as a meeting place was looked into, and the Trustees also reported that the rooms of the Historical Society, with an alcove for the library, could be obtained for $100 per annum; but as the rooms at the University had already been engaged until the following May, the change could not be made.

The Librarian had requested the Trustees to find a place other than his office to accommodate the Library. The Trustees found a room next to the Library of the University that could be secured for a consideration, but it was probably the expenses that prompted Dr. T. F. Cock to request the books remain where they were in his library for the present.

This poverty largely came from the utter neglect of the Fellows to pay their dues. A collector had been employed to collect $292 of back dues that year. Finally, after all the futile efforts to take a stand in this matter in past years, in September the Treasurer sent in a list of forty-one Fellows in arrears, and the Trustees ordered printed and sent to each of them the following:

Dear Sir:

You are hereby notified that, according to Article 3, Section II, of the By Laws of the Academy of Medicine, by a delinquency of two years in the payment of annual dues, you are liable to a forfeiture of membership one month after date hereof.

We are told later six of these forty-one paid up, and that three more called on the Treasurer, but failed to see him.

The Committee on Admissions recommended twenty-five candidates for Resident and two for Corresponding Fellow and all were elected.

1858

On February 28, Dr. Mott pronounced his Valedictory and delivered to Dr. Batchelder a copy of the Constitution.

If ten years of loyalty to the Academy, tireless energy exerted in its interests and development, regular attendance and participation in its proceedings ever entitled a Fellow to be elected President, Dr. Batchelder certainly qualified. He was sixty-three when the Academy was founded, and he was one of the "elder statesmen" invited to sign the Constitution when it was first organized. He is No. 5 on the roster of signers. Holding no elective office until 1851, when he became a Vice President for one year, he had served on the Committee on Ethics for eight years and was chairman of the Section on Surgery for four years. He it was who proposed the establishment of the scientific committees and also the formation and plan of organization of the Sections. He was always in action. He read numerous long papers before the Academy, none of which were ever published in the *Transactions*, and took an active part in many of the discussions. He always had considerable to say on any subject. He was seventy-four when elected. His Inaugural Address, published by the Academy, was not brilliant, but it was a sensible, practical appeal, emphasizing the individual responsibility of every Fellow to make the organization a success by punctual and regular attendance and participation in the Section meetings. He spoke frankly of the neglect in paying dues, which kept the Treasurer "in trouble all the while." He felt the Academy could not go on without raising the dues to $5.00. He stressed the imposition upon the chairmen in having to entertain the Sections each month at their own homes, and urged accommodations be provided, and a permanent home for the Academy.

Dr. T. Gaillard Thomas opened the year with a paper on "Prolapse of the Funis," outlining a new method of treatment. Dr. Detmold quoted a German physician as urging the immediate tying of the cord "as it was easier to resuscitate an asphixiated baby than an anemic one"! The paper "was received with marked favor" and was published in the *Transactions*.

Trouble started at once. The Philadelphia County Medical Society complained that a member of the Academy had written an endorsement of a candidate for Resident Physician of Blockley Hospital, who had been expelled from the American Medical Association for becoming associated with a drugstore which dispensed patent medicines.

This was a serious situation. Could the Academy entertain charges against a Fellow from anyone not a member? After discussing it at two meetings it was finally voted, 34 to 16:

> This Academy has learned with regret that one of its Fellows has recommended for a position of high professional responsibility an individual who had forfeited his rank in the profession.
>
> *Resolved,* That the Secretary be instructed to communicate the above to the Philadelphia County Medical Society.

The recreant Fellow was Dr. D. M. Reese, owner and editor of the *American Medical Gazette*. Dr. Reese smarted under the rebuke and expressed himself in very harsh language in his journal in April, 1858.

Our only "regret" is, that even a handful of the Academy of Medicine should render themselves contemptible by such self-stultification.

"*Mons parturiunt,—nascitur ridiculus MUS.*"

The parties chiefly concerned in this "tempest in a teapot" were: first, the *imbecile* Dr. A. [Dr. Adams], who was, once upon a time, appointed to the New York Hospital, but a compulsory resignation, followed by a necessary transfer to the Bloomingdale department, fixed the status of all concerned, "non compos mentis." Second, Dr. B. [?] the oft-defeated candidate for the presidency, whose ambitious aspirations ever lie in that direction. Third, the inevitable Dr. G. [Dr. Griscom], the standing candidate for City Inspector, Health Officer, and every other *paying* medical office, and who is ever lobbying about the City Hall and at Albany, greedy for feeding as aforetime at the public crib, and *even now is seeking to create a fat office for himself!* These, who are, *par nobile fratrum*, doctors without patients, with their toadies, uniting with the K.L.'s [Kappa Lambdas] and other cliques, all of whom have been criticized in the Gazette, make up the thirty-six whose "regrets" are duly chronicled among the archives of the Academy. Vive la bagatelle!

Dr. Reese, a Vice President of the A.M.A., had a hard time at its meeting in Washington. He was forced to apologize, and even express *his* "regrets" for his "departure from medical ethics."

This was the only unpleasant incident of the year.

Ten papers were read. Dr. J. C. Dalton made his really great contribution to the "Anatomy of the Placenta," proving that the blood from the uterine sinuses passed through the placenta to the chorion and that radicals of the fetal vessels were supplied from these pools of blood.

During the summer, puerperal fever was again brought up and another battle royal between Drs. Clark and Barker took place at two meetings. Neither added much to what had been said before. Dr. Barker summarized the French literature on the subject over the last few years, and laid particular stress on treatment: "the patient is often sacrificed by a contest between the doctor and the disease, both contributing to exhaust the vital powers." The doctor's province was to keep the patient alive till the disease was exhausted. There were sometimes cases where the stomach seemed to "give out all at once." He had "been able to persuade the stomach to resume its functions" by giving beef tea with a few drops of nitro-muriatic acid.

An essay on yellow fever was read by Dr. F. Bacon, of Galveston, which gave a clear and simple account of his experiences. He had no use for any system of treatment—mercurials, quinine, and depletion often being not only useless but harmful. He relied on satisfying the patient's thirst, sustaining his strength, and making him more comfortable by sponging with alcohol and water.

Dr. Corson read a practical paper on the importance of correct position of the shoulders in examination of the chest. Auscultation was a recent advance in medicine, and although the paper received scoffing notices, Dr. Corson brought out what is now taught every student in his first instruction in examination of the chest.

A special meeting was held to discuss the prostate gland. Dr. Van Buren opened the subject, and stated that it was properly an involuntary muscle, the true ejaculator urinae. The third lobe was the result of disease, caused by gonorrhoea and old age. It resembled fibroid tumors in the female. Drs. Parker and Wood agreed. Dr. Watson said that the gland began to develop at puberty, and retention in old men was due to twisting of the bladder by descent of overloaded bowels.

One of the exciting incidents of the year was the presentation to the Academy by Dr. Mott of a M. Groux, who "kindly exhibited himself for their gratification and instruction." M. Groux had a "congenital deficiency of the sternum" and had apparently exhibited himself all over Europe and now had arrived here to continue his activities. The Section on Anatomy examined him and he appeared a second time before the Academy. The New York Pathological Society took him in hand later and presented a long and detailed report of what they found. M. Groux was very busy and was presented with $50 by the Academy.

Some months later Dr. Peaslee presented the Academy with seven photographs of M. Groux and his deformity, which were taken in Boston. Only nine sets of these photographs were made and care had been taken "that no more shall be produced"! These photographs, taken nearly ninety years ago when photography was in its infancy, somewhat faded, mounted in a worn album ordered for them by the Academy, are still in existence. Photostatic negatives, touched up by Dr. Dickinson, show the deformity quite distinctly after all these years.

The Section on Materia Medica reported on a sample of "Vin Nutratif." It was recommended, and an endorsement must have been voted sent to the proprietors, for the *Medical Gazette* reported such an action, and the endorsement appears as an advertisement therein.

The proprietors distributed the following:

MEDICAL ACADEMY OF NEW YORK

Approval of the Vin de Bugeaud

The Medical Academy of New York adopted the following resolution on the 4th of August, 1858.

The Committee of Materia medica and Botany charged with the examination of the tonic and nutritive wine combined with quinine and cocoa, prepared by M. Bugeaud at Paris, hereby declare that the said wine has been administered by the different members of the committee in a great many cases requiring analeptic tonics and that it has constantly fulfilled their utmost expectations.

The Committee, therefore, think it their duty to recommend this wine as worthy of trial in all cases of sick people for whom tonics are prescribed, and more particularly during convalescency from ague and other febrile affections.

Have signed:
The President of the Committee,
Joel Foster, M.D.,
The Secretary of the Committee,
E. H. Jymes, M.D.

To this resolution is added in the hand-writing of the Secretary-archivist of the Academy: "While forwarding to you the above written expression of the opinion of the Committee, I feel great pleasure in adding thereto my personal approval. (*Signed*)

"*C. F. Heywood*, M.D."

This was never challenged by the Academy.

The regular meeting in September was postponed because that day had been assigned to celebrate the completion of the "Ocean Telegraph" and all scientific societies were invited to participate.

Dr. Peaslee delivered the Anniversary Address at the rooms of the New-York Historical Society, on "The Progress and Spirit of Medical Science." "The public had been generally invited and the hall was well filled by the Fellows and their families and friends."

Very important action was taken by the Academy in October. A committee of eleven had been appointed to revise and amend the Constitution and By Laws, "said committee to be chosen from the various colleges and societies that its action might be impartial." On this committee were Drs. Mott, J. M. Smith, and Horace Green for the Medical Colleges; Drs. Francis and Watson for the Hospitals; Dr. Kissam for the Trustees; Dr. Isaac Wood, Committee on Ethics; Dr. Griscom, Committee on Public Health; Dr. McNulty, representing "Young Physic"; and the President and the Secretary.

The Academy sat as a Committee of the Whole and discussed the Constitution as proposed, article by article, and then the By Laws. Their recommendations were promptly adopted and were ordered to go into effect at the stated meeting in November "provided that the present officers hold over until the new ones had been chosen."

This was in striking contrast to the revision made in 1852, when three long meetings were necessary to adopt really minor changes.

January was the date for the election of officers. Three "inspectors" took charge. While the polls were "open," Dr. Hudson showed an artificial leg, hand, and arm, and Dr. Green read an essay on the treatment of croup, with special reference to the use of silver nitrate in the air passages. He also gave a partial account of the "recent case of Mr. Whitney," the discussion of which was made the special order of business at the next meeting.

The report of the Inspectors of the Election is amusing. It was announced that Dr. Watson was elected President and also that the Recording and Corresponding Secretaries, and a Treasurer had been elected; but there was no choice for any of the three Vice Presidents, four of the five Trustees, three members of the Committees on Admissions and Ethics and two of Medical Education. There were so many vacancies that it was voted to hold an adjourned meeting January 19 at 6.30, just before the stated meeting of that date.

When that meeting was held, Dr. Hubbard, on behalf of his fellow inspectors, announced a "clerical error" in the report. There was only one vacancy for Trustees instead of four, as reported, all the Committee on Admissions had been elected, instead of two, and all but one of the Committee on Ethics; but there were still two vacancies in the Committee on Medical Education. It was voted that these three vacancies in Standing Committees be filled by electing those holding the highest number of votes at the last election. They promptly settled the three vacancies for Vice President and one Trustee, and adjourned to hold the first meeting of 1859.

Again it had been a hard year financially for the Academy. In February the Treasurer had announced a "depleted treasury." This explains many actions during the year. Dr. Hinton suggested the stated meetings of Sections be announced in the general Academy notices each month, which the President was strongly in favor of, as saving the Academy $100 per annum. Beginning in April, the Section meetings were so announced. It was very unpopular, however, with the Sections, several reporting subsequently there had been no quorum since its adoption. Later the members of four of the Sections reported they had sent notices printed at their own expense. The plan was dropped in 1859.

When Dr. Morris read his memorial address on Dr. F. U. Johnston, "permission was granted the *family* to have this address printed."

Dr. Batchelder's Inaugural Address was not voted published until September. Of the ten papers read, only two were ordered published in the *Transactions*.

Dr. Sims's Anniversary Address of the year before was voted printed, but Dr. Sims attended to its publication himself, sending 750 copies—and the bill for $140—to the Academy. This caused quite a disturbance, but Dr. Detmold thought the whole affair was only a mistake and the proper course was to accept the copies submitted and pay the bill, which was ordered done.

The moving of the library to the University was accomplished in November, and "the books were all in good condition as received from Dr. Cock, the late Librarian, and were placed in their present location without damage." The cost of moving the entire library was $3.50!

The loan by Drs. Beadle and Watson had been repaid and the Treasurer reported $171.20 in the treasury November 30, 1858. He had paid the collector $68.70 for collecting $687 of back dues.

The Committee on Admissions recommended eight candidates, all of whom were elected.

The Sections were fairly active as far as can be learned. That on Public Health requested additions to its numbers, and sixteen new names were added to it, including the President.

Although little is learned from the minutes of stated meetings, except on matters of administration, or organization, Dr. Stephen Smith tells us much in the *New York Journal of Medicine:*

> This association of the medical profession in our city is making commendable advances in fulfillment of the noble objects of its original organization. Its well-adjusted machinery of *Sections* is working admirably, and the stated meetings of the Academy are steadily increasing in practical importance and interest. . . .
>
> The Academy should occupy a position and earn a reputation second to no other medical body in the world; and with a continuation in its present career, its discussions and transactions may soon fully equal those of the Royal Medico-Chirurgical Society, or the French Academy.
>
> . . . The noble *animus* and zeal of the present venerable President, Dr. Batchelder, have done much to promote the interests and to perfect the present improved organization of the Academy. The several *Sections* are now, by their efficient labors, bestowing upon their originator honors even higher than those conferred by presiding over their combined deliberations.

Dr. Batchelder had been a good President. He was only absent from three meetings. He encouraged the younger Fellows to take a larger part in the Academy's activities. Dr. T. G. Thomas was only twenty-seven when he read his paper on prolapse of the funis. The age of the other readers of papers was in contrast with former years —Dr. Rotton thirty-two, Dr. J. C. Dalton thirty-three, Dr. Gardner thirty-seven, and Dr. Barker forty. Drs. Corson, forty-four, and Green, fifty-six, were the only *elderly* readers of papers.

1859–1860

John Watson

THE YEAR 1859 was a notable one. For twelve years the Academy had carried on in a casual sort of way. There was nothing permanent or continuing in its organization. The entire administration could be changed on a whim or by political activity. Dr. McNulty's efforts to make a clean sweep of the Standing Committees in 1857 had failed, but that incident probably had considerable influence on the committee that drafted the new Constitution. It did a good job, and the organization of the Academy is today practically the same as when put into effect nearly ninety years ago.

The President was elected for a two-year term; the number of Vice Presidents was reduced from four to three, one retiring each year. The offices of Domestic and Foreign Corresponding Secretaries were combined and, with the Recording Secretary and Treasurer, were to serve for a period of three years. The number of Trustees was reduced to five, one retiring each year, as did also one member of each Standing Committee.

A most important change was the establishment of a Council, composed of the Officers, Trustees and Chairmen of the Standing Committees. The Council is practically the same today. The Finance and Publications Committees were abolished and their duties taken over by the Council. The Council was to supervise the general affairs and interests of the Academy, to provide suitable accommodations for its meetings, to care for its movable property, to fix the annual tax and to audit the financial accounts. The Librarian and Assistant Secretary were to be appointed by it, as well as Fellows to deliver lectures, or discourses, on scientific subjects, and the Anniversary Discourse. The presentation of any paper by non-Fellows was to be decided by the Council. Selection of essays, memoirs, or reports for appearance in the *Transactions* "or in the printed account of the Proceedings and Discussions" was left to it, as well as superintending the actual printing and publication of all "papers and volumes" ordered by the Academy.

The duties of the Trustees were not much changed, but were a little more carefully defined. In general they were charged with all invested funds and real property of the Academy, just as to-day.

The ever-troublesome matter of action for nonpayment of dues was fixed by the By Laws: "Any Fellow neglecting to pay his dues for two or more years shall forfeit his membership, provided he shall have received one month's notice thereof from the Trustees." But the sending of such notice was left to the "discretion" of the Trustees.

A new Standing Committee on Medical Instruction was established and was given a difficult program. It was to have cognizance of the systems of medical instruction, private and public, in the city and state, as compared with such as were elsewhere in use. It was to "recommend such improvements in office training and office examinations, in text-books, in reading, and in practical studies proper for the students in the public courses, theoretical and practical, at the colleges and hospitals," as seemed in keeping with the advance of medical knowledge and the exigencies of the profession. They were to notice any evasion of the laws of the state that might come to their knowledge in reference to the granting of degrees and to make suggestions for rendering the system of medical education thorough, efficient, and satisfactory. Quite a job for the Committee on Medical Instruction! It is not strange it did not live up to requirements.

All candidates for election were to be on one ballot, which was to be supplied in duplicate to each Fellow before the election. The poll was to be kept open till all members had had a chance to vote. In a case of no election, an immediate second vote was to be taken, the candidate with the fewest votes being dropped at each subsequent ballot.

Dues were fixed at $4.00.

Two Stated Meetings were to be held each month, and the order of business was shortened and simplified.

At the first meeting of the year, "the officers of the past year proceeded to give place to those newly elected." Dr. Batchelder read a Valedictory Address, mainly reminiscent of the past twelve years, including his own term of office. His Valedictory was published. Dr. Watson was conducted to the seat of the President and in his Address laid particular stress upon sanitary reforms, and suggested improvements which might in time be introduced into the workings of the Academy. His Inaugural was not published.

Dr. Watson, tenth President, was of Scotch ancestry. He came from Londonderry, Ireland, to this country in 1810, at the age of three. He graduated from the College of Physicians and Surgeons in 1832, in 1837 became associated with Dr. A. H. Stevens, and was appointed Attending Surgeon to New York Hospital in 1839. He had taken a leading part in forming the American Medical Association and was very active in its discussions of medical education.

A recently discovered autobiography written by Dr. Watson for Dr. J. W. Francis tells us that the first suggestion of founding the Academy was broached by him in a conversation with Dr. Stevens in 1846. The resolutions presented by Dr. Stevens at the preliminary meeting were written by him. A member of the committee to draw up a plan of organization of the Academy, he presented one which was "not acceptable to the committee. A most objectionable plan was adopted by them," the defects of which prevented him from cooperating further with the committee. It was not until 1853, when the Constitution and By Laws had been amended, so as to "give character to the organization," that he consented to join.

He had been Orator in 1855, Vice President, 1856–1858, Chairman of the Section on Surgery in 1858, and had twice been delegate to the American Medical Association. Except for his oration, he had never presented a formal paper before the Academy. He was the first President elected to serve a two-year term, the first who was not a Founder, and was fifty-two years old when elected, the youngest President the Academy had had. Dr. Watson was a man of mark.

At the first meeting for the year, the "Whitney case" was taken up. This probably explains the large attendance noted as present. It was an unfortunate matter, and caused much bad feeling within the Academy and criticism from without. Most of our information comes from outside sources, and the records, official and others, may be summarized as follows.

Mr. Whitney, a wealthy citizen of social prominence, suffered from a severe cough and pain in his chest. Without the knowledge of his regular attendant, Dr. J. C. Beales, a Fellow of the Academy, he had consulted Dr. Horace Green, who found signs of "tubercular softening" of the left upper lobe, with an inflamed throat and "ulcerated" tonsils and epiglottis. Mr. Whitney was treated several times by local applications of silver nitrate to the throat and the interior of the larynx by the probang. He was very irregular in attendance and his throat was not well prepared for passing the catheter, which, however, he insisted on having done December 6. That was the last Dr. Green saw of him.

Later in the day Dr. Beales was called and found him in a state of "intense excitement, suffering and terror." He confessed he had been "such a fool as to go to Dr. Green to be operated upon, and the damned villain has killed me." Dr. Beales described his statements and complaints in great detail, but admitted that he had made only a casual examination of the throat, all examinations being "objected to." Shortly after, Whitney developed subcutaneous emphysema of the neck, chest wall, and subsequently most of the trunk. Dr. Mott was called in and saw him frequently thereafter up to his death several days later.

Drs. Beales and Mott made up their minds that Dr. Green, in passing the catheter, had perforated the trachea, and hence the emphysema. Without inviting Dr. Green, an autopsy was performed by Dr. Alexander Mott, but an absolutely sound and healthy trachea was found. Looking further, they found a small, ruptured cavity at the apex of the left lung, and a retropharyngeal abscess, which had also ruptured, admitting the tip of the finger. Drs. Mott and Beales now decided that Dr. Green had perforated the pharyngeal wall with his catheter and thus produced the abscess. Mr. Whitney had complained of inability to swallow, difficulty in breathing, and intense pain in the throat, but they had not suspected a retropharyngeal abscess, although, as an out-of-town commentator remarked, "the signs were as clear as an army advancing with all flags flying."

Dr. Green had fired the first shot in reporting the case in December. There is every reason to think that he rightly expected an attack on himself from Dr. Beales and Dr. Mott. They came fully prepared at the next meeting, but so was Dr. Green, and the whole picture rapidly changed from one of a defense by Dr. Green to one of defense by his detractors. Dr. Green frequently called forth applause in his statements. Dr. Sayre moved as follows:

> WHEREAS, Charges have been brought against Dr. Green, a Fellow of this Academy, which have not been substantiated by the post mortem or any evidence brought before this body, therefore
>
> *Resolved,* That in the opinion of this body, Dr. Green should be exonerated from any censure or charge of malpractice in the case of Mr. Whitney, and that the subject be dismissed.

This caused friends of Dr. Beales and especially of Dr. Mott, to fear it would not look well for them. So Dr. Gardner offered the following substitute:

> WHEREAS, Various statements by the public press and otherwise, have reflected upon the reputation of Drs. Green, Mott and Beales, as having conduced by their treatment to the death of Mr. Whitney,
>
> *Therefore* we, the Academy of Medicine, after a full examination of the reports in the case and the post mortem examination, do consider that his death was in no wise the result of any improper treatment, but was the unavoidable result of a complication of diseases.

This was unanimously adopted, and the matter was laid on the table. The affair had occupied one entire meeting and a part of two others.

When the minutes were read later, Dr. Sayre stated he had accepted the substitute motion with the distinct understanding that Dr. Mott had withdrawn his charges against Dr. Green, which the minutes, as read, failed to state. If they had not been withdrawn, he would never have accepted the substitute motion. Dr. Mott was not present, and the President suggested that the records stand till Dr. Mott could be heard from. He never was. He is never reported as taking part in any scientific session thereafter, and we hear no more of Dr. Beales.

The lay press charged it was a "whitewashing resolution." One denounced the profession as a "stupendous humbug." Another said: "If it is impossible for ordinary mortals to come to a decision on any point mooted among doctors, it would appear to be equally impossible for doctors to come to a decision on points which would be settled in twenty minutes by ordinary men."

Drs. Mott and Beales had made no attempt to shield Dr. Green from the accusations of the Whitney family. The *Medical and Surgical Reporter* (Philadelphia) commenting very unfavorably on the action of the Academy, stated: "Considering the whole affair discreditable to all participating in it, and only deserving of notice because it teaches an impressive lesson in ethics, we commend it to the oblivion which it merits."

The *Nashville Journal of Medicine and Surgery's* account of the matter occupied fourteen printed pages, and was vitriolic about Drs. Beales and Mott. It concluded: "We think Dr. Mott, difficult as it is for him to learn there is anything in medicine or surgery outside of himself, found before Dr. Green closed, that he did not belong to that breed of cocks which suffered themselves to be sacrificed to Aesculapius, or anyone else."

A little more unpleasantness started later. Dr. Corson had read a paper on "The Position of the Shoulders in Physical Examination of the Chest." He complained of remarks made by Dr. Reese in his *Medical Gazette*, and read the following:

At the last meeting, on a motion for leave to print that paper of Dr. Corson, on the gymnastics of the shoulders in physical exploration of the thorax, with which a former meeting had been bored, Drs. Detmold and McNulty brought out the fact, that it had already been printed, without leave, in the *New York Journal*, with "picters to match"; and it might have been shown that, "twaddle" as it is, copies have been bound in book form, for *popular* circulation, especially among clergymen, lawyers, etc., and it is already widely circulated. So transparent a device for seeking a specialty in practice is ludicrous enough, if it were not palpable that the paper contains nothing either new or useful. Its pictures will forcibly recall to memory the old school-books on elocution, in which the various attitudes are depicted by plates; or the recent cuts, showing the exercises of infant schools, "hands behind," "hands before," "hands overhead," &c. We are ashamed that any journal could be induced to insert it by any amount of importunity, or even by "paying for the illustrations"; and it is still more humiliating that the Academy should stoop so low as to give even a quasi endorsement. But, alas! our profession in New York seems to be doomed, and there is no telling what we are coming to.

Dr. Reese was more interested in the success of his journal than in the harmony of the Academy. Permission *had* been given for its publication.

Letters were read from two druggists, informing the Academy that they would in the future have a supply of Dr. Squibb's remedies on hand and advising that when these were desired the name of Dr. Squibb be written on the prescription. No criticism was made by any Fellows on these statements.

Dr. Squibb had been elected in 1858. He organized that year a laboratory to manufacture standard preparations of drugs "for the profession." He produced no "nostrums" or patented articles. He did a splendid piece of work, his tinctures, fluid extracts and so forth, becoming standard among the profession. "Squibb's Ether" was practically universally used for many years. By his accurate, scientific methods he rendered invaluable service to accurate medication through a long lifetime.

The Council, to which had been referred a motion by Dr. Griscom to exclude from all meetings of the Academy all reporters except those from medical journals, reported it considered it inexpedient to legislate at present on the subject. That did not please Dr. Griscom, who immediately moved to lay its report on the table, and offered the following resolution:

Whereas, The discussions and statements made at the Academy are, or should be, strictly of a professional character and import and therefore improper to be reported in the daily press,

Resolved, That the reporters, except those of medical journals, be hereafter excluded from the meetings of the Academy.

It was finally laid on the table.

A "Japanese Mission" was expected in New York, and the Common Council had appointed a reception committee for the city. It was proposed that the Academy should do something—that perhaps the two medical men in the mission should be invited to lecture. Dr. Kissam wondered what their status and attainments were in their own country. Dr. Buck, who brought the matter up, did not know, but thought that being on the staff of the Embassy ought to be proof of their being "of some standing." A committee of seven was appointed to handle the matter. Dr. Anderson, chairman, reported that, on closer acquaintance with the physicians of the medical department of the Embassy and their total inability to appreciate the proposed attentions, as well as their reluctance to accept the Academy's kindness, the Committee had terminated its activities.

In the early summer of 1860 the Academy paid a striking tribute to the memory of Dr. C. E. Isaacs, who had contributed much to its meetings. He had moved to Brooklyn, where in his fiftieth year he died of pleuro-pneumonia. A special joint meeting with the New York Pathological Society was held in the Mayor's office in Brooklyn. Dr. W. H. Van Buren read a fine tribute for the Academy.

The Legislature had passed a very cumbersome law restricting the sale of poisonous drugs, which was not being enforced. It was moved that the Academy send a copy of the law to every druggist in the city, but it was decided to ask the College of Pharmacy to take over the task.

The Academy was very active in scientific matters. In March, 1859, the Council announced a program of twelve lectures to be read in 1859 and three in 1860. The Fellows were all urged to volunteer for other papers. It is interesting to note that the readers were mostly younger Fellows. Unfortunately only two of those announced were ever read.

Thirty-four papers were read during these two years. Dr. Dalton spoke on the "Rapidity and Extent of the Physical and Chemical Changes in the Body," and Dr. Isaacs on "Milky or Chylous Urine."

Yellow fever and its personal communicability occupied much time and called forth five papers. The discussion occupied most of five meetings. The last was a most elaborate paper by Dr. Griscom, who quoted Dr. J. M. Smith's fundamental doctrines: "Contagion is a poison generated by morbid animal secretion, possessing the power of inducing a like morbid action in healthy bodies, whereby it is reproduced, and indefinitely multiplied," and infection was due "to the product of decomposition of animal and vegetable substances." From these two premises he tried to prove logically that yellow fever could not be communicated by personal contact. He ended with the introduction of resolutions passed by the National Quarantine and Sanitary Convention: "Resolved that in the absence of any evidence establishing the conclusion that Yellow Fever has ever been conveyed from one person to another, . . . personal quarantine of cases of Yellow Fever may be safely abolished, provided that fomites of every kind be rigidly restricted." As the Academy was about equally divided on the subject, it was laid on the table.

Dr. Davis of Brooklyn contributed two valuable papers on morbus coxarius, and diseases of joints in general, urging the importance of traction.

Dr. O'Reilly spoke on the nervous centers of animal and organic life (the cerebro-spinal and sympathetic nervous systems) and also on the functions of the pineal gland. At his request, a committee was appointed to study the latter subject further, but it never reported. In discussing the paper, Dr. Peaslee said it was easier to make statements in regard to the functions of the nervous system without criticism than in any other department of medicine.

Dr. Squibb read three papers, one of which, on revision of the *Pharmacopoea,* roused much interest. It was continued into a second evening, on request. The other two papers read at the same meeting were on errors in prescription writing and on a revision on medical metrology.

Dr. Watson left the Chair three times to read papers, the first he had ever presented was on the results of wounds, in which tetanus was mentioned and was considered "not invariably fatal." Another was on the efficacy of gargles in "Epidemic Sore Throat." He used a stimulating and detergent gargle "varying from Claret wine, pure or diluted, sage tea charged with yeast and sweetened, Tincture of Myrrh in Mucilage, to Chlorate of Potash." A third paper was on tetanus.

Dr. Gardner was very active. He read a paper on "Pulmonary Apoplexy," recounting two cases. Asked whether autopsies were made, he said not on the first, diagnosis having only been made after the second case ten years later. Nobody agreed with him, and he came back later with a defense based upon papers read at the French Academy.

The meetings were not all as dignified as might have been desired. Dr. Bolton, on a "question of privilege" read a paper condemning a popular article written by Dr. Gardner for the *Knickerbocker Magazine*, on the "Physical Decline of American Women." In that article he explained why woman was now "a haggard creature, dull eyed and sallow, pinched in form, an unfit mother, not a helpmeet but a drag on the energy, spirits and resolution of her partner in life." As to causes he "really thought the Polka and its variations, which so jar the frame" had done more than any single cause to injure the health of American women.

Dr. Bolton came to the defense of the women. The *American Gazette* commented, "with the merits or demerits of which the Academy had no more business than with the 'moon story' of Richard Adams Locke, but being entertained by the chair and tolerated by the members, it gave opportunity for personalities and vituperation unworthy of the body, and humiliating to its character and usefulness."

There were several long discussions which were often amusing, but space only permits their being mentioned. During one election, a paper being lacking, Dr. Watson introduced for discussion the differential diagnosis between "Diphtheria and Croup, Muguet, Measles, Putrid Sore Throat, etc." The older men believed in heroic methods, the younger in more conservative treatment. Dr. Barker summed up by saying croup was a local disease, diphtheria a constitutional one, resulting from some specific poison. In diphtheria, constitutional symptoms preceded the local disease, in croup the local symptoms preceded the constitutional. The discussion occupied two meetings.

The best and safest anaesthetic was another subject for long discussion.

Dr. Peaslee exhibited an intra-uterine stem pessary and spoke of its value. Dr. Gardner was opposed, favoring external support. Dr. Peaslee replied that external supports were as useless as trying to hold "a solid body in a definite position in a barrel of water by applying an extra hoop on the outside."

On another occasion when there was a vacancy on the program, Dr. Watson called upon the surgeons to discuss factors influencing the success of operations. Dr. Stevens thought medical after-care more important than operative skill, emphasized the importance of an empty stomach during an operation, and that hemorrhage should have ceased before the patient left the table. Dr. Batchelder considered the state of the moon of no little importance, contending that operations after a full moon were more successful than those before it.

The Anniversary Address in 1859 was delivered by Dr. W. C. Roberts, "Eulogium of Medical Science." There had been some difficulty in obtaining an Orator; five had been invited to deliver the oration but declined. Again, in 1860, when the Orator withdrew on account of ill health, Dr. Watson jumped into the breach and offered to fill in, and was accepted by the Council. It was his second anniversary address in six years. He spoke on "Medical Education." The Trustees made elaborate preparations. Five hundred circulars were sent to "medical, literary and benevolent institutions," notices were published in seven daily newspapers, and three hundred special invitations were sent to individuals. "There was a highly respectable audience of about 300."

Dr. Watson's term of office marked a tremendous advance in the affairs of the Academy. He had done his best to stimulate interest in its programs, and on three occasions had read papers. When an orator was unavailable, he had volunteered, and he had been par-

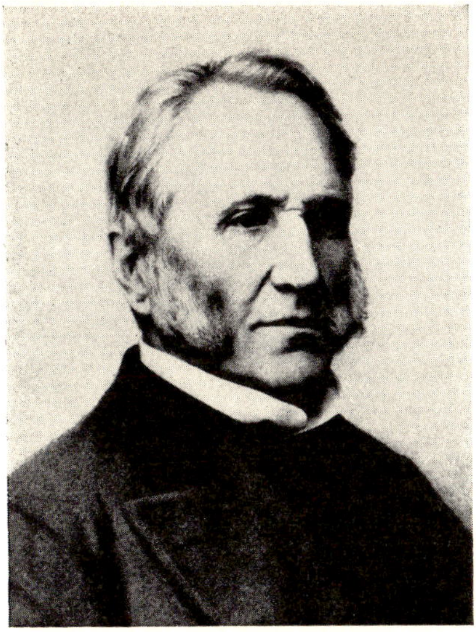

WILLARD PARKER, 1800–1884
Eighth President, 1856

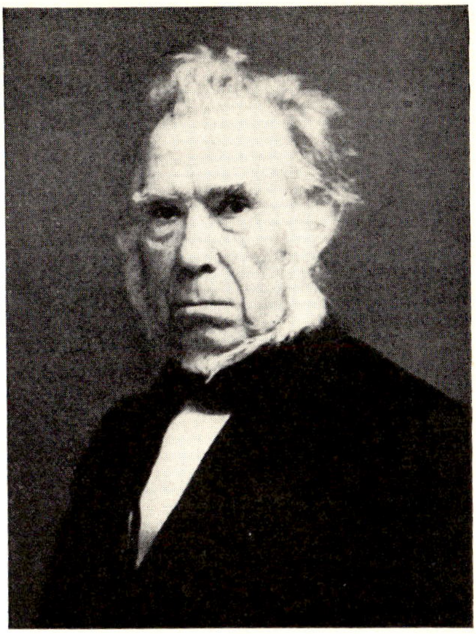

J. P. BATCHELDER, 1784–1868
Ninth President, 1858

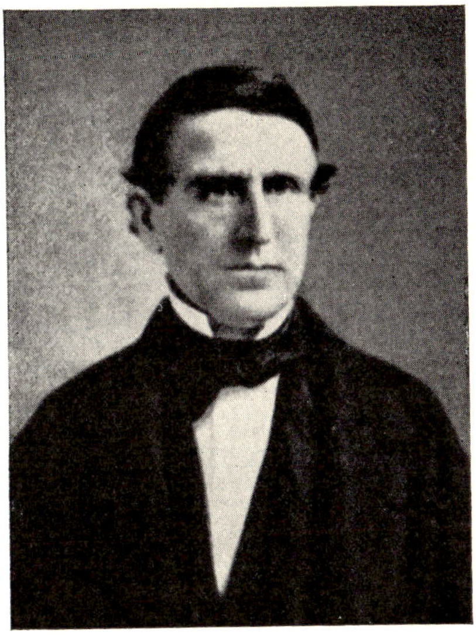

JOHN WATSON, 1807–1863
Tenth President, 1859–1860
The First to Be Elected for a Two-Year Term

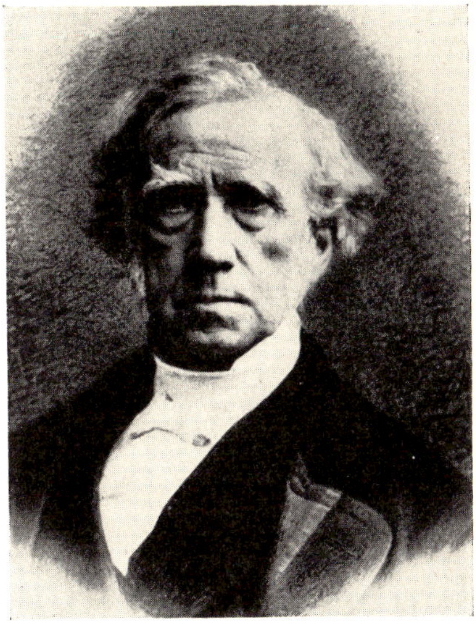

JAMES ANDERSON, 1798–1886
Eleventh President, 1861–1866

ticularly clever in filling gaps in the program with impromptu discussions. He was only absent once each year, in July.

From what little we can learn, the Sections had been working pretty well, and that on Obstetrics and Diseases of Women and Children announced it had formed a subsection on Diseases of Children, but this did not materialize. The Sections were clamoring for quarters in which to hold their meetings. The Trustees found that the Chancellor's room at the University would be available for seventy-two meetings at a cost of $200 per annum, but felt the Academy could not afford to pay rent or for special notices for the Sections.

Dr. T. Gaillard Thomas records in his annual report as Secretary that the attendance was "uniformly good" and a quorum "early obtained." And yet at three meetings there was no quorum—two in succession. As a Secretary Dr. Thomas was not accurate or painstaking.

After that hiatus, the motion was made to resume meeting once a month, but it was defeated. Later it was moved to do away with the whole system of organization and return to one meeting a month, annual election of all officers and standing committees, and a reduction of dues to $3.00. When this was voted on, it was laid on the table by a vote of 11 to 10. Twenty-one Fellows—just a quorum—to vote on a complete change of the Constitution!

For years the Academy had been complaining about the publication of its *Transactions*, or the nonpublication to be more accurate. No paper could be published except in the *Transactions*, without special permission. Several thought the Academy ought to encourage publication anywhere, because the long delay discouraged the reading of papers.

The Council took the matter up, and arrangements were made to have the proceedings published in the *American Medical Monthly*, reprints to be provided labeled *Transactions* of the New York Academy of Medicine. But that did not work out well, and the *New York Journal of Medicine* was given the job, but, finding that it did not pay, the publishers raised their price. Finally, after much delay, the Academy took on the publication itself and the *Bulletin*, a running account of papers and discussion, first appeared in April, 1860.

The Trustees finally took action in regard to delinquents. The matter had been dodged for several years. They voted the names of forty-three members, "delinquent for two years or more," to be stricken from the rolls, and an additional twenty-eight to be warned. Dr. Pond's careful records show that of the seventy-one, fifty-four were "stricken." Three had been elected in 1847 and had never paid dues. Eighteen had been in arrears for ten years or more, and twenty-two others from five to ten years. The Academy could not be accused of unreasonable action. Also it may be noted the Secretary was not overcareful of keeping the Treasurer informed, for a number of men on the list had moved out of the city years earlier. The list of Fellows, published in the June, 1861, *Bulletin*, numbered 237.

1861–1866

James Anderson

On January 16, 1861, "Dr. Watson resigned his charge, and Dr. Anderson took the chair and read his address." That's all Dr. Thomas tells us.

Dr. Anderson, eleventh President, was an outstanding figure in the Academy. Of fine presence, he came from an old Dutch family; he was born at the Battery in 1798. After studying medicine under Dr. Hosack, he graduated from P. and S. and became assistant to Dr. Hosack for several years, spending much time in instructing his pupils. He was not one of the "elder statesmen" invited to sign the Constitution, being only forty-nine at the time. His first elective office was to the Executive Committee in 1849, which resigned when Trustees were decided upon to replace it in 1850. He was among the original Trustees and served as such until his election to the presidency. He was Vice President in 1852 and 1854, and had been a member of the Committee on Medical Ethics from 1851 through 1857.

He never read a formal paper, but frequently took part in discussion. A quiet, diplomatic man, he was respected and trusted. He was always a soothing influence in the Academy's disputes and turmoils. At the time of his inauguration he was sixty-three years old. Dr. Anderson's address was a short, simple appeal to the Academy to make it what it ought to be and could be made, through the united interest and activity of every Fellow. One statement is perhaps open to question: "Its meetings have been generally well attended and the discussions conducted with gentlemanly courtesy."

At the first meeting of the year the Academy went into a Committee of the Whole to discuss and pass a rule excluding reporters of lay papers from the meetings and forbidding Fellows to provide information to them, except that the Academy at its discretion could publish anything relating to hygiene and public health.

At its next meeting it again sat as a Committee of the Whole. Dr. Cyrus Johns had been nominated for Fellowship by Drs. Dalton, Peaslee, and Watts in April, 1859. The Committee on Admissions had spent much time in investigating him, and it was not until October, 1860, that his name was finally presented for election. Action was "deferred," and then the Academy refused him election, the first time such a thing had ever happened.

When the Committee organized in February, it adopted the following resolution:

> WHEREAS, This Committee believe that the duties and functions of their office as the guardians of the portals of the Academy are of great importance and responsibility, and further believing that their exercise can not be salutory or satisfactory without their enjoying the entire confidence of the Academy, and
>
> WHEREAS, This confidence has been so signally withdrawn by a recent vote of the Academy of nearly 2 to 1 against their presentation, therefore
>
> *Resolved*, That this Committee do now resign severally and collectively their office as "The Committee on Admissions."

Dr. Anderson attended this meeting. It would have been an unfortunate matter for his presidency to have begun with the resignation of this important Standing Committee. His calm and judicious reasoning probably prevented the presentation of this "report," for the Committee met again March 4, the resolutions were reconsidered and laid on the table. In another vote on April 1, readoption was voted down.

In February, after the death of Dr. John W. Francis, a special meeting was held to take appropriate action and a committee "withdrew" to draft resolutions. These were presented by Dr. Mott and ordered published in the daily papers of the city. (This was the first time that Dr. Mott's name appears in the minutes since the matter of the Whitney case two years previously.) Arrangements were made for the Academy to attend the funeral in a body.

Dr. Francis had lived to be seventy-two years old. He had earned the respect and gratitude of the Academy. After delivering the first Anniversary Address, he was elected the second President, and was elected again, against his will, in 1855. He was always a very active and wise power in the Academy, and was recognized as one of the leaders in the profession, a man of literary distinction, and a public spirited citizen.

The regular meeting of February 20, 1861, was an innovation, for the Secretary of the Section on Obstetrics and Diseases of Women and Children gave a long report on the proceedings at its last meeting. It is a matter of interest to examine this report, for it is the first such record presented to the Academy. The older and more distinguished members of the Academy were attending the Section meetings.

A case of twin births, with flooding, was reported. The woman had been in labor eighteen hours before her physician saw her. Forceps were applied fifty-seven hours after labor started, with an easy delivery. A second head immediately presented, and the gentleman called to apply forceps left. After a few hours ergot was given, on account of severe hemorrhage. After sixty-six hours in labor, forceps were applied to the second child, who was delivered dead.

Dr. Pond reported a case of arm presentation, in which he did a version, without chloroform, because it would have taken several hours to obtain it. Dr. Foster reported a case of uterine cancer, and also asked advice on treating cracked nipples. Dr. Sims reported having seen a sound passed into the left fallopian tube. The best treatment of "nursing sore mouth" was also discussed. The lung of a seven months old child, dying of phthisis, contracted from its father, was shown. Such cases were not considered unusual.

Dr. Sewall inquired whether syphilis could produce puerperal fever. Dr. Barker scouted the idea, the virus of the latter disease being entirely different from that of syphilis, and mentioned a case of puerperal fever at Bellevue, which had recovered—the only one of several—who had serious syphilitic disease of the larynx. Dr. Bulkley reported two cases of syphilis in infants, acquired by vaccination.

The President announced the Council had decided to publish notices for the Sections, and 2,500 had been printed for them to distribute. This was a great day for the Sections!

The meeting terminated with a long account of the last illness of Dr. Francis, presented by Dr. Kissam, with all the harrowing details.

Dr. Mott was selected to deliver a eulogy, and "out of respect to the memory of the deceased, the Academy adjourned without transacting any business."

At the next meeting, the Surgical Section was heard from. Dr. Miner read a report on artificial limbs. It was long and detailed, and gave a complete statement of the most modern methods of manufacture and use, illustrated by many plates.

May 15, 1861, was an exciting evening at the Academy. Fort Sumter had been fired on in April, and the first Battle of Bull Run had occurred two days before. The meeting was called to order and the Secretary, Dr. Thomas, who came from Georgia, rose to read the minutes of the preceding meeting. Dr. Conant Foster objected on the ground that Dr. Thomas, being a known sympathizer with traitors and to have held, himself, traitorous sentiments, it was highly improper that he should be allowed to perform the functions of an officer of this body. Dr. McNulty supported this view, and spoke at length upon it. Dr. Foster then moved a suspension of the order of business and that the reading of the minutes be suspended. The motion was lost, only two voting in its favor. Dr. Foster then claimed the roll call, and at its completion declared the roll incomplete, and moved an adjournment. This was also lost. Dr. Foster had started something he could not control.

"A debate of great warmth followed," chiefly upon certain points of order, when another motion to adjourn was made, and was declared by the President to be carried.

At the next meeting the President stated that a communication had been received from Dr. Thomas. The Academy resolved itself into a Committee of the Whole, Dr. Detmold in the chair, to discuss Dr. Thomas's communication. After many warm and patriotic speeches, Dr. Thomas's resignation was tendered. The Committee of the Whole rose and reported:

"The Committee of the Whole, on the subject referred to them, has had a lengthy session and have listened to many spirited and patriotic speeches, and Dr. Thomas, Recording Secretary of the Academy, has tendered his resignation as Secretary."

The Academy then adjourned.

Two whole meetings had been spent on this matter, but between them a special meeting was held at the rooms of the Historical Society, to hear Dr. Mott's Eulogy on Dr. Francis. This was published by the Academy as a separate document. The Executive Committee of the New-York Historical Society voted to make no charge for the use of the hall on the occasion, for Dr. Francis had been an active member of the Society for many years.

At a meeting in July, 1861, Dr. Post interrupted a paper to hear a report by himself and Dr. Van Buren on Military Surgery. Dr. Post loved to talk, but as the report had been read before the Section on Surgery and therefore "a large number of those present had already heard it," it was not read. After arguing over endless trivial details as to size, number, and distribution, it was voted to print 1,500 copies as a small pamphlet, each regiment to be furnished with from three to five copies, the Academy to pay the bill. It cannot be said to have been a concise, practical document.

In July, 1861, a "summer vacation" was voted, four meetings in July, August, and September being omitted. This action was repeated the following year by "suspension of the rules" and the revised Constitution adopted in the fall of 1862 established this interval of inactivity.

Early in the fall of 1861 the Academy adopted Dr. Griscom's resolution: that a committee of five be appointed to cooperate with the New York Sanitary Association in endeavoring to obtain a reformation in the laws pertaining to public health in this city and in their administration. This was the beginning of the effort which resulted in the establishment of the Metropolitan Board of Health, the precursor of our modern Department of Health. Dr. Griscom had been very active in this direction for years, and the following article, printed in the *American Medical Gazette*, April, 1861, was obviously directed at him:

PUFFERY AND THE ACADEMY OF MEDICINE

The attention of the Academy of Medicine has, by some of the morning papers, been called to the fact that, contrary to its standing rules, and in defiance of its recent resolutions forbidding any of its Fellows to report its meetings for the daily press, or to do anything akin to puffery or advertising, one of the most prominent of these gentlemen has lately been running about from one city editor to another, trying to get them to endorse and advertise a certain health bill which he has concocted, and by which, if passed at Albany, he hopes to get money. Now, as no member of so respectable, learned, and influential a body as the Academy of Medicine can, under penalty of expulsion, "advertise his health-pills, or puff his health-bills," in the public press, we hope proper action will without delay be taken by the Academy to prevent a repetition of such forbidden manoeuvres, and to put an end to such unprofessional and reprehensible practices by every one over whom it has jurisdiction or control.—*New York Evening Paper.*

Dr. Foster, Orator-elect, wrote urging the Annual Address be omitted (1861) owing to "the troubled condition of our country." It was so voted.

Dr. Richard S. Kissam, one of the Founders and regular attendants at meetings, died in the fall of 1861. He had served on the Committee on Admissions, and had been a Trustee since 1853. A chronic husky voice made him hesitate to speak much, but he was universally respected.

A special meeting was called on his death. Resolutions were adopted, the wearing of mourning for thirty days was ordered, and a committee appointed to make arrangements for attending the funeral in a body.

The minutes of the Trustees contain this black-bordered note on a separate page,

With sorrow we record the loss of a beloved associate Richard S. Kissam, M. D., who died Thursday, November 28, 1861.

By order

S. T. Hubbard, SECRETARY

In the fall of 1861 several French frigates arrived in the Harbor, and at Dr. Detmold's suggestion, a committee was appointed to invite the Medical Officers to attend the Academy meetings. The committee was appointed and the following comment on this action appeared in the *American Medical Monthly*, January, 1862:

The extending of the right hand of fellowship, and of professional hospitalities, to the Surgeons of the French war-ships in our harbor, on the part of the Academy, was a refreshing little act of genuine courtesy, for which we are indebted to the nice perceptions of Dr. Detmold. We only hope that in case these gentlemen accept the invitation of the Academy to be present at its meetings, they will not be asphyxiated by the foul air of the room in which its deliberations are held, or shocked by the ungentlemanly air of many of its members.

The *New York Times* of June 21 carried a story of the courtesies exchanged.

VISIT OF THE NEW-YORK ACADEMY OF MEDICINE
TO THE FRENCH FRIGATE LA BELLONE

On Friday last a Committee of the New-York Academy of Medicine, consisting of Drs. Detmold, Watson, Woods, and a son of Dr. Anderson, paid a visit to the French frigate *La Bellone*, now lying in our harbor. Accompanying them were Drs. Marmon and Ceccarini. On arriving on board, they were met by Dr. Manger, the principal Surgeon of the frigate, who conducted them to the cabin of the Admiral, M. Reynaud. After an interchange of compliments, the company sat down to an elegant repast, toasts were made, and the whole affair was one of evident satisfaction to all. Dr. Detmold, on behalf of the Medical Academy, presented the freedom of that Institution to the Surgeons of *La Bellone*. Dr. Manger in replying, said that he was pleased to have such a distinction conferred on him and his colleagues, and that when he returned to France he should mention the honor as an evidence of the good-will of the New-York Medical fraternity.

Thursday, Dr. Manger, accompanied by his Assistant Surgeons visited the house of Dr. Anderson, the President of the Academy of Medicine. Yesterday the same gentlemen visited the various hospitals in the City, and were hospitably entertained by the Committee of those institutions.

An interesting minute of the Council is recorded October 3, 1861. "This meeting was in place of one that should have taken place on September 26th; this being the day appointed by the President of the United States as a day of fasting and prayer, the Chairman of the Council advised the convening of the Council be deferred one week."

Dr. Anderson's first year had been an eminently successful, if not peaceful one. The Council were somewhat averse to papers by "outsiders." It reflected on the Academy's ability to produce papers themselves. This caused the temporary shelving of three papers, but Dr. Anderson won, and they were all read.

Nine papers were read. Dr. Barker's on the use of anaesthetics in midwifery emphasized the difference between its use in such cases and in surgery. In surgery it was used for anticipated pain, in obstetrics for existing pain. In surgery it weakened nerve force and depressed vital power. In obstetrics it stimulated and supported those forces. He preferred chloroform to ether because it was more pleasant, quicker in action, and easier to regulate the degree of anaesthesia.

The discussion lasted through three meetings. Dr. Watson was very critical of the use of chloroform, and did not believe Dr. Barker thought it was the safest, as he had implied. He was none too polite in his remarks. The *American Medical Monthly* commenting, stated: "Dr. Watson animadverted very strongly upon the same point, as well as upon instrumental interference in obstetrics. We must submit that the charging of one fellow-Fellow with malpractice, and another with deliberate falsehood, is a procedure scarcely consistent with the dignity of a grand scientific body, and one that ought not to have been passed over in silence by the Chair."

A paper was read on "Moral Insanity in Relation to Criminal Acts" by Dr. Parigot of Belgium. It was considered so important that its discussion was continued at a later meeting, for which the Council authorized the President to send out 100 invitations to outsiders, with a copy of the *Bulletin* containing the paper.

Dr. Buck described a new method of treatment of fractures of the thigh (by traction), which occupied two meetings. Dr. Church described and showed the laryngoscope. Dr. Wynne (guest) read on "Diphtheria," and Dr. Martin on the "Mechanism and Treatment of Face Presentation."

From the Section on Public Health Dr. Griscom reported the work for cretins done by Dr. Guggenbühl of Switzerland, who had recently been elected a Corresponding member. He had organized the first institution for infant cretins. Dr. Griscom thought "the discovery in a being of that order of a mental ray which might be nurtured and developed to reflect and memorize, indicates a genius not surpassed by that of Columbus or Copernicus."

In discussing the report, Dr. Detmold said that a French Commission had reported one cause to be a deficiency in iodine in the water drunk.

The Trustees reported a long list of delinquents. The Academy took strong action, ordering their names stricken from the rolls. Twenty-nine had been delinquent since 1859, twenty-seven since 1860, and six since 1861. At least five of these gentlemen, however, had left the city several years before.

Early in 1862 Dr. Mott wrote proposing resolutions to be presented to both Houses of Congress, protesting against the efforts to have homeopaths appointed surgeons in the Army. He said a "broken metatarsal bone" prevented him from presenting them himself. The resolutions were passed.

Dr. Stevens presented resolutions which were adopted and sent to every medical journal in the country. The *American Medical Times* (January 29, 1862) stated:

> The action of our army surgeons upon the field and elsewhere during the present war have frequently called forth the unqualified approbation of their professional brethren at home, but in no instance has so high a compliment been paid to their bravery and their devotion to humanity as is set forth in the following preamble and resolutions offered by Dr. A. H. Stevens at the last meeting of the New York Academy of Medicine:—
>
> WHEREAS, During the present unhappy war, many of our professional brethren in service among the combatants have risked their lives and gone into voluntary captivity, rather than to desert their sick and wounded, and have exercised their skill alike on friend and foe; therefore be it
>
> *Resolved that,* In such conduct this Academy recognizes the true spirit which shall ever animate the ministers of humanity and in testimonial thereof it is further

Resolved, To welcome to this city those who have acted under these self-sacrificing and generous impulses.

There had been organized an "association of volunteer surgeons" who undertook to answer any request for help in the care of the wounded at the call of the Surgeon General of the Army. In September the reading of an important paper was interrupted by Dr. Detmold who had just received a telegram from Surgeon General Hammond, asking for twenty surgeons to attend wounded soldiers in Maryland. The proceedings were interrupted in order that arrangements might be started.

From the *American Medical Times* we learn that in May Drs. Parker, Stephen Smith, and Kissam of Brooklyn, had been ordered to report at Fortress Monroe, and had left with Drs. N. C. Husted, and Robert Watts, Jr., as Assistants; also that the "Corps" had responded to an unnecessary call and had been placed in charge of the Capitol Hospital in Washington. When relieved, at the request of the Surgeon General the Corps pledged themselves to continue ready to render service when called upon. The Executive Committee of the organization consisted of Drs. Detmold, J. O. Stone, and Thaddeus M. Halsted, all active members of the Academy.

From its organization, the Academy had been interested in improving the sanitary condition of the city and in efforts to secure an efficient health department. A bill was now before the Legislature, and it unanimously adopted the following: "Resolved that the members of the Academy heartily approve of the Metropolitan Health Bill, which is now before the Legislature of their state, and do hereby respectfully ask for the enactment of the same."

This was sent to each member of both houses of the Legislature. The bill was passed by the Assembly, but Mayor Opdyke changed his attitude and it was defeated in the Senate. A city newspaper stated the employees of the Sanitary Inspectors Staff were assessed one month's salary to defeat the bill.

But the Academy had occasion to rejoice over the passage of a law by this same Legislature "to prevent the adulteration of milk and prevent the traffic in impure and unwholesome milk." It had been much interested in this since 1847, and in 1858, a committee had presented a brief report, backed by a separate one from Dr. Percy citing in detail the conditions existing. This was published and received considerable notice. It was now given credit by the *American Medical Times* for the legislative action.

The Academy appointed a committee of three, Drs. Parker, I. E. Taylor, and Percy to attend to the enforcement of the law.

The Secretary having announced that copies of the Constitution and By Laws were nearly exhausted, a committee of five was appointed to make recommendations for alterations, and incorporate those already made. In the fall of 1861 the Academy sat as a Committee of the Whole on its recommendations and they were adopted. Few changes were made, the most important one making the President eligible for reelection.

A new office was established, that of Statistical Secretary, whose duties were to "keep tabular record of the names of every former and present Resident Fellow of the Academy, with their places and dates of birth, education and graduation, their social condition, the number, names and dates of birth and death of the family of each, also the date, place and cause of death of each Fellow, with such other circumstances as will fully illustrate the vital statistics of the Academy. He shall report to the Academy, as early as practicable thereafter, the decease of each fellow with such facts relating to the life and death as may be obtainable." This office was continued until 1899.

The summer recess was made official.

The Annual Address, omitted in 1861, was given, and the *American Medical Times* reported,

The Annual Oration before the Academy of Medicine was delivered Tuesday evening at Dodsworth Hall, by Dr. S. C. Foster. The audience was large and select. The president, Dr. Anderson, was in the chair, and first introduced the Rev. Dr. Vermilye, who opened the exercises with an appropriate prayer. The Orator was then introduced, who discussed at length, the many sided character of the medical profession, its duties, its labors and its rewards. The address was attentively listened to and will soon be published by the Academy.

Dr. Anderson's second year was almost wholly given over to scientific matters, chiefly due to his enthusiasm in forwarding this feature of the Academy. While only thirteen papers were read, the discussions carried over several meetings.

Albuminuria was the real subject of the year. Dr. Clark spent three evenings presenting his views. Dr. J. M. Smith read on its therapeutics and Dr. Barker on its relation to pregnancy, parturition, and the puerperal state. These papers were extensively discussed.

A really important paper was that of Dr. I. E. Taylor on "Non-shortening of the Neck of the Uterus up to the Full Term of Pregnancy." It had been generally taught that the process began in the late months of pregnancy. The paper was illustrated with diagrams and specimens.

Other papers were read by Dr. S. C. Foster, on "Human Monstrosities," being a compilation of all cases in the literature; by Dr. Noeggerath on "Inversion of the Uterus"; Dr. Gardner "Amputation of the Cervix Uteri"; Dr. M. H. Ranney on "Epilepsy"; Dr. O'Reilly "On Strangulated Hernia"; and Dr. Underhill, "Delphinium in Vomiting of Pregnancy." Drs. Byrne and Noeggerath also read on "Pelvic Haematocele," which caused long discussions.

Dr. Barker's statements regarding chloroform, presented the previous year, were brought up for a decision. The *American Medical Monthly* states:

> On motion of Dr. Griscom, however, the whole matter was tabled. The ground which the doctor took in offering the motion, viz, that the Academy of Medicine is not competent to decide upon purely scientific matters, and that such decision does not come within the scope of its powers, we consider at least debatable, if not utterly unsound. . . . We were somewhat surprised that no Fellow attempted to dispute the point.

A number of interesting cases were presented and discussed. Dr. Post reported a tumor of the thyroid with marked protrusion of the eyes, and "did not recollect to have seen a similar case." Drs. Parker, Detmold and Hinton each related one.

The only trouble of any moment was caused by Dr. Percy. He

had read a series of papers on the physiological action, upon animals, of veratrum viridi, its alkaloids and resinoids. After some delay the first part was ordered published in the *Transactions*. But it was stated that Dr. Percy had submitted it for an A.M.A. prize. The previous action was therefore laid on the table and Dr. Percy was informed why. He promptly "protested" and the Secretary was instructed to send him a copy of the By Laws dealing with the matter and "allowing him to withdraw his communication of June 15th." At the same time the Council barred all discussion of the paper from the *Bulletin*.

Evidently nothing was heard from Dr. Percy, and several months later the Secretary was instructed to notify him that "if his paper was not in the hands of the Council before October 29th" the matter would be referred to the Academy. On October 29, true to its warning, the Council voted to refer the matter to the Academy, which promptly turned it over to the Committee on Ethics. On December 2, Dr. Percy asked if the Committee on Ethics was ready to report, because if it did do so promptly, he would offer some resolutions.

The minutes of December 16 tell us:

> The Committee on Ethics made a report on the case of Dr. Percy, which on motion was accepted. As the question upon the adoption of the report was about to be put, Dr. Percy objected to its adoption in terms indecorous both to the President and the Council, during which Dr. Detmold expressed the wish that he might be called to order; further on in his remarks Dr. Purple moved, seconded by Dr. Watts, that the matter be laid on the table. The question was put by the President and declared carried, which Dr. Percy questioned and called for the ayes and nays. The question being again put, twenty voted in the affirmative, and five in the negative. The matter was again declared tabled, whereupon Dr. Percy offered his resignation as a Fellow of the Academy.

At the annual election there were six candidates for President, and eight for Vice President. For the other officers there were few nominations. Dr. Anderson was reelected by a large majority.

Dr. Anderson started his second term with no quorum present, so he postponed his Inaugural till the meeting of February 4th.

The death of Dr. G. H. Tucker was announced by Dr. Roberts. He read a memoir and offered resolutions, which were about to be acted upon when the Secretary stated that Dr. Tucker had never signed the Constitution and was therefore not a member. Dr. Roberts said he considered himself one (he had been elected very recently). The President called attention to a similar case, when Dr. Watson had signed the Constitution and paid the initiation fee for the late Dr. Ray, so Dr. Roberts obligated himself to fulfill these formalities, and the resolutions were passed.

In September a special meeting of the Council was held to arrange to offer a welcome to the Medical Staff of the Russian Fleet now in the Harbor, and a special committee was appointed "to offer such courtesies as they deemed proper." The *American Medical Times* tells us:

A deputation of the New York Academy of Medicine visited the Flagship of the Russian Squadron in our Harbor on Monday the 5th instant, and was most cordially received by the whole medical staff assembled by previous appointment. After mutual greetings, the company proceeded to the Admiral's cabin, where refreshments were provided. The Chairman of the deputation made a brief address in French to the Staff, welcoming them to our city in the name of the Academy, inviting them to be present at the regular meetings during their stay among us, and tendering such personal services as might render their visit agreeable and useful. A response was made in the same language by one of the Staff, heartily reciprocating the fraternal sentiments expressed by the delegation. An hour was then most agreeably spent in conversation and the exchange of mutual good wishes; another member of the Staff also addressed the deputation in English, reiterating the fraternal feelings which all present shared in. After being shown through the ship and admiring the completeness of her equipment and the admirable order everywhere conspicuous, the deputation took their leave, highly gratified with their visit.

On October 7, a "memorial address was interrupted by the Medical Staff of the Russian Fleet, and Dr. Mauger (?) of the French Fleet, accompanied by the delegation from the Academy. They were introduced to the President by Dr. Buck, Chairman of the Committee, and the President addressed them at some length.

"After the address, he asked that the Academy might be adjourned that he might receive our guests and the Academy at his house."

Among the bills ordered paid by the Council at its next meeting was "carriage hire for the Russian Committee $15.00."

While only nine papers were read this year, they were long ones and called forth much discussion. Dr. Lewis Smith's on "Cyanosis" occupied two meetings. It was an analysis of 191 published cases of Cyanosis due to "some permanent abnormal state of the economy, and therefore continuing until the close of life." It occupied fifty-three pages in the *Transactions.*

Dr. Squibb announced the completion of the new *Pharmacopoea,* after seven years of hard work, and he was requested to give a digest thereof, which he did during *four* meetings. Very dull reading now, but the Academy was deeply interested.

"Topical Treatment of the Larynx and Neighboring Organs under Sight" by Dr. Elsberg was a brilliant paper, most flatteringly received. Its closing remarks are worth recording:

> In concluding, I should do violence to my sense of justice, if, speaking in this Academy, in which the subject of one of the Committee-Reports to which I have already alluded, still lies slumbering upon the table among undisposed of business—I should withhold from a fellow-member the oft-contested, hard-earned meed of credit for having guided the "probang and tube" through the laryngeal cavity, in the darkness of ignorance and despite the overshadowing gloom of prejudice, long before the path had been illuminated by the genius of others. If justification of the practice, or confirmation of his assertions, was still needed, laryngoscopy must have appeared to him a very godsend to defend the right and prove the truth! And though the means at our command at present are more in conformity with the exact and scientific requirements and discriminate indications of Pathology and Therapy, it cannot be denied that the name of Horace Green is inseparably and most honorably connected with the history of Topical Medication of the Larynx; and his methods and his success will for ever remain a brilliant monument of his intrepidity, perseverance, and skill.

Dr. Green was still alive. He was always an optimist, and often told his friends he could "afford to wait."

Dr. Blumenthal read an excellent paper on "Vulvo-Vaginitis, or Leukorrhoea of Infants and Young Children." Dr. Austin Flint's paper on "Management of Tuberculosis (Pulmonary) with Special Reference to the Employment of Alcoholic Stimulants" was a long and cool analysis of thirty-five cases. The finding was that alcohol taken regularly had had an influence in causing "arrest" of the disease. With the appendix containing the history of the cases, the paper occupied seventy pages in the *Transactions.*

Dr. Vedder read on "Inhalations of Steam in Croup and Diseases of the Air Passages." Dr. Van Buren discussed "Certain Points in the Surgical Treatment of Diseases of the Rectum," the discussion of which was continued into the next year. A paper on "Surgical Treatment in Hospitals at Frederick, Maryland," read by Surgeon Hewett, U.S.A., was "a private document" of the Surgeon General and therefore could not be recorded.

Altogether this was a very creditable group of papers; all of them are recorded in the *Bulletin* or *Transactions.*

Dr. Anderson had worked indefatigably in procuring papers for the Academy. In May, 1863, he printed a personal letter to all Fellows which went out with a list of thirty-one promised papers, urging them to be prepared to discuss, and to send in their names as discussers so that the program would be complete. It must be confessed that not all of the promised papers were delivered.

There were formal discussions on hernia and hospital gangrene and the treatment of the latter by Bromine and its compounds.

Dr. Batchelder, now seventy-nine, exhibited a fully equipped medicine case for the "self cure of Gonorrhoea."

The records of the Academy are silent about the work of the Sections. We rarely hear more than that this or that Section "reported." The *American Medical Times* of November 23, 1863, says:

At the next meeting of the Surgical Section of the Academy of Medicine, which will be held at the house of Dr. James R. Wood, a subject of unusual importance is to be brought forward. We refer to the discussion on Amputation in Gun shot Fractures of the Thigh. Professor Hamilton will give his experience in detail while in the Army. It is anticipated that the surgeons of the foreign ships in the Harbor will be present, and take part in the discussion. No question in military surgery has received more attention than this, and still it remains unsettled. If this discussion shall elicit the opinion of our most experienced surgeons an important chapter will be added to the history of the subject.

Because the Secretary of the Council forgot to notify the Orator, Dr. J. W. Draper, of his appointment until September, the Anniversary Address was not delivered till December. The *American Medical Times* tells us: ". . . The subject was the Influence of History upon the Medical Profession, and it was treated by the distinguished Orator with the most consummate ability. His study of history enabled him to illustrate his subject with many exquisite sketches, and enrich it with philosophical deductions. The audience was large and select, and received the address with great favor."

During the year occurred the deaths of six Resident Fellows. That of Dr. John Watson was the only one which affected the Academy closely. He had been a most active President and had continued his interest for two years thereafter. He died of cancer of the rectum. Although Dr. Cammann had been a member only one year, he was highly thought of and Dr. Mott presented the resolutions. His last illness was also reported in detail to the Academy. Dr. W. W. Miner had been one of the Founders of the Academy and was one of the "elder statesmen" invited to sign the Constitution. He was the oldest practitioner in the city at the time of his death.

The American Medical Association was to hold its annual meeting in New York in 1864, and Dr. Bulkley, the Academy's delegate on the Committee on Arrangements, asked for an opinion whether a public dinner should be given the delegates. The general opinion was that it was "inexpedient" to do so, but unwise to vote openly against it, so the matter was left on the table.

In the Fall the Executive Committee of the Committee on Arrangements voted to give the balance of the funds raised for entertainment to the Academy, and the Treasurer received a check from Dr. Post for $671.82 to be applied to the building fund. This was the second time this had happened, the building fund having been established in 1854 by the balance turned over from the meeting of the year before. The Academy's action was probably wise!

In February, 1864, the Committee on Public Health offered a memorial to the Legislature regarding the sanitary condition of the city; it was ordered sent, and was signed by the President and Officers. There is no record of what its contents were.

The Trustees presented a list of delinquent members for action. Three of them, including Dr. McNulty, were *thought* to be serving in the Army, so their names were not presented. Those reported were ordered dropped from the rolls. Later Dr. Rockwell, who had been dropped, was found to be in the Army also, and he was promptly reinstated. Dr. Hinton was a distressingly uncommunicative Recording Secretary and that is all he tells us of the activities of 1864.

Thirteen papers were presented. Dr. Wood reported on "Necrosis and Reproduction of Bone." The *Bulletin* was held up for some time awaiting this paper, but in vain. Dr. Wood was a great extemporaneous talker as well as a very busy man, and he probably never wrote his remarks out in full. Dr. Peaselee read two papers; the first on the "Diseases of the Ovary and Their Treatment, not Including Ovariotomy." It was a carefully written detailed account of the various modes of treatment. The second paper was on "Ovariotomy."

Cerebrospinal meningitis occupied a large part of three meetings. Interest had been aroused by a small epidemic which occurred in New Jersey. Papers read by Drs. Detmold, Draper (at two meetings), and Scriven, were extensively discussed. Dr. Sayre read a letter from a doctor in Illinois, who proved to his own satisfaction the disease was caused by the coloring matter of candy distributed widely at a fair in his locality. No case developed in which the candy had not been eaten. (Thousands of others who ate the candy did not come down with it.)

Dr. Noyes read a valuable paper on "Strabismus" and the approved modern treatment thereof. Papers were read by Dr. Dalton on "Trichina Spiralis" with illustrations; Dr. J. C. Draper on "Insensible Perspiration"; Dr. Bumstead on "Venereal Diseases of the Rectum"; Dr. A. K. Gardner on "Non-Specific Character of the Disease called Gonorrhoea"; and Dr. A. N. Bell on "Non-Contagiousness of Typhus Fever." All these caused much discussion.

A Mr. Gunning read a paper on the treatment of fracture of the lower jaw by means of vulcanized dental plates. He was asked to continue his experiments.

The *American Medical Times* stated:

The meetings of the New York Academy of Medicine have of late, chiefly through the exertions of the President, been unusually interesting and instructive. Many of the most prominent physicians in the city have been enlisted in the preparation of papers to be read before the society or in the discussion of topics already presented to it; and the largely increased attendance of members shows that the privilege which they enjoy is not unappreciated.

Announced discussions were held on "Malignant Disease of the Rectum," opened by Dr. Parker; "Fistula in Ano" by Dr. Post; and "The Ulterior Effects of Anaesthetic" by Dr. F. H. Hamilton, which latter occupied much of the time of two meetings.

Dr. Buck demonstrated a case of plastic surgery of the face in a man who had serious and extensive necrosis after overuse of mercury, and Dr. Conant showed a calcified extra-uterine foetus removed from the mother thirty-five years after term, three living children having been born in the interim.

No Anniversary Oration was delivered this year. No one seemed willing to be Orator.

The Annual Election was quiet but occupied the entire meeting of January 4. Nominations were surprisingly few. Dr. Anderson was elected for a third term.

When the Academy met April 19, 1865, the death of President Lincoln was on everybody's mind. The following resolutions were passed:

WHEREAS, Our Nation has been bereaved by the sudden and violent death of its Chief Magistrate at the hands of an unprincipled assassin:

Resolved, That in common with our fellow-citizens of every class, the members of this Academy mourn over the loss which our Country has sustained.

Resolved, That we cherish with grateful hearts the memory of the virtuous life of our late President, and the remembrance of the distinguished services which he has rendered to the Nation in the trying times in which he was called to preside over our destinies.

Resolved, That we regard with abhorrence the wicked and brutal violence which has deprived the Country of his valuable services, and which has cast a gloom over every loyal house and heart throughout the land.

Sending a copy of the resolutions to the family was proposed, but it was felt that if every society were to send resolutions, the family would be simply overwhelmed. Dr. Van Kleek remarked "This Nation mourns as no nation ever mourned before, and the occasion for, and the depth and universality of the grief has never before had a parallel in the history of the world. It is certain that no twenty millions of people were ever before swayed to such an extent by an emotion of grief springing as it did from a single source."

The meeting then adjourned without transacting any further business.

Nine days later a special meeting was held to take action on the death of Dr. Mott. The resolutions said, in part:

Resolved, That our common country has reason to cherish the memory of Dr. Mott, not only as the greatest surgeon ever produced in America, but as one who has taken rank with the first of this century in any part of the world; as one whose reputation was indeed, world-wide, and whose name is known and revered wherever our profession are found. . . . .

Resolved, That we will attend the funeral in a body, and that we invite the surgeons of the Army and Navy, and the members of our profession generally, in this city and its vicinity, to unite with us in paying this last tribute of respect to the memory of our lamented colleague.

The resolutions were ordered published in four morning and two evening papers. The Academy was to meet at the Presbyterian Church, 22d Street and Fourth Avenue, and proceed to the funeral in a body. Crepe was to be worn on the left arm.

At the first May meeting Dr. Flint described, in detail, the last illness of Dr. Mott. In October the Department of State forwarded through the Consular Service in Spain resolutions passed by the Academy of Medicine of Barcelona, expressing its great regret and sympathy with the Academy on the death of Dr. Mott. A eulogy was delivered by Dr. Post at the Chapel of the University, November 30th. The meeting was largely attended. The address was printed by the Academy.

Nine papers were read before the Academy in 1865. Dr. Loomis spoke on typhus fever, with discussion of cases in Bellevue, with particular reference to the avoidance of alcoholic stimulants in treatment. This was not generally endorsed. The discussion, long and unusually friendly for the Academy, was continued during four meetings. Drs. W. H. Draper and Loomis were the most active combatants.

Another important paper was on "Pyaemia," by Dr. Krackowizer. Pyaemia was a "specific" disease, caused by a "miasma"; its effects different from those induced by injecting "putrid matter" into the blood, and therefore it and septicemia must be "two distinct affections." Discussion occupied a large part of three meetings.

Dr. Alonzo Clark started what was to be a long series of papers on pneumonia, and the discussion occupied most of another meeting. Dr. Kingsley read on "Cleft Palate," advocating mechanical occlusion rather than operation, which caused discussion, and Dr. Parigot (by invitation) read on "Lunacy Legislation."

War matters occupied considerable time. A confidential report on the work of the Medical Department of the Army of the Ohio was read, and Dr. Post gave an abstract of a report for the Sanitary Commission on "Gunshot Fractures of the Thigh," which was discussed by Dr. Tripler, U.S.A., who urged the Academy not to make up its mind at once but to await the surgical history of the war. He said a great change was taking place in regard to primary amputations. Dr. E. Harris gave his "hygienic experiences" in New Orleans during the war.

Smallpox, prevalent during the year, and dislocations were other subjects of discussion.

Of the work of the Sections we still hear little. Their meetings were not mentioned in the *Bulletin.* The *American Medical Gazette* reported that the Section on Surgery had a most interesting meeting in April at the home of Dr. J. R. Wood, "to which many outsiders had been invited." The exsection of joints was discussed at great length, demonstrated by specimens, drawings, and sometimes by patients. "A social entertainment closed this meeting which throughout was interesting and profitable."

The financial condition of the Academy was so good that $350 were voted transferred to the Building Fund. During the year the University having raised the rent, the library was moved and obtained temporary shelter at the home of the Librarian, Dr. Hinton.

A very important event of the year of 1866 was the establishment of the Metropolitan Board of Health. Dr. Anderson announced that the "Health Bill" was a legitimate offspring of the Academy, and suggested a history of the event be prepared. A committee of two was promptly appointed, but there is no record of their having produced the history.

At a later meeting, it was voted:

> WHEREAS, The Metropolitan Board of Health has been called into being mainly through the instrumentality of members of the profession,
>
> *Resolved,* That the Fellows of this Academy will cordially cooperate with the Board of Health in carrying out their plans for the improvement of the Metropolitan District.

The next month Dr. Sayre moved this motion be reconsidered because the Board of Health had endorsed homeopathic practitioners, which was contrary to the Code of Ethics of the American Medical Association, under which the Academy worked.

Dr. Harris stated the medical members of the Board of Health had all protested at this measure, but Dr. Sayre said that made no difference. The measure was passed and the homeopaths gloated over their endorsement by the Academy. As a matter of courtesy the subject was laid on the table until those who were present at the meeting of the Board of Health could answer in person. But, at the next meeting, Dr. Sayre was in action again, and the matter was taken from the table. The *Medical Record* reports very bitter remarks concerning Drs. Parker and Stone, Commissioners. Dr. Van Kleek thought the original resolution of the Academy was not to endorse everything the Board did, but only its sanitary measures, and this hubbub was unnecessary. "Supplemental resolutions" were, however, adopted: "Whereas at a previous meeting the Academy by resolutions offered its cooperation with the Metropolitan Board of Health, it hereby expressly disclaims having approved or countenanced so much of that action of the Board as relates to the admission of Homeopaths to practice in the public hospitals."

To satisfy Dr. Sayre, copies of this explanatory resolution were ordered sent to Drs. Stone and Parker.

In April the Academy adopted a proposal from the Council that a committee be appointed to consider and report upon "the expediency of immediate action in reference to a building for the Academy." The committee was appointed and reported, after the vacation, that with the means at the command of the Academy immediate action was inexpedient. The matter was referred back to the Council, which promptly recommended that the Committee now report on the expediency of at once raising funds to erect a building. The Committee could not seem to make up its mind, and the Council had to work out the details for it:

"Resolved that the Council recommend to the Academy that it should appoint a *Committee on Ways and Means* to adopt and prosecute a method for securing funds for the purchase of a site and the erection of a building."

The Academy promptly adopted the resolution, and the President appointed Drs. Willard Parker, S. T. Hubbard, Jared Linsly, Ernst Krackowizer, and Samuel Purple to serve on the committee. Dr. Anderson was later added and was made chairman.

And so began nine long years of discouraging and hard work to eventually obtain a modest home for the Academy.

In April, 1866, Dr. Joseph M. Smith died at the age of seventy-seven. The Academy met at the church at the corner of 19th Street and Fifth Avenue, adopted resolutions, and attended the funeral in a body, wearing the "usual badge of mourning." The Academy voted its thanks to the Trustees of the church for the gratuitous use of its lecture room.

Scientifically it was a very busy year for the Academy. Nineteen papers and reports were read. Dr. Anderson's efforts had produced results. Dr. Elliot read an elaborate paper on the induction of labor, which concluded: "I may venture to prophesy . . . that the day may come when it may not be considered an objectionable procedure to assign a day for bringing on the labor at close of pregnancy in favorable cases, even for consideration of personal convenience to the pregnant woman or to admit of her receiving under peculiar circumstances the attendance of a selected physician."

From February, 1866, until September an expected epidemic of cholera occupied unbroken attention. Dr. Metcalfe was appointed to open the discussion. He said:

I am confident that I do not err in saying that an epidemic visitation of our dreaded antagonist is to be reasonably looked for between now and the end of summer. Its approach is discerned afar off as distinctly as a storm foreseen by the rising of the clouds from the horizon in the direction of the wind. The storm *may* pass around, or burst before reaching our home. Nonetheless it is our duty to act in such a manner as shall enable us to avert the calamity if possible, or to diminish its dangers if the advent is inevitable. The profession and the public have a right to expect this at our hands.

Dr. Griscom read a formidable paper on "The Where, the When, the Why and the How of the First Appearance and Greatest Prevalence of Cholera in Cities." He was a non-believer in its contagiousness, but a firm believer in the necessity of city cleanliness. Dr. Sayre spoke on his convictions of its "portability and portability alone," and the necessity of an absolute quarantine. Dr. Clark exhibited and explained Cruveilhier's and Pirogov's plates on the pathology of cholera.

When a new disinfecting agent was presented and referred to the Section on Public Health, Dr. Anderson stated there was no longer a Section on Public Health. To fill the gap a special committee of five was appointed, which by subsequent additions was increased to thirteen members. This committee was kept very busy.

In Dr. Griscom's opinion the cholera outbreak was not because two ships had arrived with cases of cholera on board. He thought the *ships* themselves were the cause of the disease: due to "a peculiar condition of the atmosphere combined with filth and bad ventilation. With proper sanitary care, the disease could not have broken out. If there had not been a 'tendency to Cholera' we would have had 'Ship Fever.' "

The Public Health Committee presented three reports, all of which are interesting as showing the attitude toward cholera. Dr. Stephen Smith presented the first, recommending that (1) Boards of Health should provide gratuitous medical relief in homes, during the early stages of the disease; (2) inhabitants of infected areas be provided with temporary "refuges" while their homes were being disinfected; and (3) small hospitals should be opened near the cholera focuses. All were adopted.

Dr. Squibb reported on disinfectants. Cleanliness, ventilation and preliminary "scavenging" were essential. The best disinfectants were heat, and chlorine for control of effluvia, together with lime, and a mixture of lime and charcoal. For disinfection of cellars, smoke from green wood was the best. This report fills eighteen pages of the *Bulletin.*

Dr. Harris, an experienced health authority, reported on "Sanitary Police Measures." He insisted that cholera was spread through the diarrhoeal discharges of patients, that disinfection was a simple matter, and rigid regulations should be enforced to disinfect permanently all ejecta, and to provide strictest cleanliness of person and premises, including privies, water closets, and cesspools. If this was done there should be no fear or hesitancy in caring for the sick.

All these reports were ordered published in the medical press.

"Superheated Steam" was endorsed as a disinfectant, and "Rankin's disinfecting chamber pail" was considered so valuable that a committee was appointed to make suggestions to increase its usefulness. The full printed records of these reports and discussions occupy 123 pages of the *Bulletin,* and constituted the chief subject of attention at eleven meetings—nine stated, one adjourned, and one special.

The epidemic was over in the fall. When the Academy reassembled it resumed its general program. An excellent paper on "Inflammation of the Cavitas Tympani in Relation to Exanthematous

Diseases" was read by Dr. Pomeroy, and another on "Medical Jurisprudence, Department of Malpractice" by Dr. Ordronaux, who was invited to continue at another meeting.

Dr. Dalton spoke on "Vivisection" and what it had accomplished, and Dr. Lidell read a memoir on "Osteomyelitis" based on a report for the United States Sanitary Commission. Two special meetings were held to hear Dr. Brown-Séquard of Paris on the pathology of the nervous system.

The meeting of December 19 was given over to the Anniversary Address. "The Orator of the occasion, Dr. John Ordronaux, having been conducted to the rostrum by the Vice President and Trustees, delivered a discourse on 'Prophylaxis.' "

During the year nineteen papers and reports were read. A long discussion lasting two meetings was held on "Chronic Metritis."

Twenty-two cases were reported in detail and six forms of apparatus were exhibited.

The death of Dr. Horace Green was announced in the fall. He had had a slight stroke several years before and had given up much of his practice. Up to that time he had been a very regular and cooperative member of the Academy, in spite of rather rough usage. Dr. Peaslee spoke at length, reminding the Academy of what had been done on the two occasions when Dr. Green was before them, and emphasizing his claims as to what he had accomplished, claims that had been proved without doubt. Drs. Stevens, Richards, and Sims also spoke on his contributions to medicine. The resolutions which were then adopted are a fitting close to Dr. Green's hectic career in the Academy. He had said he "could afford to wait."

Resolved, That the New York Academy of Medicine proudly claims the late Dr. Horace Green as one of its most distinguished Fellows, recognizing him as one of its active and most useful members, as an accomplished physician, a bold and independent writer, a successful teacher, a courteous gentleman, and an honest man.

Resolved, That with unfeigned grief we regret his loss, as one of our associates, as a member of our noble profession, and as a fellow man; and we hereby tender to the bereaved family and friends our sincere sympathy and condolence.

Resolved, That these proceedings be entered on the minutes of the Academy, and that a copy be transmitted to the family of the deceased.

On motion of Dr. Griscom, the Academy also passed, unanimously, this resolution:

Resolved, That the Academy hereby extends a cordial welcome to its associate member, Dr. J. Marion Sims on his recent return from abroad, where, by his genius, skill, and industry in his specialty, he has raised the character of American medical science and art to an eminence before unattained.

When the Academy came to elect officers for the next year, it was found the Secretary had failed to announce the list of candidates, so the election had to be postponed a week. Dr. Post was elected President.

On January 19, 1867, Dr. Anderson read his Valedictory Address. He told of the foundation of the Academy, and outlined its accomplishments. He took particular pleasure in mentioning the fact that cholera, which had appeared in a small way during the summer, had been held in check by the Board of Health, whose foundation the Academy could claim as its own, and also that it had carried out largely the recommendations of the Academy in controlling cholera. He made a strong plea to every Fellow to unite and make an organized effort to secure a home for the Academy, without which it could never reach the influence it should exert.

Dr. Anderson had been a splendid President, giving untiringly of his time and effort. As President of the Council, he guided the Academy wisely and constructively. A member of all Standing Committees ex officio, he attended a large proportion of all their meetings. He rarely missed a Trustees' meeting, and failed to preside at the Stated Meetings of the Academy only once in six years. There was a marked decrease in unpleasant incidents during his tenure, and the scientific activities increased immensely. Ten of the thirty speakers announced as promising to read definite papers before the Academy had complied, and three others read papers on other subjects. Dr. Anderson deserved the vote of thanks he received, and he continued undiminished in his influence and activity on behalf of the Academy for more than ten years after ceasing to be President.

The Academy passed the following resolution:

Resolved, That the thanks of the New York Academy of Medicine be tendered Doctor Anderson for his faithful, energetic, and eminently successful administration as presiding officer for the last six years, as well as his urbane and courteous manner to all its members.

The Council also rendered its own merited tribute, as follows:

Resolved, That on his taking leave of the Council of the New York Academy of Medicine, over which he has presided with so much courtesy and impartiality during the last six years, Dr. James Anderson is entitled to the thanks of his associates, and those thanks are hereby tendered for his long and faithful services in this capacity, as well as in that of President of the Academy itself—services which have contributed greatly to the success of that association, and must have involved many sacrifices on his part.

Resolved, That the Secretary of the Council be requested to communicate to Dr. Anderson the above expression of the feelings of the Council, with their best wishes for his continued welfare and prosperity.

1867–1874

Alfred C. Post · Henry D. Bulkley
Edmund R. Peaslee · Austin Flint

After Dr. Anderson's retirement as President ensued eight years of steady growth.

1867–1868

Dr. Post, twelfth President, was sixty-one when he took office. He was a small man with a tremendously heavy beard. "The clever nephew of a clever uncle" (Dr. Wright Post, 1766–1828), and possessed of ample means, he had been graduated from Columbia with honors at the age of sixteen, and immediately began the study of medicine. After graduation, he "flitted about" in England, Paris, Berlin, and Italy, acquiring amongst other things a good working knowledge of foreign languages. He was a tremendous reader, had a prodigious memory, and was always ready on any subject, rarely failing, as President, to discuss a paper or a case. A very religious man, he is quoted as saying his two greatest pleasures were performing an operation and attending a prayer meeting. He made a good President and failed to preside only five times in his term of office.

Essentially an operative surgeon, he was personally much more interested in clinical cases than in long papers. The President had a great deal to do with the character of the program. In 1859, the Council had appointed a committee on "Lectures and Addresses," whose activities were chiefly confined to deciding upon papers to be read by non-Fellows. To go outside the Academy was considered bad policy, as admitting its inability to provide suitable material. Dr. Anderson's personal influence had rather overcome that attitude and he was responsible for the establishment of a planned yearly program, including several outside speakers.

Under Dr. Post, interest fell off to some extent. Only eight formal papers were read in 1867 and at several Stated Meetings there was no quorum. Many cases were shown and discussed, however. From 1868 on, probably due to Dr. Anderson's continued influence, the Academy developed renewed energy, and there was rarely a break in the regular, semimonthly series of papers, except when a "discussion" was substituted.

The Academy's attention was called to the habit of druggists of refilling prescriptions without an order from the physician. Legal opinion was obtained, which stated that druggists were liable to suit if they did so. The matter was finally voted to be referred to the State Society for its action.

The subject of vaccination was brought up and a committee of five appointed to report measures best adapted to "promote universal and perfect vaccination."

During 1867 the Academy seems to have become particularly sensitive to ethical matters, and more charges against Fellows were presented that year than in any previous five-year period. Dr. Krackowizer brought charges against Dr. Griscom. A sample of Hoff's Malt Extract had been submitted to a special committee. Drs. Griscom and Bulkley reported in favor of endorsing it, but Dr. Krackowizer opposed. The Academy adopted Dr. Krackowizer's report. Dr. Griscom, however, gave a copy of the favorable report to the agent on condition that he would not publish it, which of course he did in a very exaggerated form. The Committee on Ethics reported, giving all the details, and concluded, "We do not believe that Dr. Griscom, in thus compromising the Academy, intended to degrade it or to defy its laws. We are annoyed that the Academy has been used by Mr. Hoff to subserve his private ends and are assured no one regrets this more than Dr. Griscom himself." When the Academy accepted this report, Dr. Krackowizer resented the action and wrote a very critical letter to the Academy, which was "returned to him for further consideration." The "endorsements" of

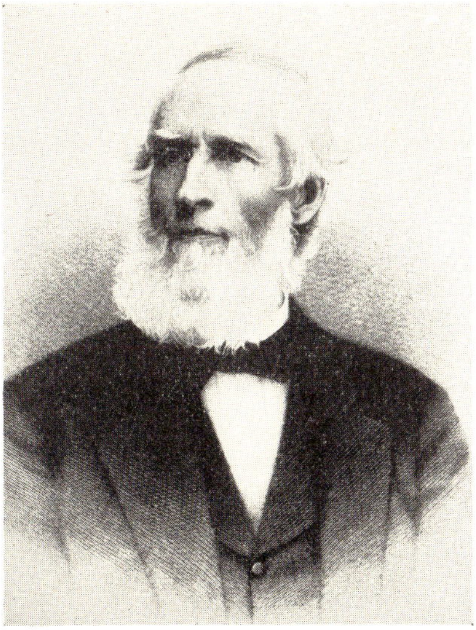

EDMUND R. PEASLEE, 1814–1878
Fourteenth President, 1871–1872

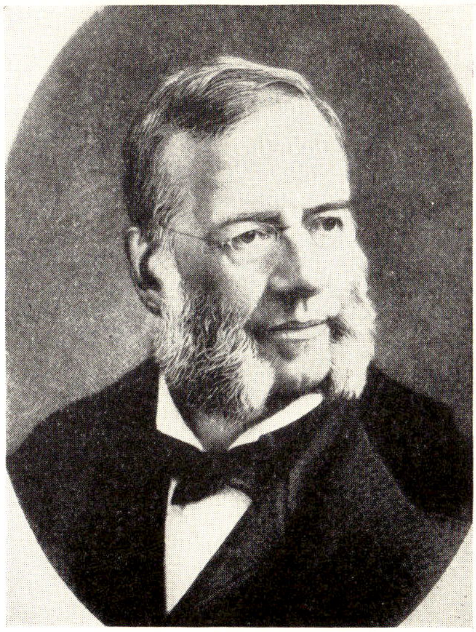

AUSTIN FLINT, 1812–1886
Fifteenth President, 1873–1874

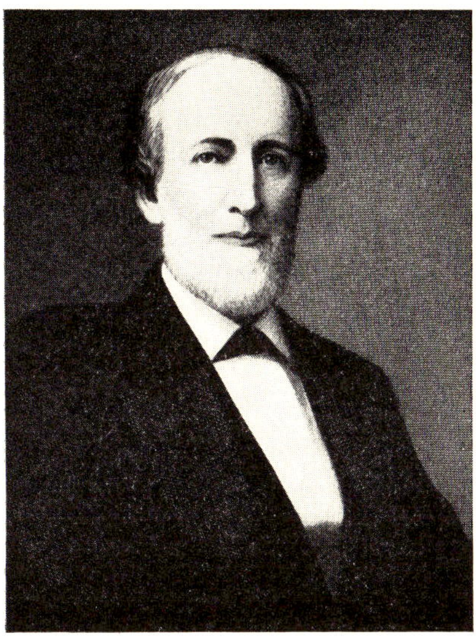

SAMUEL S. PURPLE, 1822–1900
Sixteenth President, 1875–1878

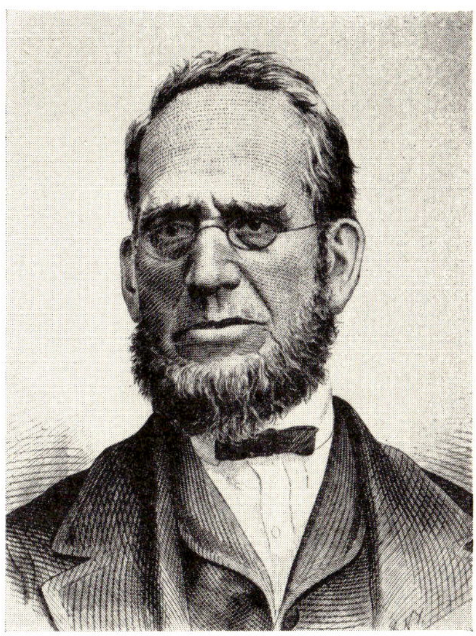

JAMES O. POND, 1790–1881
Treasurer, 1848–1876

Hoff's Extract continued, and the Academy later was forced to publish an official denial of their authenticity.

About this time, resolutions were passed making it the duty of every Fellow to report to the Committee on Ethics any consultations with abortionists or homeopaths. Shortly after, the Committee on Ethics, after investigating certain charges, recommended that Dr. A. K. Gardner, one of the Founders of the Academy who had taken an active and important part in its development, should be suspended for consulting with a homeopath. Dr. Gardner was neither polite nor politic in his answers at his hearing, and he was promptly suspended. Probably owing to his attitude, a motion for immediate reinstatement was lost. The medical press endorsed the action of the Academy, but the *New York Tribune* and *New York Times* came to Dr. Gardner's defense. The former stated,

> His parchment is of no more use to him than if it had been cut out of a drumhead. Whatever may have been his services to the sick and suffering during his twenty-three years' practice, whatever his accuracy of diagnosis, his skill in prescription, his faithfulness to duty, his success, his reputation, his general standing among the physicians—there is no doubt about him now; he is a pariah and an outcast. He need not expect any more fees. He may take down his sign and sell his gig.

Several years later Dr. Gardner appealed for reinstatement, but action was deferred, and he died in 1876 un-reinstated.

Another charge was brought against Dr. Elisha Harris of the Board of Health. The accusing physician had signed a death certificate for a baby dying in a very questionable "foundling home." Dr. Harris was after these places, and as the death certificate was unsatisfactory ("convulsions"), he ordered an autopsy without informing the attendant physician. Dr. Harris was adjudged innocent "of any feeling of malice or unprofessional conduct . . . having acted in his official capacity as he believed it to be his duty." The Academy agreed to this verdict. The Fellow bringing the charges ceased paying his dues and was dropped three years later.

Still another charge, never officially brought before the Academy, was made by Dr. C. F. Taylor against Dr. L. A. Sayre in April, 1867.

Efforts were made to have a hearing, but Dr. Sayre was ill. In October the Committee reported that it had decided to act as a "Court Medical," and that both parties had had a complete reconciliation and exchanged a warm handshake. "Thus the matter was closed to the great gratification of the Committee and also, as they believe, the parties interested."

The final explosion of charges in 1867 was when in open meeting, a Fellow charged the President with doing him "an injustice in refusing him credentials to the International Medical Congress in Paris, the previous summer." He was told to present formal charges, which he did. They were considered too absurd to be acted upon by the Committee.

On the whole, things remained quiet until 1870, although in 1868 the Academy was quite disturbed by the action of the American Medical Association declaring it ethical to consult with anyone having evidence of a regular medical education. Many practicing homeopaths were graduates of regular medical schools. It was explained, however, that the purpose was to permit consultation with *female* regular practitioners.

In 1867, the South was stricken with yellow fever. The Academy passed resolutions of sympathy and the President and Council were appointed a special committee to ask for and receive contributions for the relief of the victims. During the summer recess over $2,500 was received and forwarded, most of it contributed through the churches.

Always very friendly with, and appreciative of, the Army, the Academy later passed resolutions eulogizing the members of the Medical Corps who had died of yellow fever while caring for its victims. A list was read at the Anniversary Meeting, and recorded in the minutes. Eight names are therein inscribed. It was also proposed to memorialize the Congress to appropriate funds for a representative medical commission to study yellow fever and propose a plan for its control. This motion died on the table.

After having met on Wednesdays for twenty-one years, the day was shifted to Thursdays for reasons which were "explained" to

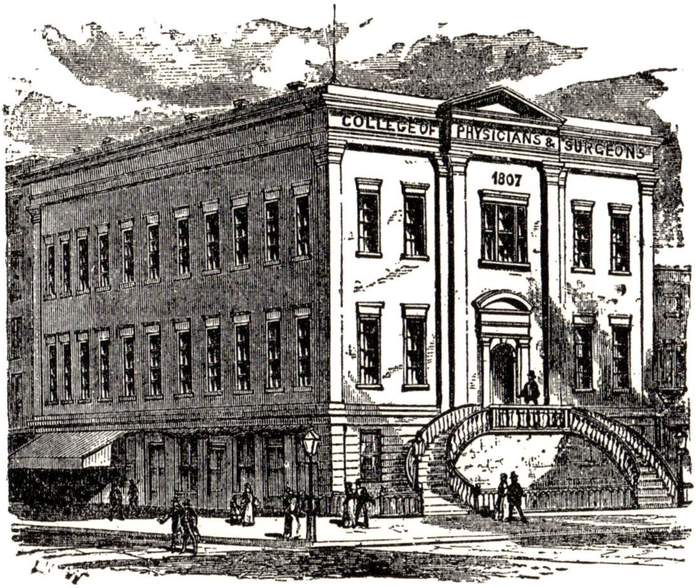

COLLEGE OF PHYSICIANS AND SURGEONS,
23D STREET AND FOURTH AVENUE
Meetings Held Here from May 7, 1868, to April, 1875

them, but not to us. Therefore, since April 16, 1868, Thursday has been the Stated Meeting day of the Academy.

Meetings had been held at the "small Chapel of the University" since July, 1850. The original rent was $7.00 per night—including light, heat, and routine janitor services. But the University had been slowly raising the rent, and it now cost $250 a year, or $12.50 a meeting. The "Church at Twenty-ninth Street and Fifth Avenue" offered its lecture room at "very liberal terms," but it was decided to rent the lower lecture room at the College of Physicians and Surgeons for $75 a year, and notices were sent out for a meeting there on May 7, 1868. The minutes tell us there was no quorum. Perhaps the members got lost going so far north as 23d Street and Fourth Avenue, instead of to Washington Square. A number of times in 1868 the lack of a quorum necessitated starting the meeting "informally."

In March, 1868, Dr. Isaac Wood, twice President of the Academy, died, aged seventy-four, and in April Dr. Batchelder, Father of the Sections, aged eighty-three. Neither had been active in Academy affairs since their retirement, and the Academy passed brief formal resolutions.

The Anniversary Addresses were delivered, in 1867, by Dr. Stephen Smith, on "The History of Surgery in New York City during the last Century"; in 1868 by Dr. Austin Flint, on "The Past, Present and Future of Medicine."

1869–1870

Dr. Henry D. Bulkley became thirteenth President. He was born in New Haven and was in business there for several years before he took up the study of medicine. He graduated from the Yale Medical College in 1828. After returning from study abroad, he gave a course of lectures on diseases of the skin, the first ever given in this country. A Founder of the Academy, he had been active in its affairs continuously. He had served on the Committee on

Publications for a number of years. Like Dr. Post, he was a man of small stature, and was sixty-five years old when he assumed office.

Dr. Bulkley's term of office were particularly active years for the Academy, and relatively very peaceful ones. There is very little on the minutes except the briefest of notes regarding papers.

In 1869 a prize offered by (the late) Dr. John O'Reilly for the best essay on "The Vital or Ganglionic Nervous System, the Oxygen and the Blood, and the Cerebro-Spinal Nervous System" to be competed for by "Medical students of the United States and Medical practitioners of three years' standing," was awarded to Dr. Robert P. Edes of Boston Highland. It was ordered published in the *Transactions* and occupied 152 printed pages, together with a large folded plate of the nervous system, central and ganglionic.

The history of that prize is rather unfortunate. Dr. O'Reilly was deeply interested in the subject and had read a paper thereon in 1860. In 1866 he turned over a bank account of $600 to the Academy to be used as a prize as noted above. The Academy accepted the gift, and appointed a Prize Committee of three to issue an announcement and the terms of the prize. In November, 1867, the Council suddenly remembered this had never been done. "Someone had blundered." The notices eventually appeared. But in 1868 Dr. O'Reilly died. It was announced that he had left a sum to the Academy for a permanent prize fund, but in a subsequent will, "which would probably be declared invalid," he had canceled the bequest. The will was apparently not declared invalid, as there is no record of such a fund. It is not strange that, after more than two years without any results from his first prize offer, he should have changed his will.

In 1870 harmony was broken briefly by charges, which now seem rather absurd, brought against Dr. J. Marion Sims. They were: "1, In betrayal of the secrets of a patient; 2, In resorting to public advertising."

The charges were made by Dr. Finnell, a member of the Committee on Ethics, who sat in judgment on them. The first charge was based upon a letter to the New York *Times*, one of whose reporters had written that Miss Charlotte Cushman—a very popular actress—was "at the point of death" at Malvern, England. Dr. Sims wrote to the *Times* that he had seen her in Paris—that she had a small indurated gland, and that he had advised her to forget it. She had, however, gone to Dr. Simpson of Edinburgh (Dr. Sims did not state to whom she had gone) and it had been removed contrary to his advice. Knowing what she had, he believed she must have developed erysipelas after the operation, which was a self-limiting disease, and as no notice of her death had been received, he advised her friends to cheer up. (That was the "betrayal of the secrets of a patient.")

Dr. Sims had operated in Paris for vesico-vaginal fistula on the invitation of many of the most celebrated surgeons of that city, with spectacular results. He had been awarded the Legion of Honor. He disclaimed acquaintance with any reporter and had spoken to none. Yet he was charged with advertising because he had written to the *Times*.

The Committee found (he had returned to Europe a few days after submitting his defense) the charges "fully sustained," and recommended "the mildest penalty . . . reprimand of the offender by the President of the Academy, be administered without delay." The motion to adopt was seconded by Dr. Finnell, and carried. It was finally decided the "reprimand" should be a copy of the report signed by the President and Secretary, to be sent to Dr. Sims.

It may be remembered that, four years earlier, resolutions had been passed welcoming Dr. Sims on his return from Europe, where he had "raised the character of American medical science and art to an eminence before unattained." The Academy could be fickle at times!

In March, 1869, Dr. Alexander H. Stevens died at the age of seventy-nine. He was the last of the three original callers of the "meeting of regular Physicians" in 1846. Appropriate resolutions were adopted, and his ardent admirer, Dr. John G. Adams, was delegated to read a eulogy at a special meeting in 1871, which he did, and which he published.

In 1869 the Anniversary Address was delivered by Dr. Gouverneur M. Smith, on "Inherent Difficulties which have beset Medical Progress." Dr. R. C. Stiles was elected Anniversary Orator for 1870, but he was prevented from delivering it by illness.

Dr. Bulkley had made a most excellent presiding officer and had been present at every meeting during his term of office.

1871–1872

Dr. Edmund R. Peaslee was fifty-seven years old when he became the fourteenth President. Born in New Hampshire, he had moved to New York in 1858. He had been a teacher all his life. After graduation from the Yale Medical School, he was called back from an intended stay of two years abroad, to become Professor of Anatomy and Physiology at Dartmouth, succeeding Oliver Wendell Holmes. He taught at Dartmouth, his Alma Mater, continuously for thirty-eight years until his death. During these years he filled the chair of every recognized department of medicine, except chemistry. Even in the seventies it was still not unusual in the schools in rural districts for professors from New York and other cities to crowd into three brief weeks a course of lectures, often giving two each day.

There is no printed record of Dr. Peaslee's Inaugural Address. His administration was particularly peaceful—in fact so peaceful that frequently the minutes state "the meeting started informally, no quorum being present."

The Commissioner of Pensions in Washington had issued an order excluding all irregular physicians from serving as "examining pension surgeons." This called forth a storm of protest from the homeopaths. The Academy passed resolutions approving the action of the Commissioner and urging the Secretary of the Interior to sustain him.

Two notorious abortionists were tried before Judge Gunning S. Bedford, son of Dr. Gunning S. Bedford of New York University Medical College, and convicted. Judge Bedford's speech in pronouncing sentence drew attention to the frequency of the crime, the inadequate penalty, stated that all offenders coming before him need expect no clemency, and urged the law be changed to make the offense punishable as first degree murder. This called forth long resolutions of appreciation of the Judge's stand, and the Academy's recorded approval of his recommendation to change the law.

The Academy also passed resolutions authorizing the appointment of a committee to study the question of quarantine and to prepare a statement concerning the necessary sanitary measures to be taken to control "exotic diseases."

A matter came to a head during Dr. Peaslee's administration which had been a thorn in the side for many years—the publication of papers read before the Academy. A volume of *Transactions* had been published from time to time since 1851, but there was great delay in its appearance. In 1860 a bulletin had been established, which came out in parts, was supposed to be up to date, and print the papers and discussions. The important papers were usually reserved for the *Transactions*—which meant further delay. There was a rule that no papers read could be published elsewhere than in Academy publications without special permission and that permission was often given only when the Academy did not itself care to publish the material.

As applied to the Section Meetings, these rules were even more unfair. No stenographic reporting was provided, but although papers were not supposed to be published in the journals, occasionally this was done, and nothing was said.

When the *Bulletin* was started in 1860, Dr. George F. Shrady had been made the reporter; he was a very efficient one, but when he left trouble began. The various subsequent incumbents did well for a time, but soon lost interest, although they received $10 a night. There were periods when the *Bulletin* contained only the briefest notes of the Recording Secretary, and there were long periods when nothing was printed, the Council, owing to financial difficulties, deciding to suspend publication of the *Bulletin* for several months.

In May, 1871, the Constitution was amended to permit Fellows to publish their papers wherever they pleased, and the *Bulletin* was discontinued. In lieu, a "new series" of *Transactions* was begun. This was continued for thirty years, with varying degrees of completeness, but was planned on the lines of the *Bulletin.* From 1872 the journals contained many papers read at Stated Meetings and Section Meetings.

In fairness to the Council Committee on Publications, it faced a very difficult situation. It had to consider the cost of publishing presidential and valedictory addresses, anniversary and memorial addresses. In 1867, the memorial addresses were neglected. That of Dr. Mott was printed by a "committee of medical gentlemen," of which Dr. Anderson was chairman. Dr. Anderson presented the Academy with a "sufficient number of copies," and proposed one should be sent to each graduating member of the three medical schools in the city. This was promptly approved and Dr. Anderson announced he had already taken the step, and proceeded to read letters of appreciation from the various presidents of the colleges!

The memoir of Dr. Joseph M. Smith, another former President, was voted sent to his family that they might publish it. Dr. Stephen Smith's and Dr. Flint's Anniversary Addresses were not published by the Academy. Even at that, during those eight years publications cost the Academy $4,192.19.

In November, 1871, a report to the Council showed the Treasurer was in trouble. There were outstanding bills for $833.49, with $104.42 in the Treasury. Nearly $600 was due for printing. As assets, the Treasurer listed back dues $555, classified as follows:

Probably collectible	$320.00
Doubtful value	120.00
Believed of little value	115.00

There is no official record of what was done to meet this emergency, except that in the account book of the Treasurer there are listed seven "loans" of $30 each, between November 29 and December 4, 1871, "for which the Treasurer gave his receipt." The Treasurer himself was one of them. The loans were all repaid by January, 1873. It is perhaps understandable why anniversary, presidential, and memorial addresses were not published. In 1872 the dues were raised to $5.00.

In 1872 Dr. H. D. Bulkley died. It had only been two years since he was President. Very appreciative resolutions were adopted and the Academy voted to attend his funeral in a body.

There was no Anniversary Oration in 1871. It had been customary, when an orator was prevented by illness from delivering his oration, to reappoint him the following year. This may have been done in this case, but Dr. Stiles was evidently unable to deliver it. He died in 1873. In 1872 Dr. E. S. Dunster was the Orator and spoke on "The Logic of Medicine."

On Dr. Peaslee's retirement as President, instead of the usual resolutions of thanks for "impartial, dignified and successful" term of office, the Academy voted:

Resolved, That the New York Academy of Medicine, in separating from their late President, Dr. E. R. Peaslee, upon the expiration of his term of office, beg to convey to him their high sense of his faithful, urbane and zealous services while in the Chair; their warm appreciation of his attainments as a classical and medical scholar, physiologist, pathologist and practitioner, and assure him of their affectionate regard and best wishes for his future health and prosperity.

Resolved, That this resolution be entered on the minutes to remain a lasting record of the sense of the Academy.

He presided over all but four meetings of the Academy during his two years. He was a very lovable character.

1873–1874

Dr. Austin Flint became the fifteenth President. Although only sixty-one years old, he was probably the best-known clinician in the country. He had contributed much to medical literature, and his writings were a real contribution to medical knowledge. A native of Massachusetts, with a long list of medical ancestors, he had taught, written, and practiced, at Buffalo, Chicago, Louisville, and New Orleans before he came to New York in 1859. He devoted practically all his time to teaching and consulting work. He had been Orator in 1858. His term was most successful, and he presided at all but two meetings in his two years. Under his guidance, the Academy made further strides. The minutes record less often "no quorum," and matters of public concern were handled promptly.

A resolution was sent to each New York Member of Congress urging measures to increase the efficiency of the medical department of the Army by granting them rank—and pay—commensurable with their duties and responsibilities; another urged Congress not to cut the appropriation for the Army Medical Museum and Library from $10,000 to $5,000.

The Academy also sent resolutions to the Legislature, endorsing bills to establish a State Board of Health, and one on "general drainage." The State Medical Society was urged to combat the proposed legislation to forbid the use of animals in vivisection. And finally a committee of three was appointed to cooperate with the College of Pharmacy to appeal to the Commissioners of Parks to establish and maintain a *botanical garden* in one of the parks!

Only one charge was brought against a Fellow, a Dr. Justus J. Spreng, by four Fellows. At the meeting to which he was called to defend himself, Dr. Spreng did not appear. His accusers did. He was accused of public advertisement, several being submitted, and publishing a pamphlet on diseases of the liver, which he sold for ten cents. He sent a copy of this pamphlet, by request, to Dr. Rogers, with the inscription, "With the compliments of the author to be independent and make money." The Committee recommended his expulsion, although he had, since the charges were made, resigned. He was unanimously expelled.

In 1873 Dr. J. C. Dalton, the Orator, spoke on "The Origin and Propagation of Disease." A committee had been appointed to arrange a supper after the address, at the Ashland House, just across the street from the College. The supper was not to cost more than $2.00 per head and "about 100 Fellows" adjourned to the festive board. The menu indicates a generous supper. The *Medical Record* tells us:

The toasts were as follows: "The New York Academy of Medicine una fides altare commune—gathered on this twenty-sixth anniversary its Fellows to renew their expression of veneration of the wisdom of its founders and renew their pledges to maintain the noble purposes for which it was designed," responded to by President Flint.

"Divinity, Law and Physics, triplets nurtured by faith, animated by hope, inspired by charity," responded to by Dr. Post [Dr. C. E. Post, son of Dr. A. C. Post?] for the Clergy, Edward S. Van Winkle for the Bar, and Dr. A. N. Bell of Brooklyn, for the physicians.

"The Building Fund," responded to by Dr. James Anderson.

The festivities closed shortly before midnight.

In 1874 the Anniversary Address was delivered by Dr. D. B. St. J. Roosa, "The Coming Medical Man."

Ever since the founding of the Academy, the subject of delinquents in dues had been a troublesome one. The rule was clear enough in the By Laws, but the Trustees had to pass on who should be dropped and notices had to be sent each delinquent, informing him that if he did not pay within a month, he was *liable* to be dropped. In 1874, the Council requested the Trustees to ascertain which Fellows were delinquent and to "take without delay" such steps as necessary.

It also called the Trustees' attention to the fact that they themselves had established the custom of waiting a year before finally reporting delinquents for the action authorized by the By Laws. The chairman of the Trustees replied that he had, at the request of the chairman of the Committee on Publication of the Council, made a complete list a month before and had reported it to the Recording Secretary, but Dr. Pond had not been sure that they had all been given the necessary one month's warning. The Trustees later voted that the Council be informed that the names had already been submitted to the chairman of their Committee on Publication, and that the list would be submitted to the Academy according to the By Laws. During eight years only nine Fellows had been dropped, and resignations of three, long unacted upon, were finally accepted.

The progress in the scientific function of the Academy during the eight years is striking. More than seventy Fellows contributed 127 papers. Dr. W. C. Roberts was the most communicative, contributing seven; Drs. G. M. Smith and Dalton five each; and Drs.

Buck and C. A. Leale four each. A striking feature was the number of recently elected Fellows who contributed.

The character of these contributions was really very high, and they were carefully prepared. It was still the custom, in presenting a subject, to go back to the earliest records of cases, and describe at length the views of the ancients.

Looking over the list, gynecological papers were most widely presented, and many were read by Drs. Peaslee, T. G. Thomas, I. E. Taylor, Joseph Kammerer, W. C. Roberts, E. Noeggerath, A. Underhill, W. T. Lusk, and W. M. Chamberlain. Bright's Disease was extensively discussed by Drs. G. M. Smith (two papers), A. L. Loomis, W. M. Chamberlain, A. S. Church and J. H. Griscom. Pulmonary tuberculosis attracted much attention, and long papers were read by Drs. Flint, W. H. Draper, W. C. Roberts and E. D. Hudson. Dr. J. R. Leaming contributed two interesting papers, on respiratory murmurs and on pleuritis. The latter brought Dr. H. P. Bowditch "all the way from Boston" to discuss and urge the early resort to thoracentisis. Another paper on "Thoracentisis" was read by Dr. C. A. Leale. Dr. Buck read a valuable paper on the treatment of "Abscesses of the Right Iliac Fossa," urging their early evacuation.

Plastic surgery was much talked of by Drs. W. Detmold, F. H. Hamilton and, especially, Dr. Buck. He at one meeting described an operation he had performed, demonstrated it on the cadaver, and then showed the result in the patient!

Dr. Herman Knapp (by invitation) read on "Physiological and Pathological Asymmetry of the Eye"; Dr. E. G. Loring spoke on the "modern" operation for strabismus, and Dr. H. D. Noyes gave "magic lantern" pictures illustrating the "Fundus of the Eye in Health and Disease." Dr. T. R. Pooley spoke on the causes of sudden blindness.

Orthopedics was taking a place, the cure of clubfoot by mechanical measures frequently discussed, and Dr. C. F. Taylor read a paper (two evenings) on lateral curvature of the spine and its treatment.

Electricity in the treatment of diseases interested Drs. A. D. Rockwell and G. M. Beard (two papers).

Public health and vital statistics were well taken care of by papers on "Statistical Medicine" by Dr. W. F. Thoms; "Causes of Disease and Death in New York City," Dr. W. C. Roberts; "Mortality in the Various Cities of the United States," Dr. Stephen Rogers; "Mortality in the Various States of the Union," Dr. C. P. Russell; "The Economy of Life" (that is, expectancy of life), Dr. A. N. Bell; "The Hygiene of the Primary Schools," Dr. R. J. O'Sullivan; and "Relapsing Fever as It Occurred in New York," Drs. Alonzo Clark and E. Harris.

Dr. W. B. Neftel read a paper on "Exact Methods of Medical Treatment," mentioning particularly the value of the clinical thermometer. This was apparently little in vogue, but Dr. Bulkley said at the New York Hospital it had been in use for two or three years, and the temperature of every case of typhoid fever was taken regularly and recorded on a paper at the foot of the bed (1868).

A number of strictly scientific papers were read. Dr. Dalton was the most active on these subjects. He spoke on "The Glycogenic Function of the Liver," "On the Spectrum of the Bile," and "A New Method of Determining the Absorption Band in the Spectrum of Organic Liquids." "Spectrum Analysis" was also discussed by Drs. A. H. Gallatin and Waterman (by invitation). Dr. J. C. Draper spoke on the "Relation of Urea to Muscular Action" and Dr. A. Flint, Jr., on "Cholesteraemia." Dr. S. F. Speir wrote on "The Use of the Microscope in Differential Diagnosis of Morbid Growths"; and Dr. Dalton exhibited "Trichina Spiralis" under the microscope.

Dr. Hanbury Smith read a paper on the use of mineral waters, urging they be taken in limited amounts—about two pints a day—in divided doses and, to get full effects, after each draught moderate exercise should be taken.

The use of carbolized catgut sutures was brought to the attention of the Academy by Dr. Peaslee and strongly recommended by him.

During these years the Fellowship had steadily increased, 116 Resident Fellows being elected.

But death took a fairly large toll; thirty-five Resident Fellows died—twelve in one year, alone. Many of them had been very active and valuable members up to their deaths, especially Drs. W. B. Bibbins, G. T. Elliot, J. G. Sewall, and J. H. Griscom.

1875–1878

Samuel S. Purple

On January 21, 1875, Dr. Flint made an excellent Valedictory Address and Dr. Purple became the sixteenth President. The son of a tanner in upper New York, at the age of seventeen Samuel Purple was left the sole support of a family, with nothing but a business burdened down with debts. He paid off the debts and, through the influence of two medical uncles, he accomplished his ambition and attended, free, a course of medical lectures at Geneva Medical College and then, a free course at New York University, studying under Valentine Mott. He secured his M.D. in 1844.

Coming to New York, he obtained a position at the old Marion Street Maternity Hospital until he was appointed Physician to the New York Dispensary. He prospered and, being of a literary nature, became an editor of the *New York Journal of Medicine*, serving as such for ten years.

He was one of the Founders of the Academy and from 1851 had been active in its affairs. He had served on the Committee on Publications from 1851–1857, Committee on Admissions 1859, 1860, and 1865, and as Statistical Secretary in 1863.

The first Committee on Ways and Means found him a member, and he was elected Secretary and served as such until he was elected President, when "for obvious reasons" he resigned that post.

Among his papers is a draft of a letter addressed to the President, Dr. Anderson. A verbatim copy follows:

New York Christmas December 1866

Dr. James Anderson
President of the New York Academy of Medicine

Dear Sir through you permit me to say that with some dilligence during the past twenty years I have been collecting a medical refference library which now comprises several thousand volumes. I propose to donate the same to the New York Academy of Medicine (on such terms relating to its preservation and increase as shall be mutual to each)—the conveyance to be made as soon as the Academy shall erect a fire proof building sufficiently commodious to contain said library with its prospective additions and which building shall also be suitable for the purposes of a Museum and a Hall in which the meetings of the Academy and the profession can be held.

For the purpose of aiding the Academy in the accomplishment of such an undertaking it may consider me as pledged for two thousand dollars towards the construction of the proposed building.

With earnest wishes for a great and glorious future for the Academy I am faithfully yours in the bonds of Aesculapius

Samuel S. Purple

Whether this letter was sent is not known, but the minutes of the Committee on Ways and Means state under date of December 29, 1866, "Dr. Purple announced his readiness to donate portions of his medical library to the Academy when it had a permanent home under suitable restrictions for their preservation." Those books are among the most prized possessions of the Academy today.

The year 1875 began a new era for the Academy—the humble beginnings of the modern Academy. In 1866 during the last year of Dr. Anderson's presidency, and probably at his instigation, the Council recommended that a committee be appointed to take action regarding obtaining a Home for the Academy. This Committee reported it did not consider it expedient, at the present time, owing to the financial status of the Academy, to attempt the matter. The Council replied that was not what the committee was appointed for and referred the matter back to it again, adding Dr. Anderson to its membership. Informal meetings were held and the whole matter was again thrown back on the Council "where the matter originated."

The Council then did a little thinking of its own and recommended a "Committee on Ways and Means" to work out a plan for securing a lot and erecting a building for the Academy. Drs. Willard Parker, S. T. Hubbard, Jared Linsly, Ernst Krackowizer, and S. S. Purple were promptly appointed by President Anderson, and he was added to the Committee by the Academy.

The Committee met the day it received notice of its appointment. Their first action was to search for an "available site" and they decided three lots, the area considered necessary, on West 42d Street "opposite Reservoir Square" were the best. Each would cost about $35,000!

The "Building Fund" of the Academy, established by the donation of the surplus from the Entertainment Fund for the American Medical Association in 1853, amounted to $1,736. This was made a round $2,500 by appropriation from Academy Funds and had slowly increased to $7,524.22. It was invested in a mortgage at 7 percent and in U.S. Government Bonds and Notes. A second contribution from another surplus from an A.M.A. entertainment fund had been received, and the Academy appropriated some of its surplus, from time to time.

The Committee asked and received from the Academy "full power to raise funds, select a site, and if necessary, erect a building."

A subcommittee was appointed to search for Fellows who would be willing to head a subscription list "liberally." The subscription form adopted pledged the subscriber to pay the amount in four semiannual payments. In case of death it was optional for the heirs to cancel the unpaid balance.

From February 18, 1867, to April 24, 1868, no record exists of a meeting. Drs. Stephen Smith, and C. L. Mitchell of Brooklyn were added to the committee. In November a circular appeal was issued, emphasizing the need of a central organization and modestly announcing on account of "a prestige of age and respectability, a liberal charter and an accumulated fund of over ten thousand dollars," it had taken the initiative in obtaining a home for the profession, and hoped it would respond liberally. Two thousand copies of this circular were printed. If the fund was now "over ten thousand dollars," the Committee had raised around $2,500 in about two years.

There is no record of another meeting till January, 1870. The Committee had not been idle, however, for Dr. Hubbard announced he had nearly $4,000 on his books, and $3,571 had been *collected.*

In June, 1870, it was decided to hold a "meeting of a social character" at Dr. Anderson's house (he had been chairman from the start), which thirty or forty members of the profession and laity should be invited to attend. This is the first time the idea of enlisting the laity had been mentioned. There is, however, no record of any meeting till January, 1873, and as at that meeting it was explained why the "social gathering" had not been held, there probably was none. In these three years the Committee had collected some $3,000, and its bank account showed $6,697.85.

Drs. John G. Adams and Gouverneur Smith were added to the committee to take on the subscription books of Drs. Parker and Linsly, who were too busy to make personal approaches. Another circular was prepared and sent out in 1874, practically identical with that of 1868 except that the accumulated building fund was now announced as "over $24,000." The Committee passed a resolution to "act with renewed vigor" in an attempt to secure a building before the end of 1874.

These two circulars are the only ones mentioned in the minutes, but there is another among the Purple papers, which, headed with a cut of the front of a classical building of two stories, reads:

AN APPEAL

The great and noble profession of Medicine in this city needs at least one benefactor. The College of Physicians of London had its Harvey, who in his lifetime laid the foundation for "a library and repository for simples and rarities," which is to this day the great centre of the profession in that city. The College of Physicians of Philadelphia had its Mütter, who in his lifetime also laid a foundation for its hall, library and museum, which stands out prominent among the notable institutions of that city. And shall the profession of the Metropolis of American any longer remain without a home and a benefactor, A HALL AND LIBRARY, which shall serve as a rallying-point where medical men may meet together and hold communion with each other? Is there not at least one among those who have had the favored confidence of the profession who will say it shall be done? If so, the work will be accomplished. The present is the occasion —now is the auspicious time for a Harvey, a Radcliff, or a Mütter to rise up here, and, while he does good to the cause of Medicine, immortalize himself through all time in the memory of his professional brethren.

In commenting on these endeavors the *Medical Record* remarked, in less than complimentary fashion:

The most pretentious of our societies—the New York Academy of Medicine—a society which calls its members *fellows*, which publishes transactions at irregular intervals and which is said to have a library in the garret of one of its members, has been engaged during the last ten or a dozen years in picking up subscriptions for the purpose of erecting a building, of which the glory of name and ownership shall belong to itself; while the County Medical and Pathological Societies with the Journal Association and a lot of smaller and special organizations, such as the Obstetrical and Ophthalmological may, if they chose, get admission in a strictly subordinate way.

In November, 1874, the Committee was informed that the Academy would like a report at their meeting of December 3, which, after a summary of its long activities, closes as follows:

The urgent need of the Academy, as also that of sister organizations, for a fixed habitation, has led your Committee to canvass the propriety of purchasing a building in a central location, and at a moderate cost, cause such alterations to be made as will for some time to come answer the purposes of the Academy.

In this view of the question the Committee would suggest that an expression of the wishes of the Academy be made on this occasion. It is the opinion of your Committee that a united response from the profession and particularly from the Fellows of the Academy, would lead to the immediate accomplishment of this object, for in the prosecution of their labors they have been generally received with cordiality and instances are not wanting where liberal responses have been made to their solicitations. The kindly feeling with which they have been received and the general success of their efforts, have left on the minds of the members of your Committee the belief that the object contemplated by the Academy may and of a right ought to be in some form soon realized.

That the profession has not been mistaken in the wisdom, determination and ability of the body which the Committee represents, will be shown in the subjoined exhibit of the amount of the permanent fund of the Academy available at the present moment for the building purposes, which is as follows:

Total amount in the hands of the Trustees, invested in U.S. Bonds, bearing interest at 6% in gold	15,009.36
Present premium on the U.S. Securities	1,402.20
Total amount received from subscriptions obtained by the Committee and deposited in the bank	9,532.44
Accrued interest on deposit in the bank	206.00
Sum total of amount now available	26,150.00
Total amount of unpaid subscriptions	2,342.00
Total	28,492.00

During the years 1868, 1869, and 1870 the Academy had transferred to the Building Fund $1,400 from its income.

After receipt of this report the Academy took a "recess" of an hour, to hold a "recess" meeting, at which Dr. Oliver White presided and Dr. Eliot was Secretary. It was voted that the Committee on Ways and Means should, with as little delay as possible, procure a building for the accommodation of the Academy and other medical organizations of the city, and that, if necessary, a debt of $10,000 or $15,000 might be incurred.

The Committee immediately secured an option on No. 12 West 31st Street, and after many negotiations, searching the title, and other necessary matters were attended to, on December 24, 1874, had signed this contract:

Cash on signing the contract	$1,500.00
End of 30 days, on passing title	31,000.00
On Bond and Mortgage	10,000.00
Total	$42,500.00

Dr. Flint announced this at the last meeting over which he presided, January 7, 1875.

The Committee worked very hard to raise the nearly $4,000 still required, and after delays, waiting for the "papers" from the owner, and so on, early in March the transaction was completed, and the Academy owned a HOME, a brown stone, high stoop house of four

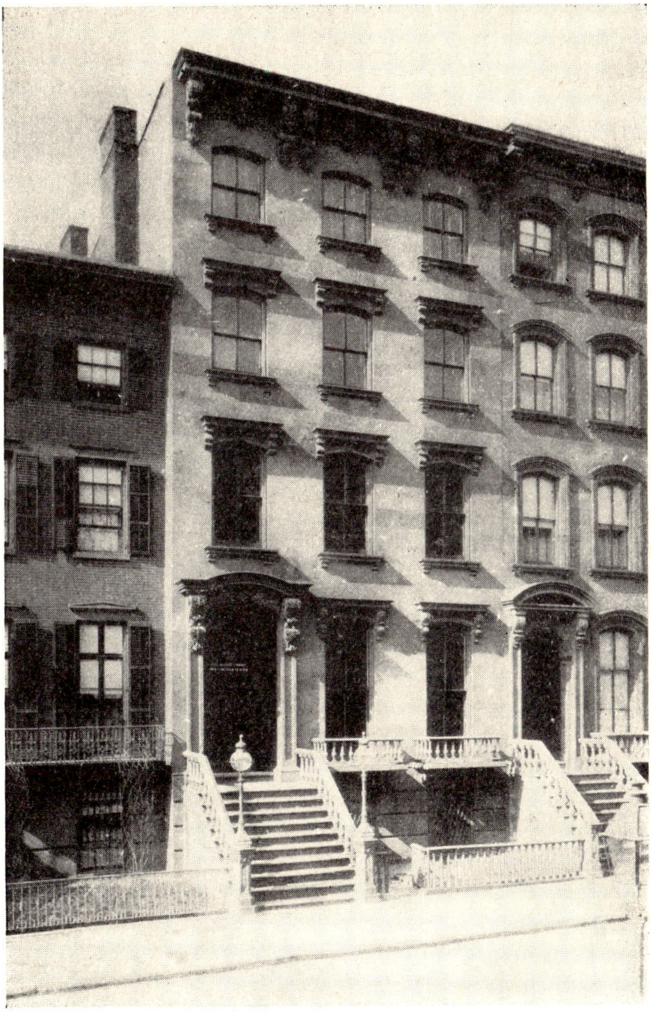

FIRST HOME OF THE ACADEMY
12 WEST 31ST STREET
Meetings Held Here from May 20, 1875, through May, 1890

stories, 28 feet by 60, on a lot 100 feet deep. Dr. Anderson reported the good news March 4, 1875, and also the receipt of $250 from Mrs. Hartley in memory of her father, Dr. S. P. White, one of the Founders.

From what we know of the general arrangements of such houses and of the use made by the Academy of the rooms, the basement floor contained a kitchen in the rear, and a dining room in front. The first floor consisted of two parlors, probably connected with large folding doors, so that both could be thrown into one. The upper floors (three) had two large rooms, and two small "hall" rooms, one of which was a bathroom. On the second floor, there were closets between the rooms, and a basin with running water. From somewhere the Committee secured sufficient funds to "furnish" the house.

On May 20, 1875, the Academy had the formal "opening." It was quite a celebration, as well it might have been.

The President, Dr. Purple, after words of greeting and congratulation, introduced Dr. James Anderson, the Chairman of the Committee on Ways and Means. For nine long years he had been its chairman, and had worked tirelessly. After detailing the history of the Academy, from the first meeting of "Regular Physicians" in December, 1846, to the present time, he presented to the President the abstract of Title and Deed, two policies of insurance, *and* the mortgage. The subscriptions received, after paying for the house, had enabled the Committee to pay the interest ($350) and insurance premiums, and was also sufficient to pay for carpets, cleaning and renovation, leaving $1,000 for improvements and repairs to be raised within three months.

With all formality the President received the documents and officially transferred them to Dr. Oliver White, the Chairman of the Board of Trustees, who equally formally accepted them on behalf of the Trustees, and offered a vote of thanks to the Committee on Ways and Means for their activities in securing "this pleasant and commodious home."

A letter was then read from the children of the late Galen Carter, presenting a portrait of Dr. John Stearns, the first President, and also one of Dr. Galen Carter, an early Vice President. After the usual vote of thanks, Dr. Purple left the Chair and read a memorial of Dr. Stearns. It is interesting to note that on the death of Dr. Stearns in 1848, Dr. Francis had been appointed to prepare a memorial, but he died in 1861 without doing so, and Dr. Purple was appointed to take his place. The memorial was perhaps a little late.

Dr. Post made a few remarks on Dr. Carter. A letter was then read from Dr. Gouverneur M. Smith, presenting a portrait of his father, Dr. Joseph M. Smith, "painted expressly for the Academy." He was its President in 1854. Dr. Elisha Harris made some remarks on Dr. Smith. Dr. Charles D. Smith then presented, by letter, a portrait of his father, Dr. Gilbert Smith, one of the Founders and a very active early member. Dr. J. G. Adams was prepared with some remarks on Dr. Smith.

A letter was read from Dr. J. G. Adams asking the Academy to accept "busts of those ancient masters of our art, Aesculapius and Hippocrates. Give them a resting place among our '*lares and penates*' and let them be handed down to posterity in commemoration of this auspicious inauguration." They are still at the Academy.

A letter was read from Dr. Austin Flint, expressing regret at his absence:

> The circumstances preventing my attendance were beyond my control, but I claim the privilege of imposing on myself, for my absence, a fine, which I hereby inclose. . . .
>
> A minor cause of regret in not being with you tonight is the loss of hearing the "three cheers and tiger" which, as the Chairman of Ways and Means has assured me, the occasion will call for. I do not doubt that Dr. Anderson's voice and vigor will render the cheers effective, and I am sorry that the absence of our honored Fellow, Dr. Peaslee, will prevent him from leading off with the "tiger."

After this the cheers were "heartily given." (Dr. Flint's "fine" was $50.)

Dr. Detmold, called upon to speak on the origin of the Building Fund, described the early meetings of the Academy "in a dingy room over a coal yard, I think somewhere in Wooster Street near Houston," and remarked that the discussions of those days bore the same relation to those of today "as that dingy room bears to the elegant hall in which we are assembled tonight." In describing the origin of the Building Fund, he stated that most of the Committee of Entertainment of the A.M.A. in 1853 were in favor of giving the residue to the Society for the Relief of Widows and Orphans of Medical Men, but he had persuaded them it was better to contribute it to something "which would benefit the whole profession," and thus it came to the Academy.

After announcing that if through inadvertance any Fellows had not been called on to contribute they could now do so, they were all invited to partake of a collation, which had been provided for the occasion (by the President). And so the Academy started on the first period in the new environment.

Almost the first thing the Academy did, after moving in, was to establish a Standing Committee on Library, which was to supervise its operation, report upon its condition annually, and furnish a statement of needs for the ensuing year. There was to be a Librarian and an Assistant Librarian, one of whom was to be on duty from 9–12 A.M., and 1–4 P.M. daily, Sundays excepted, and from November through March from 7–10 P.M. (No salary was provided.)

Section 3 states: "The Librarian shall have charge of all the books, manuscripts, anatomical or pathological specimens, apparatus, instruments, portraits, medals, coins and other scientific property of the Academy and shall attend to their preservation, arrangement and cataloguing. He shall fix to each donation the name of the donor."

The Librarian was also to arrange for access to all journals and new publications. No book was to be taken from the building.

The Library occupied the two large rooms on the second floor. Dr. Hinton, the incumbent, was reappointed Librarian.

The By Laws relating to hours were suspended, almost as soon as adopted, and it was not until October, 1875, that the Library was really opened, and then only from 2 to 5. In September it was announced Dr. Purple, true to his word, had contributed 2,000 bound volumes of journals and monographs.

The Academy was hard pressed financially that year, although several very welcome contributions were received from Fellows and friends. Unexpected expenses kept coming up. The roof leaked and had to be repaired, as did also the gas pipes; and the plumbing was frequently out of order. The interest on the mortgage had to be paid, but worst of all the city insisted on imposing a real-estate tax of $823 the first year! There was always the expense of printing the *Transactions*, and the Academy ordered 750 copies of the proceedings of its opening meeting printed. A committee was appointed to try to have the tax on the real estate removed, but it was unsuccessful for two years.

The New York Medical Journal Association rented most of the third floor for its library, and the Medico-Legal Society also was permitted to rent a room for its meetings, and a "small room" for its books. The Society for the Relief of Widows and Orphans of Medical Men, and the Physicians Mutual Aid were given the use of rooms for their meetings, free.

In November, 1875, there was $20 in the Treasury, and the Academy promptly raised its dues for the next year from $5 to $10.

The postcard announcements of the meetings of June 3 and 17 contain this footnote:

☞ Fresh vaccine virus may be obtained at all hours of the day, on application to the Janitor of the Academy.

Scientific meetings were held regularly all year, eight at the College of Physicians and Surgeons and eight at "The Academy's Hall." Papers were read by Dr. Flint on pneumonia and on functional murmurs of the heart with infrequent pulse; Dr. Leaming on the same subjects; Dr. Buck on migration of pus, and perityphlitic abscess successfully treated by incision. Sixteen papers were presented, of which six were ordered printed in the *Transactions.*

The Anniversary Address was given in November, by Dr. E. D. Hudson, Jr., "Doctors, Hygiene and Therapeutics." Dr. Hudson had only been appointed in October, *vice* Dr. D. Tilden Brown, who was ill, and the Academy voted its thanks to him for his "promptness in preparing his interesting anniversary discourse."

During 1876 the Academy memorialized the State Legislature

for a bill to record births, marriages and deaths, and vital statistics in general, which it had also done, unsuccessfully, in 1847. It also joined with the Medical Society of the District of Columbia in protesting to Congress the incorporation of a "National Surgical Institute" which was another diploma mill. Senator Conklin presented this protest, and the Institute was not incorporated.

The Library was growing very fast, and there were frequent requests for more shelf room and for more help. It was voted in 1876 to appoint at $300 a year an assistant librarian, who would also collect dues. Even in its new home the Academy was having the usual difficulty in this matter, and a number of names were "stricken from the rolls," but only after careful investigation. The following is interesting:

"WHEREAS, Dr. Stephen Wood, having been unfortunate and being unable to pay his back dues in money, has offered to pay them in books, and having retired from the profession, therefore

"*Resolved*, That the Trustees accept the offer, but in so doing determine their action shall not be adopted as a precedent."

His back dues amounted to $45 and Dr. Purple estimated the books were worth $50.

The "tenant" societies were a source of considerable trouble. They were very slow in paying rent, and the Medical Journal Association was not only remiss, but demanded a good deal. For example:

Dear Doctor:

In pursuance of a resolution adopted by the Board of Directors of the Medical Journal Association of the City of New York, the Executive Committee is instructed to notify the Academy of Medicine of the desire of the Association to place a suitable sign bearing its name at the door of the building No. 12 West 31st Street, and further, that the Association proposes to place a sign bearing its name on its own portion of the building in case it does not by the end of two weeks receive the assent of the Academy to placing one at the door as desired.

Yours respectfully

J. H. Emerson, SECRETARY OF EX. COM.

The Trustees replied with this resolution:

WHEREAS, The letter from the Executive Committee of the Medical Journal Association of the City of New York, addressed to the Secretary of the Academy, having been referred by the President to this Board, therefore

Resolved, That inasmuch as the subject of the communication has been hitherto under consideration and since the letter above quoted contains a menace to the Academy, the Secretary be instructed to return the said communication to the said Executive Committee.

Resolved, That permission be given to any society or association, regularly holding its meetings in the Academy building, to place a bulletin upon the walls of the hall by the side of, or opposite to, the Academy's bulletin.

Resolved, That no permission be given to any society or association to place any sign upon the exterior of the Academy building.

Signed *W. T. White,* SECRETARY PRO TEM.

The Academy had appointed a committee of three to cooperate with the Centennial Exhibition in Philadelphia. This resulted in two papers: "Hospitals and Their Development during the Century of the American Republic," by Dr. W. Gill Wylie, and "Epidemics of the Century and Lessons Derived from Them," by Dr. G. M. Smith. Eighteen papers were read during the year, many of them emphasizing the changing ideas of the day. Dr. I. E. Taylor discussed "Destructive Operations vs. Caesarian Section in Pelves of 1½–2½ Inches in Diameter," Dr. Peaslee "Incision and Discission of the Cervix Uteri," and Dr. Flint, Sr., "Studies Relating to Phthisis."

The Anniversary Address by Dr. W. T. White was "The History of Medicine in the Century of the Republic." He stated there were forty-six medical journals being published in the United States, survivors of the 198 that had been started. He also stressed that the "Germ Theory" was now under discussion.

Dr. Barker moved a vote of thanks, which was given, for his "cool, cautious and temperate relation of facts, and the excellent taste manifested in his discourse by avoiding everything like extravagant pretensions or claims."

Dr. Purple was renominated for President and Dr. Pond declined to serve another term. He had been Treasurer of the Academy since 1848, twenty-nine years, and was now 86 years old. Dr. Pond's accounts, all in his own hand, are interesting reading. Every transaction was in "*Cash*"; no matter how large the sum. Of course the Building Fund was in the hands of the Trustees, who had their own Treasurer. Dr. Pond had been through difficult times, and the Academy had often been in the red, but he always managed to get through—somehow. The following resolutions were adopted and, properly framed in oak, were presented to him.

WHEREAS, Dr. James O. Pond, having attained the age of eighty-six years, and having concluded a service of twenty-nine consecutive years as Treasurer of the New York Academy of Medicine, has declined to be a candidate for re-election; therefore,

Resolved, That the Academy desires to place on permanent record its warm appreciation of his long and faithful interest in the Association.

Resolved, That as one of the founders of the Academy in 1847, as one of the incorporators in 1851, as Treasurer since 1848, he has, from the inception of the Association to the present moment, manifested a zeal in the welfare of the Society which has contributed largely to its success.

Resolved, That in the onerous duties of the Treasurership he has always held the unbounded confidence of the Academy, and his example for courtesy, efficiency, and integrity, will ever remain as a model for future incumbents of the office.

Resolved, That the Academy wish him length of years, with health to enjoy the close of a long and honorable career.

Resolved, That a copy of this preamble and of these resolutions be entered in full on the minutes of the Academy, be published in the medical journals of this city, and that a suitably engrossed and authenticated copy be presented to Dr. Pond.

In 1880 it was voted that Dr. Pond, "having faithfully served the Academy as its Treasurer for twenty-nine years, and now being incapacitated for professional labor by reason of advancing age and bodily infirmities," be exempt from dues, after January 1, 1879. He died in 1881.

The Academy now modernized its system of finance. It was voted:

Resolved, That a bank account be opened in the Second National Bank or bank approved by the President and Treasurer of the Association in the name of the New York Academy of Medicine.

Resolved, That the Trustees and the Treasurer procure a checkbook, each check to contain the name of the Academy on its border.

Resolved, That all money received by the Treasurer shall be immediately deposited in such bank, the checkbook to show with each deposit the source of such income.

Resolved, That all moneys withdrawn from the bank shall be withdrawn by the checks above designated and the stub corresponding with each check to designate the use to which the money is applied.

Nine of the ten papers read through June 15, 1876, were published in the *Transactions* at a cost of nearly $800. Thereafter the Academy ceased publishing *Transactions* until April, 1881.

Dr. Purple, reelected President, delivered his Inaugural, and after a brief account of Academy progress, gave a most interesting account of the development of medical libraries in New York. This is an important historical document today.

During 1877 the Academy continued its fairly peaceful course. The Committee on Ways and Means had collected since March, 1875, $2,135, which had all been expended on repairs, furniture, and fixtures. It announced that one contractor had deducted $9.90 from his bill, and another $3.55, as a "donation" to the Academy. Also Mr. Hawes, the legal gentleman who had searched the title to the building, sent in a bill for $100, *receipted,* requesting the amount be turned over to the use of the Library. Five hundred and forty-five dollars in subscriptions were still due, and the Committee felt the Fellows should recognize their obligation to pay, "as the expenditures of the Academy were based upon their liquidation."

It was announced that the Legislature had amended the Charter, granting the Academy power to hold in trust permanent funds and property, the income of which should not exceed $10,000, which income should be spent for the advancement of medical science in general, or as specified by the donors. "This act will keep intact any bequests for all time." It was voted that 1,000 copies of the act be printed "for the use of the Academy"(?).

As recommended by Dr. Purple in his address, the Committee on Ways and Means were empowered to solicit subscriptions for a Permanent Library Fund.

The names of all candidates for fellowship were ordered printed in the notices of meetings as soon as nominated. This has accordingly been carried out for sixty-nine years.

Dr. Laurence Johnson was appointed Librarian to the Academy. A young, active and enthusiastic man, he served for six years, greatly improving the usefulness of the Library. This was enriched by the gift of Dr. J. C. Peters of his collection of books on Asiatic Cholera, "the largest in existence."

Fifteen papers were read during the year. Dr. Herman Knapp, by invitation, reported results in 200 operations for removal of cataract. Dr. Flint, Sr., discussed rectal alimentation, Dr. Flint, Jr., reported his experiments on respiration, and Dr. Barker read a paper on the use of the obstetrical forceps. A most surprising case was reported by Dr. V. P. Gibney,—one of "Tuberculous Meningitis Successfully Treated by the Use of Ergot"!

The Anniversary Address was delivered by Dr. T. Gaillard Thomas, who spoke eloquently on "The Influences Which Are Elevating Medicine to the Position of a Science."

In 1878 the Academy was saddened by the sudden death of Dr. Peaslee, and the Stated Meeting of February 7 was held at the vestry of the "Church at 29th Street and 5th Avenue." After the minutes and election of new members, Dr. Barker read a long biography of Dr. Peaslee and the following resolutions were adopted:

That by the death of our late fellow and ex-President the Academy of Medicine has lost one of its most distinguished and useful members, who was ever zealous for its interest, usefulness and reputation; who by his great success as a Teacher of various departments in several medical colleges has done much for the education of a large class of medical practitioners in all parts of the country now working in the interests of humanity; who by his important papers either read before the Academy or published in different medical journals and by his learned and able works has added much to the science of medicine and greatly improved its practice in many important departments, and has left an imperishable name, greatly to the honor and reputation of this Academy and of the profession this city and of this country; and who by his personal character won our warm esteem and high respect;

That these resolutions be entered in the Minutes of the Academy of Medicine, sent to the Medical Journals of this city for publication, and that an engrossed copy be sent to the bereaved family.

Signed *Fordyce Barker*
James L. Banks } COMMITTEE
Austin Flint

In seconding the resolution, Drs. Thomas, Flint and O'Sullivan spoke feelingly of Dr. Peaslee. No papers were read that evening. Dr. Peaslee's portrait was presented to the Academy in June, as directed in his will.

The committee appointed to try to have the taxes on the building removed reported in March that in spite of the adverse opinion of Mr. Elial F. Hall, retained to give legal advice, it had approached the Commissioners of Taxes and presented the claim for exemption on the ground that the property was "used as a public library and for the elevation of the standards of medical education, the promotion of public health, and instruction of the medical profession and the public." The Chairman of the Committee, Dr. Purple, had been "cordially received," his declarations "attentively considered," and the Academy's property was officially adjudged exempt from taxation. The Academy was saved seven to eight hundred dollars yearly. Legal Counsel made a gift of the fee for his adverse opinion, plus $25 as a contribution to the Library!

The Academy granted the use of the "Hall" to the New York Academy of Sciences for forty meetings during the year, and the majority of the third floor ("except the small room in the rear") to the Medical Journal Association. The use of rooms was also given for meetings to the New York Neurological and Medico-Legal Societies, the Public Health Association, and the Therapeutical Society. These organizations contributed $758 toward the upkeep of the building during the year.

Mr. E. R. Purple, brother of the President, had been appointed Assistant Librarian, but had been ill and unable to attend to his duties. Dr. Purple gave much time to the work and presented to the Library Fund, in his brother's name, a check for $375, the amount of the salary from October 1, 1876, to June 3, 1878. Mr. Purple resigned as Assistant Librarian; he was later elected a Benefactor of the Academy.

In September, 1878, the Academy voted, as recommended by the President, to open the Library to the public, from 10 to 5 daily, and in October this was done. The Library has therefore been open to the public for seventy years. At the same time a new Assistant Librarian was elected, Dr. Robert Campbell.

The Academy passed resolutions protesting the proposal to diminish the area of parks in the city by building an armory in part of one. A copy was sent to the Legislature. It also appointed a committee to cooperate with the School of Mines in an attempt to prevent the adulteration of foods and drugs.

Fifteen papers were read during the year. Dr. L. S. Pilcher of Brooklyn was invited to read one on "Injuries to the Wrist Joint, Particularly Colles' Fracture." Dr. Gaillard Thomas read four, one on "Elytrotomy, as a Substitute for Caesarian Section." Almost all were practical papers and called forth considerable discussion.

Dr. Piffard explained and demonstrated the use of some pills which, when diluted with water and boiled, would detect the presence of sugar in the urine.

Because "of the exceedingly severe storm, but few Fellows were present" in November. The Anniversary Address was therefore postponed until December, when Dr. W. H. Thomson delivered it. Its subject was "one of the most widely felt trials which the active practitioner of our day is called upon to experience." He stated:

There are but few physicians of fifteen or twenty years' experience in practice who would not be glad to take advantage of a law or custom which would oblige the whole medical fraternity to go back, once every ten years, to their educational institutions and take an entirely new course in all branches, not excepting the most elementary ones. . . .

[The physician] must expect to find that much of the freight which cost him so much trouble to collect and stow away, is constantly becoming wholly unsalable or going out of market. He must even be circumspect how he displays his wares, lest he be ridiculed for their antiquated character. As well might he enter a circle of modern astronomers discussing a transit, as to mention laudable pus to those who are discussing the migration of white curpuscles.

He also paid his compliments to Medical Schools:

They are chiefly isolated and strictly private institutions, generally owned by a portion of their faculties, and less known to the general public, and certainly less cared for, than many second-class female seminaries. As their support is wholly derived from their pupils, the exigencies of the average medical student's purse prescribes the length of the course of instruction. The result is, that the young mind must be stored as rapidly as possible with the effect of rendering our five months of medical lectures, at the rate of eight a day, altogether too suggestive of the five minutes for refreshments at our railway stations, where some of the most varied viands are bolted simultaneously, with much that is paid for left forever behind.

Dr. Purple was a very efficient President, his main interest being in the Library. He presided at every meeting held, and was very regular in attendance at Council and Trustees' meetings.

1879–1884

Fordyce Barker

IN FEBRUARY Dr. Purple, after two terms of office, delivered his Valedictory Address, in which he announced that $5,000 had been promised the Academy to build the much needed addition to the building, *if* the Fellows would raise $3,000 more.

Dr. Fordyce Barker, seventeenth President, was the son of a physician. He entered Bowdoin College at the age of fifteen, and that same year delivered the Fourth of July address in his native town of Wilton, Maine. For two years he studied medicine in Boston, and then returned to graduate from the Medical Department of Bowdoin in 1841. After studying in Paris for a year, intending to take a degree there, he started practice in Norwich, Connecticut, making the trip from Maine on horseback. "Always cheerful and gentle in the sickroom, very social, telling a good story, singing beautifully, and playing the piano, organ and trombone, he was welcomed everywhere socially, and his success was immediate."

He moved to New York in March, 1850, to become Professor of Obstetrics in the New York Medical College. A successful operation for submucous fibroids on a socially prominent lady made his reputation. Ultimately he acquired an enormous practice among the wealthy and cultured population. He was appointed to the Staff of Bellevue Hospital and served there till his death. He was also Consulting Physician to the Woman's Hospital and Nursery and Child's. He was made a Fellow of the Academy in 1854, and took a leading part in its professional activities. He had been Vice President during three years before his election as President at the age of fifty-seven.

After Dr. Barker's Inaugural, which was full of optimism over the future of the Academy and pride over the position the Academy had attained, resolutions were offered thanking Dr. Purple for the great success of his administration, the high position attained by the Academy as a scientific body, especially in its library and reading room, "to which he has personally contributed so largely, and which have grown up under his fostering care. The Academy have reason to thank him for his distinguished and self-denying service."

Dr. Austin Flint then immediately became active, suggesting that a subscription to raise the $3,000 mentioned by Dr. Purple in his Valedictory be immediately started. Before the evening was over $850 was promised, and a committee was appointed to solicit further subscriptions. By mid-April the full sum was raised, and the conditional $5,000 was promptly paid by Dr. Abram Dubois, who was not a Fellow of the Academy. Resolutions were passed, thanking Dr. Dubois for his generosity, declaring him a "Benefactor" and making him an honorary Fellow. The class of Benefactors, on payment of $1,000, open to the laity as well as the profession, had been established at the previous meeting.

Dr. Dubois certainly was a Benefactor. When the sum was raised, he added another $3,000 to be part of the Library Fund, and he requested Dr. Purple to purchase for the Library such recently published books as would place it in as complete working order as possible, at his expense. By mid-October Dr. Purple had expended $1,318.33 for this purpose. Dr. Dubois continued his contributions for new books until 1884.

No meetings were held between May 15 and October 2, by which time the alterations were completed, and the "new Library Hall" was dedicated. The minutes state:

The meeting was one of deep interest to the academicians and to the profession of the city. The President, Dr. Barker, occupied the chair, while on the platform with him were the three Vice Presidents, Drs. W. T. White, T. Gaillard Thomas, J. R. Leaming, and five ex-Presidents, viz: Drs. Willard Parker, A. C. Post, James Anderson, Austin Flint, Sr., and S. S. Purple. Also the following invited guests: Sir Henry W. Acland, Regius Professor of Medicine, University of Oxford; Dr. Samuel D. Gross, Honorary Fellow of Philadelphia; Dr. Shattuck of Boston, late Professor of Medicine in Harvard University; Dr. John S. Billings,

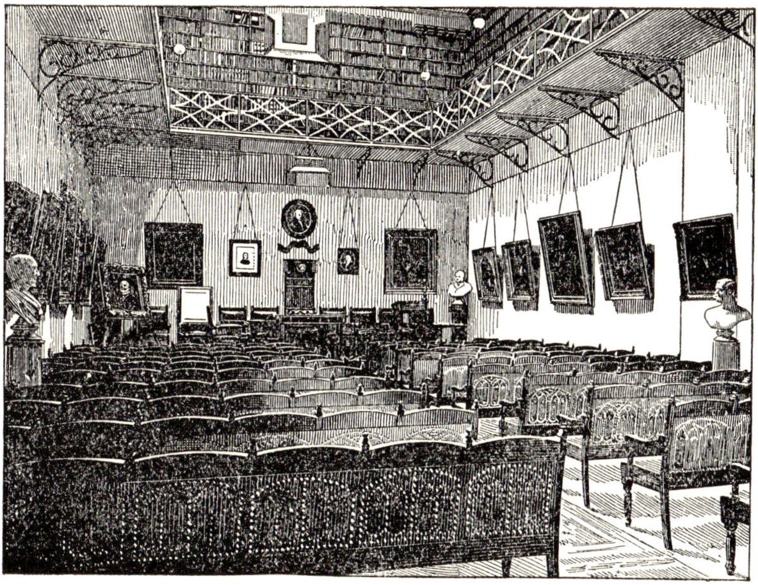

DU BOIS HALL, 12 WEST 31ST STREET
Addition Built in 1879, Showing Library Stacks

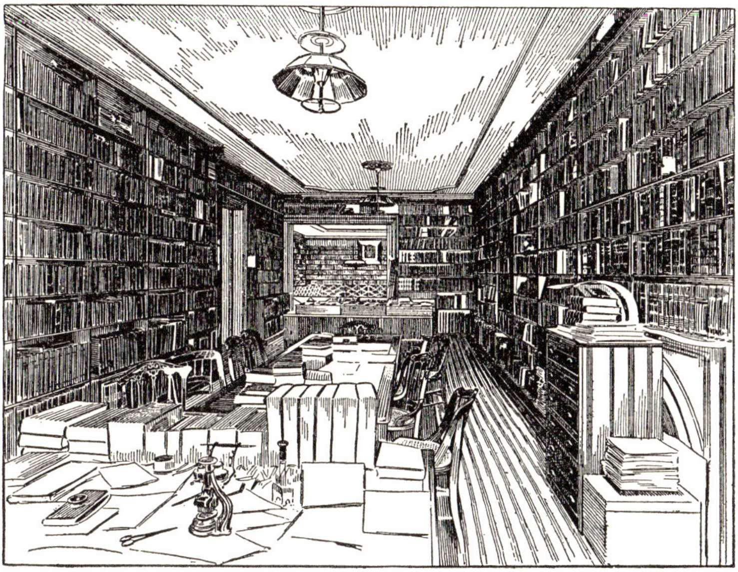

MAIN READING ROOM, 12 WEST 31ST STREET

U.S.A., Librarian of the Surgeon General's Library, Washington, D.C.; also the President of the Medical Society of the County of New York, Dr. F. J. Bumstead; and Dr. R. F. Weir, President of the Medical Journal Association of the City of New York. There were also present a very large number of the Fellows and members of the medical profession of the city.

The walls of the new hall had been decorated with numerous portraits of the Founders of the Academy, many of these having been loaned for the occasion.

Dr. Purple, chairman of the Building Committee, reported that $12,573 had been collected and $12,566 had been disbursed. This, however, included Dr. Dubois's additional $3,000.

The President then delivered an address and at its close he unveiled a beautiful marble bust of T. Spencer Wells, and presented it, together with the President's Chair and Table, the Reading Desk, and the Secretary's Table, which were upon the platform, to the Academy.

Remarks were made by Drs. Acland, Gross, Billings and Shattuck.

Dr. Willard Parker, the senior ex-President, in a congratulatory speech, presented the following resolutions, viz:

Resolved, That the opening of the new Library-Hall on the present occasion, is a demonstration of the wisdom and zeal of the founders of the New York Academy of Medicine, for the education and culture of the profession.

The resolution was duly seconded by Dr. Austin Flint, and unanimously approved by the Academy.

The President, Dr. Barker, then invited the Fellows and guests of the Academy to the lower rooms, where an elegant collation had been provided through the generosity of the President.

The Academy then adjourned.

In his address Dr. Barker emphasized that this building was, after all, only the *temporary* home of the Academy, and envisioned a building similar to the Royal College in London. He remarked that four years earlier the library consisted of 400 volumes—now it had over 9,000. He said "no time is now frittered away in the discussion of parliamentary usage and motions and amendments. No cheap notoriety can now be gained by frivolous speeches on such matters, by those who from incompetency or from a just self-appreciation, fortunately never take part in our scientific discussions." In closing, he said that when in London, he had been shown a golden goblet and was told it was a "loving cup"; he thereupon invited all present to remain and "to take a loving cup, and only regretted that it must be one of glass instead of gold."

T. Spencer Wells was a great English ovariotomist, the greatest in his day. The bust was by Richard Liebreich, an eminent ophthalmologist, which had caused much comment in London, where Dr. Barker had purchased it.

The speeches were reported very fully in the *Medical Record*, and the *Boston Medical and Surgical Journal* tells us something about the building.

The new audience-room measures twenty-eight feet in width by fifty feet in length, and is two stories in height. It forms an extension to the building purchased by the Academy four and a half years ago, and this now covers the entire lot of one hundred by twenty-eight feet. . . .

The floor is composed of Georgia pine, covered with a handsome carpet, and forty settees have been provided for the use of members attending the meetings of the academy and other bodies. These will seat two hundred persons, but by calling into requisition the seats in the gallery and the old meeting hall in part, an audience of five hundred can be accommodated, as on this occasion. The ceiling is lofty, having been carried up to the height of the third floor of the main building, and there is a gallery extending around all four sides of the room, which communicates with the second floor of the latter through a wide archway, and contains a considerable portion of the books of the library, arranged on neat shelves. The acoustic properties of the new hall are perfect, and the most approved plans of heating and ventilating the rooms have been adopted. In the centre of the ceiling is a large, double skylight, with a space between the upper and lower sashes of about five feet; while the lower sash bears the seal of the academy (the principal feature of which is the head of Hippocrates), beautifully finished in colored glass. Around this lower sash is a space about six inches wide, just beneath which a border of gas-jets, sixty-four in number, is placed. By means of this arrangement the room is beautifully lighted, and the burning gas producing a current, the foul air of the room rushes upward and outward through the upper sky-light, while its place is supplied by fresh air admitted through ventilators near the floor. . . .

On the evening of the dedication of the new hall the walls were decorated with portraits (most of them life-size) of all the presidents of the Academy since its organization, and of many of the founders in addition. . . . The portrait of Dr. Dubois had the place of honor directly over the head of the president's chair, and still higher up on the wall was the motto of the Academy, "*Una fides altare commune*," just above which there was a black mural tablet with the inscription in letters of gold, "This Hall, the Gift of Abram Dubois, M.D., Generous Benefactor of the New York Academy of Medicine, was erected A.D. 1879."

Dr. Purple, as chairman of the Building Committee, had suggested the stained glass medallion of the Seal of the Academy, and at a meeting of the Trustees he had been permitted to provide it "at his own expense"!

During the next month the Dermatological Society presented its collection of books on its specialty to the Library. Mrs. John Jacob Astor, through Dr. Barker, gave two hundred dollars for books, and "the president announced and showed $25.00 in gold" from a friend of Dr. Eliot for the same purpose.

The Academy raised the initiation fee from five to twenty dollars, "to those who applied for admission after the first meeting in January." There were an unusually large number of candidates recommended for election, or announced as "before the Committee" before the deadline was reached.

The Anniversary Address of Dr. L. M. Yale, "The Academy as an Educator," was read by Dr. Castle, Dr. Yale being ill.

Another very important action occurred at the close of the year. The Medical Library and Journal Association of New York had been founded in December, 1864, "to provide immediate access to all current medical literature in the department of medical journals and monographs," so the *Medical Register* tells us. It had purchased 1,200 volumes from the library of the late Dr. G. T. Elliot. During the winter regular Friday evening "re-unions" were held, at which digests of all new and important matter in the journals were presented and discussed. The Association subscribed to seventy domestic and foreign journals and allowed duplicate copies to be taken out. Its annual dues were $10, to medical students $5. It had been assigned rooms on the third floor of the Academy soon after its opening, but as has been indicated, things did not run very smoothly.

The Association turned over all of its property to the Academy on the first of January, 1880. All members of the Association were to become Fellows of the Academy, if eligible, without paying an initiation fee, and the Academy was to start, as soon as practicable, a circulating department of medical journals, similar to that of the Association. This was a sensible, practical arrangement and was of great value to both organizations.

Not long after Dr. Barker's reference, in January, 1880, to the glass "loving cup," the Academy received a check for $200 for its Library from "a lady whose earnestness in every good word and work, and whose interest in and sympathy with, all the benevolent labors of our profession is universally known and acknowledged in the city." To do better justice in its reading, he asked Dr. Thomas to read the following letter:

Dear Doctor Barker:

I beg your acceptance, as President of the New York Academy of Medicine, of the accompanying cup, which if you will oblige me by using as a "*Loving Cup*" on the occasion of your next anniversary meeting, will owe all of its grace to words spoken by yourself in the early autumn. It comes to you as a messenger of a true sympathy in the purposes of the Society and it is engraved with words that I believe touch equally your *ideals* for its work and your *personal* feelings toward all of your associates; and I shall feel a sincere gratification if its occasional use —in agreement with such kindly sentiments—may procure a moment's pleasure to those whose days hold necessarily so large a measure of care and sacrifice.

Always, my dear Doctor, with faithful regard,

Your friend

Augusta Astor

Dr. Barker said the Cup had been designed by Mrs. Astor herself, and continued: "Its surface is ornamented by the acacia, symbol of friendship and love. On the front is the seal of the Academy, its

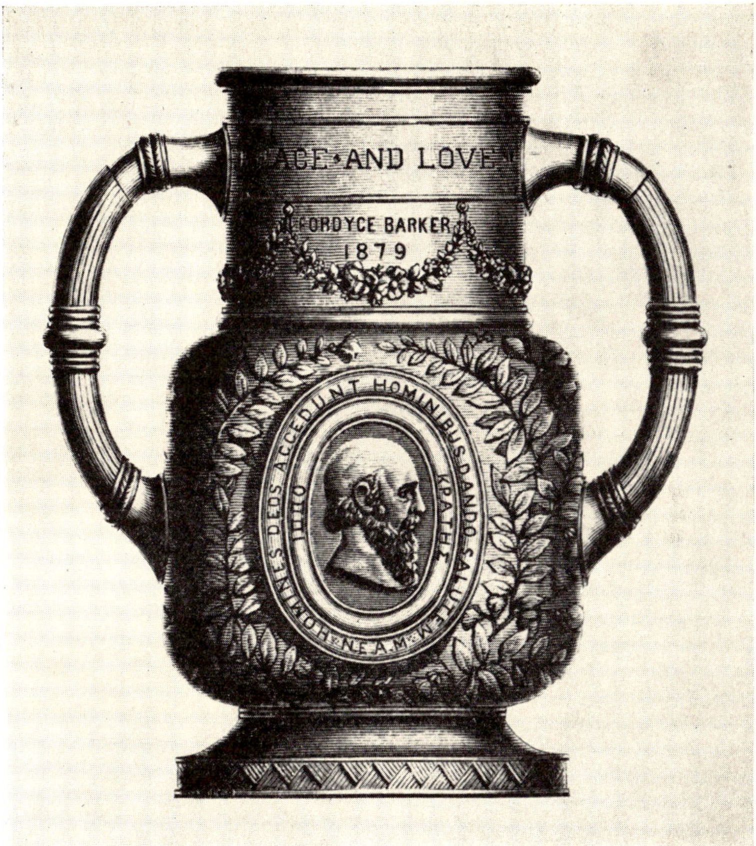
AND LOVE
FORDYCE BARKER
1879
HOMINES DEOS ACCEDUNT HOMINIBUS DANDO SALUTEM
N.E.A.M.

LOVING CUP PRESENTED BY MRS. JOHN JACOB ASTOR

motto, and the head of Hippocrates. Above is the name of the President and the date of his election, with spaces left for the names of his successors, while on its upper part is engraved a sentiment in which I am sure that all of us will most heartily sympathize. When we adjourn, I shall ask you to make use of this 'Loving Cup' in the room below. It has already been consecrated by the lips of woman, the aroma of which let us hope will ever remain to perpetuate the beautiful sentiment engraved upon it. 'May peace and love be multiplied unto us.' "

Dr. Sayre and Dr. Thomas, in proposing and seconding the thanks of the Academy, spoke at length and with much feeling, emphasizing that the gift marked a new era in New York—one of interest in the profession by the wealthy; "it is an olive branch held out to us by an appreciative public and it comes to us through the hand of a noble woman . . . Let us hope that it will prove an earnest of the future . . ."

"The Academy adjourned to partake of the Loving Cup."

So reported the *Medical Record*, and it added, editorially: "The sentiment engraved upon the cup is most appropriate, and, we trust, will find a response not only in the heart of every Fellow of the Academy, but in that of every member of the profession throughout the country. If all medical communities could lift the 'loving cup' above the little prejudices and jealousies of professional competition, in how much clearer atmosphere the usual pledges could be offered, and how often would 'peace and love be multiplied unto us!' "

Later Mrs. Astor contributed $500 for the benefit of the circulating and journal departments of the library to be expended in 1881 "at the discretion of the President, Dr. Barker."

It was voted to omit the first June meeting, the A.M.A. being in session in New York at that time, and that the use of the building ("when not otherwise occupied") and the Library be tendered to the delegates. The Hall and supper room were granted to Drs. Barker and Thomas for use in "receiving" members of the A.M.A.

In December, Dr. Barker sent to each Fellow copies of a printed circular letter appealing for funds and asking that the recipient distribute the copies among his clientele. The letter, which occupied three large pages, emphasized the importance of the Library, explained what the profession had done to maintain it, and asked for a contribution of at least $100 to expand its usefulness. Dr. Barker also enclosed a copy of a personal letter sent to possible contributors and suggested that each Fellow send out a letter "in similar spirit and tone, although it will doubtless be expressed much more felicitously."

The Constitution and By Laws were amended. Duplicate copies of books, pamphlets and periodicals, including periodicals of the current year (except the last number) could be taken out. Compounding of dues, after having been paid for five years, was established, at various amounts, according to age, from $150 at thirty years of age to $65 at seventy.

Great care was being exercised in finances. The building committee had removed the bathtub on the third floor, and put up more shelves. They sold the old tub and some old doors, and the Academy netted $12.07 on the transaction. At the end of the year there was $98.28 in the treasury.

During these two years the scientific sessions were very active. Seventeen papers were read in 1879 and twenty-two in 1880. They were all interesting and profitable papers. Dr. Barker was taking an interested part, and presided at every meeting but one. The library had increased tremendously; it now had 17,000 volumes exclusive of pamphlets. The acquisition of the Medical Journal Association Library had been partly responsible for this, and Dr. Bumstead had left the Library his books, "the most complete and valuable collection of works and writing on syphilography . . . to be found in any public medical library in the world." His portrait was presented to the Academy by a group of his friends.

The Academy had taken part in numerous public health matters. Dr. Nachtel, by invitation, read a paper on the night medical service in Paris, and a special committee reported that with some modifications it would be beneficial for New York. They recommended the matter be referred to the Board of Health. A bill was passed in the Legislature establishing such a service in New York.

The Academy also, with the County and State Societies, the New York Medical and Surgical, New York Pathological, the Albany and Elmira Academies of Medicine, the Rochester and Buffalo Medical Societies and the Brooklyn Anatomical and Surgical Society, presented a strong joint memorial to the Legislature protesting against a bill to prevent vivisection.

A committee of three, appointed to attend the convention to amend the *Pharmacopoea* in 1880, reported back that after a long session a committee has been appointed with definite instructions as to how to make the *Pharmacopoea* a useful compendium.

1881–1882

Dr. Barker was reelected President without opposition. His inaugural address was *discussed*—an unusual event—by ex-Presidents Parker, Flint, and Purple, and by two visitors from Utica and California. He had urged greater activity in public health matters, and his address was ordered sent to Senator William Astor "indicating to him that the sentiments therein are fully endorsed by the Academy."

The President "invited the Academy and its guests to the dining hall where they were bountifully entertained." The postcard notice of the meeting contains a notice that after adjournment all were invited to partake in the Loving Cup. The *World* describes the incident: "The cup bearer appeared before the President's chair holding the large embossed silver cup before him in both hands, and followed by the President and ex-Presidents and the Fellows of the Academy in double file, led the way to the hall below, where the cup was sent around, and luncheon was eaten."

The present whereabouts of the cup is a mystery. Its history is given and it is shown in an illustrated "feature" article in the New York *Herald Tribune* in 1925 (see p. 252). Perhaps it was lost in moving to 103d Street. No trace of it can be found.

One of the first things the Academy did in 1881 was to pass resolutions on the filthy condition of the streets. The meeting was called to discuss pneumonia, and Dr. Loomis, after speaking of its unusual severity and mortality that year, proposed the following which were passed:

WHEREAS, It is our opinion that the uncleanly condition of the streets of this city is an efficient factor in increasing the malignity of many diseases, and thus contributes to the present alarming death rate,

Resolved, That, acting under a deep sense of our responsibility as members of a profession whose chief duty it is to check the development of disease, we earnestly warn the public against the danger of allowing this state of things to continue.

Resolved, That we are heartily in accord with the call for a citizens' meeting, to be held at Cooper Union, Friday evening, March 18th, to demand relief from the Legislature.

A medical mass meeting was held at Chickering Hall on the 13th of March. Drs. Willard Parker, Barker, W. H. Draper, and Loomis spoke, and long—very long—resolutions offered by Dr. Roosa were adopted. The meeting at Cooper Union on the 18th was much influenced by this meeting and by the resolutions of the Academy which were presented by Dr. Loomis.

In May, Dr. Barker showed the Academy a sheaf of checks from twelve *lay* individuals totaling $1,250 to be used in paying off the mortgage. At the same meeting it was voted that "the congratulations of the New York Academy of Medicine be transmitted to T. Spencer Wells, Esq., foreign associate of the Academy, for his remarkable and unprecedented achievement of 1,000 operations of ovariotomy, by which the lives of 769 women have been saved."

In the fall much time was occupied by Dr. J. G. Adams reporting on the International Medical Congress in London. It was a full meeting and Drs. Déclat of Paris, Meyer of Copenhagen, Gelbke of Dresden, Major Gardner, U.S.A., Didama of Syracuse, Sabal of Florida, Newell of New Brunswick, N.J., Shine of St. Augustine, Cushing of San Francisco, and Mussey of Cincinnati were introduced and invited to sit on the platform. It must have been rather crowded. The Academy's meetings were attracting visitors from other cities, and Dr. Barker's reputation was helpful to that end.

That Dr. Marion Sims was to speak on abdominal surgery was responsible for the attendance at this meeting.

The question of reporters of secular papers being present at Stated Meetings had been again referred to the Council, which reported that the matter had been decided (adversely) January 16, 1861, and that regulations then adopted were still in force.

Mr. J. S. Brownne, Assistant Librarian at the Astor Library, was appointed Assistant Librarian at the Academy in January, 1880. A number of candidates were seen and their ability tested by, among other things, verbal translations of German and French literature. Mr. Brownne was not in residence at first, but in 1881 the rooms on the top floor were put in order and he moved in. He was in residence until 1925.

In 1880 and in the previous year there was a great deal of difficulty with the janitor. One was discharged and another appointed only to be discharged promptly. The Trustees now arranged with Mr. Brownne to take general charge of the building, and a man was hired to keep it clean for $25 a month and board ($3.00); he was to board with Mr. Brownne.

Dr. Barker's fourth year was a busy one. In January he announced that next meeting's paper would be of special interest to the public, and asked someone to move suspension of the regulation, so that reporters of the secular press might be present. The regulation was suspended. Mr. Charles F. Wingate, Consulting Sanitary Engineer, spoke on "Practical Points in Plumbing; Knowledge Necessary for Physicians for the Protection of Their Patients." The paper was discussed by Professor Doremus, who demonstrated the facility with which air would pass through a brick wall and common illuminating gas through brownstone, and also demonstrated the passage of hydrogen gas through porous earthenware and other porous substances, without pressure, and of ammonia against the pressure of a 30-inch column of mercury. He also showed the methods of decomposing some of the poisonous gases.

The Academy then listened to a communication and voted its

warm sympathy "with the efforts of the State Charities Aid Association to instruct all classes of society in giving intelligent aid to the injured before the arrival of the surgeon or physician, and heartily commends the movement both to the profession and the public."

The matter of plumbing was brought up at a later meeting, and after more demonstrations by Professor Doremus, the Academy went on record as opposing, with the Sanitary Reform Association, any modification of the recent law requiring registration of plumbers, which would modify its force.

In March the delegates to the State Medical Society reported that their credentials were refused because the Academy had not paid its dues for two years; they therefore had to pay $50 to be received!

Then Dr. Adams described, in some detail, the action of the State Society in discarding the old Code of Ethics of 1823, for which it had substituted a short, simple one, but not without long and earnest discussion and protest. This was the beginning of a twenty-year struggle, which split the profession into two camps. Action was deferred until the next meeting, and then unanimously "indefinitely postponed."

The Council proposed that Fellows in arrears forfeit the right to take out books from the Library. This was referred to the Library Committee for an opinion, which opposed the idea, on the ground that the Library was made a means of discipline. It suggested those in arrears be "suspended from the privileges of the Academy," but this was not adopted. At a third meeting the subject was again discussed and it was voted that Fellows in arrears be deprived of the right to take books from the Library.

The years had been very active professionally. Dr. Barker did a fine job getting papers read. Nineteen papers were offered in 1881, and twenty-one in 1882. Most of them were excellent, and some were of unusual interest and value. Drs. S. W. Gross of Philadelphia, and H. J. Bigelow of Boston were among the contributors.

The Library was increasing rapidly and was obliged several times to ask for more shelving. Funds were inadequate, and a special appeal was made for contributions to bind pamphlets and books sorely needing it, and to purchase books. Considerable money was donated for these special purposes, including a contribution of $100 from the Medical Society of the Northwestern Dispensary, from their "surplus." Dr. Weir had contributed $250 to the Library Fund and Dr. Wiener had collected $125 for binding. Dr. E. L. Beadle, a Founder, left his library and $5,000 to the Academy. Mr. Brownne, accompanied by the janitor, was sent to Poughkeepsie to pack and ship the books. He was allowed $30 for necessary expenses.

At the end of 1882 the only unfortunate thing was the state of the Treasury. In October bills of $200 were outstanding with $125 in the Treasury to pay them. The Academy had a strange system of finances. The Treasurer of the Academy (elected) paid for certain running expenses, and the Treasurer of the Trustees (appointed by them) paid other bills chargeable to the permanent funds. So when one Treasurer got into difficulties, the other was authorized to lend him such amounts as were available. On this occasion the Treasurer of the Trustees was authorized to loan the Treasurer of the Academy $150. The Academy paid off $2,000 of its mortgage, and the Trustees had $58.40 in the bank.

1883–1884

Dr. Barker read his third inaugural address in February, and painted a very rosy picture of progress and the future. He emphasized the growth of the Library, which now contained over 19,000 volumes, and from five to six thousand pamphlets. The scientific work had been very creditable: "We have rarely been compelled to listen to platitudes or crude statements of facts already well known to every intelligent and educated man. I can say that we have never been compelled to listen to the flippant loquacity of garrulous pretensions and assumptions." Many papers were declined, because the program was already completely full. Dr. Barker urged the younger men to take greater part in the discussion: "It is from them that I get the most useful knowledge and most valuable suggestions."

He emphasized the financial difficulties which prevented the Library from being kept in proper state. Means must somehow be provided for binding pamphlets and keeping bound volumes in repair.

After the address and remarks by ex-President Post, ex-Vice President Detmold, F. Seymour Haden of London (better known as an etcher than a surgeon), and Vice President Weir, Dr. W. M. Carpenter's resolution was unanimously adopted:

> WHEREAS, To those of us who have been accustomed to attend the meetings of this organization, the concise and comprehensive résumé of the history and present condition of the New York Academy of Medicine, to which we have listened, has passed before us like a pleasing and edifying panorama, Be it
>
> *Resolved*, That we hereby express our hearty appreciation of the fidelity and untiring industry of our president for the welfare of this institution.
>
> *Resolved*, That we are ever ready to respond to his call, and indulge the hope that whatever we have received from our most worthy founders, whether it be physical or scientific, constructed of brick and stone, we shall be able to transmit constructed of solid marble.

The Academy then adjourned to partake of the Loving Cup.

Although things started so harmoniously, trouble was brewing, and Dr. J. G. Adams, the seventy-five year old Corresponding Secretary lit the fire by reporting in detail that part of the meeting of the State Society which dealt with the Code controversy. Attempts were made to repeal the new Code (which had been adopted by a vote of 52 to 18 for the profession of the whole state), to re-adopt the old Code, or appoint a new committee to review it and report the next year, final action to be taken in 1885. All were laid over till 1884, after four hours of discussion.

Dr. Adams had recorded with the State Society his protest: "As a delegate from the New York Academy of Medicine, I beg leave to record my protest against the recent action of the Society of the State of New York in regard to the Code of Ethics, and I charge that the Society by its action in this matter has assumed an attitude and adopted a policy in direct and open hostility to the honor as well as the best interests of the medical profession."

The Stated Meeting adjourned without electing delegates to the A.M.A., it "being deemed inexpedient for the present." The A.M.A., since the action of the previous year, required delegates, before being recognized, to sign a statement in support of the old Code. The discussion, pro and con, occupied much space in the medical press.

A Committee on Ways and Means to devise plans for reducing the expenses of the Academy and raising means to meet them were elected: Drs. Austin Flint, J. G. Adams, E. Herrick, W. F. Cushman, and Willard Parker, Jr. Dr. Barker had declined to serve.

In April real trouble started. Dr. Austin Flint, Jr., offered the following:

WHEREAS, The New York Academy of Medicine has adopted in its By Laws as its standard of medical ethics the Code of Ethics of the American Medical Association, and

WHEREAS, Each newly elected Fellow of the Academy is required to sign its Constitution and By Laws, Be it

Resolved, That the Committee on Admissions be, and is hereby instructed to report to the Academy for election as Resident Fellow no physician who is known to the Committee to be in opposition to the Code of Ethics of the Academy and who as a consequence cannot consistently sign the By Laws of the Academy.

Resolved, That these instructions to the Committee on Admissions be continued in force until the American Medical Association shall have modified or repealed its Code of Ethics and such modification or repeal shall have been adopted by the Academy, or until the Academy shall have modified or repealed its By Laws referring to Medical Ethics.

Remarks were made by Drs. Agnew and Roosa, advocates of the new Code, and Dr. Purple, an "old Code-er" and others. The motion to lay the resolutions on the table was lost. After more discussion the resolutions were then adopted, 57 to 26.

Dr. Flint then offered the following, which was also adopted: "That the Academy hereby disavows any sympathy to the action of the State Medical Society, which has put the profession of the

State, through its State and County Societies, in an attitude of opposition to the medical profession of the rest of the United States."

At the suggestion of the President, it was moved that the Academy adjourn till the first Thursday in October; the motion was lost. Dr. Barker then announced that in consequence of the vote, at the close of this session, he would resign the office of the President, as he felt he could no longer perform the duties of the office with advantage to the Academy or satisfaction to himself.

Resignations were then offered by Drs. C. R. Agnew, W. F. Cushman, Treasurer, R. F. Weir, Vice President, and St. John Roosa. No action was taken.

It was then voted, as had been suggested by the President, that the By Laws be suspended and the Academy adjourn till the first Thursday in October, after which the President withdrew his proposed resignation.

The minutes only give the motions and votes, nothing about what was said in discussion. But a stenographic report printed by the *Medical Record* showed very discreditable action. It was without question—and without denial either—a packed meeting, under the leadership of Dr. Flint, Jr., assisted by Dr. Gouley. Very bitter remarks were made, and were answered as bitterly. It is not necessary to go into details.

The *Medical Record* commented editorially:

The proceedings at the Academy of Medicine on Thursday evening of last week were of a character to bring the blush to the cheek of every honorable member of the profession, whatever opinion he may hold concerning the Code or the question that was before the meeting.

Certain resolutions, designed to commit the Academy to a decision in a matter concerning which its members hold widely differing views, and which is seeking its legitimate solution elsewhere, were prepared in secret, brought without notice before a regular meeting, secretly packed with partisan supporters, and rushed without debate to a hasty adoption. Members who asked only for time to discuss the question and for notice to other members of the question to be discussed were received with hisses and the protests with jeers.

The trick, worthy of a machine politician, carried with the manners of a ward primary in a society one of whose declared objects is "the advancement of the character and honor of the profession"!

And then . . . a motion was made to reconsider, and then another to lay this one on the table, this being a parliamentary device to dispose finally of a motion. As if any final parliamentary disposal of a *motion* could prevent reconsideration of a *subject.* Such a move might avail to delay where long preliminary proceedings were necessary before a motion could be brought to a vote, but in such a case as this it would be gross flattery to call it even puerile. It served, however, to bring out the two following remarks, as reported elsewhere:

Dr. Agnew asked: "Then the object is to throttle this Academy?"

"Undoubtedly it is," said Dr. Flint, Jr.

The members of the Academy may well cry "Pause," and hesitate to sanction such methods—to follow such leadership. And we believe there are many, even among those who are heartily in support of the old Code, who will not allow their honorable reputation to be smirched by a tacit acceptance of the acts to which we have referred.

But a respite of over five months had been secured, during which something might be done. Dr. Barker sent out this letter to every member of the Academy:

Dear Doctor:

I assume that every Fellow of the New York Academy of Medicine must regard it as a most unfortunate event that anything should occur to interrupt its fraternal harmony, its useful work, and its progressive growth. While we cannot shut our eyes to the fact that this is the present condition of the Academy, it would be both useless and unwise to discuss the causes which have brought about this state of things, because, from their nature, they involve questions on which the most able, the most loyal, and the most conscientious men in the Profession honestly differ. Let us accept this fact as inevitable, and that the Academy can do nothing which will effectively advance the interests of the Profession by way of discussions, which irritate, but do not change convictions, or by arbitrary regulations, secured by shrewd tactics, but which carry no moral force.

The Academy of Medicine is not fulfilling its mission when it is engaged in warm discussions of questions of casuistry, in polemical controversies, or in medical politics.

The *Ephemeris* of Dr. Squibb quotes with approval an editorial from the *Boston Medical and Surgical Journal*, which contains the following sentence: "The lesson also is so obvious that he who runs may read, that the more our Societies confine themselves to their proper field—the joint cultivation of medical science and good fellowship—and the less they meddle with medical politics, the better will it be for their own future and the common good of the Profession." [Dr. Squibb was one of the most active supporters of the old Code and the *Ephemeris*, his own paper, was full of articles supporting it.]

It seems to me that the truth of the above sentiment has been unfortunately, but clearly, demonstrated by our Academy of Medicine.

The question which we have now to meet is: What measures can be taken to secure for the Academy a return of its prosperity? by which I mean a restoration of its fraternal harmony and good fellowship; a renewal of its active scientific work; an increase of its funds for the growth of its library and the adequate support of its journal department.

Since our last meeting this question must have occupied the minds of all our Fellows, who appreciate the importance of the Academy, which should represent the highest scientific work of the Profession of this city. All must feel that the character of the Profession and the grade of individual reputation is deeply involved in a wise settlement of this question.

I trust that no one will suspect me of a wish to force my individual views upon the Academy, but that, in consideration of the experience which I have had in its affairs, each will understand the spirit in which I venture to offer a few suggestions to be discussed, amended or improved at our first meeting in October. I do not feel it necessary to apologize for expressing the hope and the belief that every Fellow of the Academy who feels a proper sense of his personal responsibility and what he owes to the Profession and the public, will be present, and contribute by his voice or his vote to a satisfactory adjustment of our present difficulties.

It must be obvious to all, that to attain this end we must make a new departure on certain questions, to which it is unnecessary to refer more definitely. There is an "irrepressible conflict" of views and opinions which cannot be settled by parliamentary tactics or a majority of votes but must continue until in the progress of time the moral sentiment of the Profession is crystallized in a public opinion which will have the force of law. No possible good can come from profitless and irritating discussions of these questions in the Academy of Medicine. It therefore

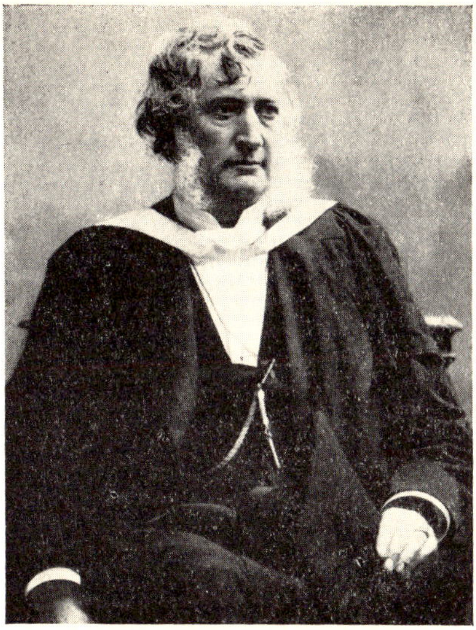

B. FORDYCE BARKER, 1818–1891
Seventeenth President, 1879–1884

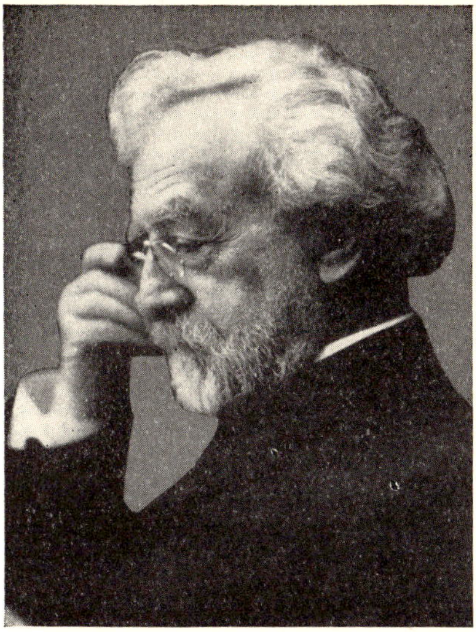

ABRAHAM JACOBI, 1830–1919
Eighteenth President, 1885–1888

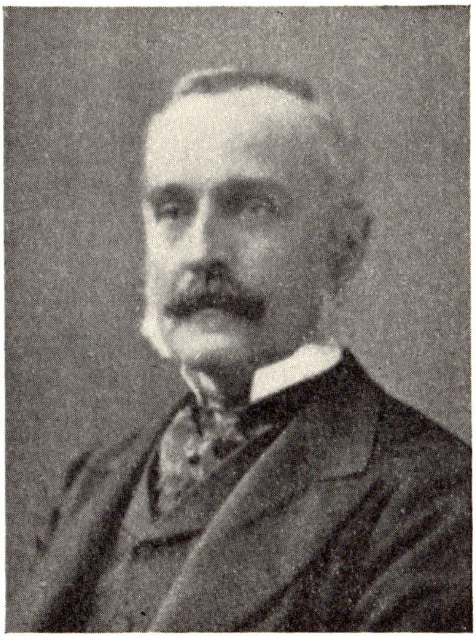

CORNELIUS R. AGNEW, 1830–1888
Trustee, 1884–1888

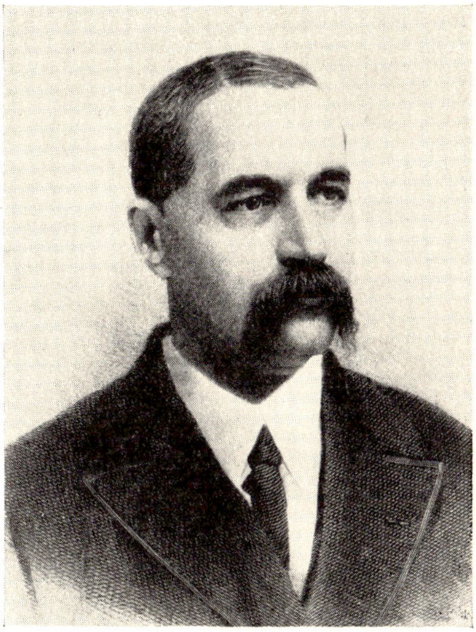

ALFRED L. LOOMIS, 1831–1895
Nineteenth President, 1889–1892

seems to me of vital importance that now, in making a new departure, everything in relation to them should be buried in the past and forgotten. No unhappy differences can be settled, no principle or cause can be advanced, no society or individual can be benefited by keeping up a galling wakefulness and feeding the living ulcer of a corroding memory of the past. The anodyne draught of oblivion is the first specific remedy for healing such ills as those under which the Academy is now suffering.

The next point to be secured is by such a change in our organic laws as to make it impossible that trouble and danger can ever occur again in the Academy.

At our first meeting in October, certain amendments to the Constitution and By-Laws will be proposed for discussion, and at the following meeting they will be submitted to the vote of the Academy.

Every change proposed has been the result of a most careful study of the subject, and has a distinct purpose which will be obvious to all.

I think that it will be apparent that the whole intent of the proposed amendments is to make the Academy of Medicine a purely scientific society, independent of all other organizations; to place its standard of ethics on a higher plane than before; and to prevent the possibility of any future troubles by the introduction of matters foreign to its advanced objects.

Respectfully submitting the above suggestions to your candid consideration,

I remain

Very sincerely yours

Fordyce Barker

As a result of this letter, the other side issued the following statement:

Dear Doctor:

The Council of the Organization for Upholding the National Code of Medical Ethics in the State of New York, begs to call your attention to a circular recently issued in which are proposed certain amendments to the constitution and by-laws of the New York Academy of Medicine. The Council cannot but regret the issuing of this circular as a covert movement, under a plea for harmony, in behalf of the organized effort in opposition to the National Code of Ethics. The proposed amendments, were they adopted, would eliminate from the constitution and by-laws everything relating to ethics, and surrender the Academy to those who advocate the abolition of all ethical codes. The Academy would thereby be deprived of the right to representation in the American Medical Association, and of affiliation with other medical organizations out of the State of New York. It may be assumed that there is no disposition on the part of those who are for upholding the National Code of Ethics to raise any discussion respecting the Code in the Academy. The Code has never been made a subject of discussion in the Academy by any one in favor of upholding it, and there is no ground for the supposition that it ever will be, unless it becomes necessary in the way of defence. The resolutions presented and adopted at the last meeting of the Academy had for their object the prevention of any future discussion relating to the Code. Every true friend of the Academy is earnestly requested to attend its meetings in order to resist the introduction of discussions and controversies in relation to ethics, by simply maintaining, in their integrity, the time-honored constitution and bylaws of this institution, to which it owes its origin and prosperity.

(*Signed*) Abram Dubois, Austin Flint, Austin Flint, Jr., J. W. S. Gouley, John H. Hinton, Samuel T. Hubbard, Wm. T. Lusk, Samuel S. Purple, T. Gaillard Thomas, *Council.*

In the meantime steps had been taken to form State and County Medical *Associations*, in opposition to the State and County *Societies.* A statement signed by 277 physicians was printed and circulated: "We the undersigned, agree to form an association to uphold the National Code of Medical Ethics, and to resist any modification of this Code that does not emanate from the body in which it originated." Of the 277 signers, 155 were members of the Academy, including four ex-Presidents.

When the Academy met again in October, things were still in a very troubled state. Dr. Barker had submitted to the Council a series of amendments to the Constitution and By Laws. The Council did not approve of them, and advised their withdrawal. This Dr. Barker refused to do, and the Council then voted "that the Council after careful and meticulous consideration do not approve of the proposed amendments. . . ." This was reported to the Academy. In spite of this, Dr. Keyes moved their adoption, solely because it would eliminate all controversy over the Code and medical politics. Dr. Loomis seconded the motion on the same grounds.

After many attempts to postpone action, the Academy sat for two meetings as a Committee of the Whole and finally recommended the amendments be adopted. But they did not receive the necessary three-fourths vote. The President expressed his regrets at the Academy's action and then, after much acrimonious discussion, the vote of the previous April, which had caused all the trouble—requiring the Committee on Admissions to find out whether a candidate subscribed to the Code of Ethics before recommending him for Fellowship—was *rescinded.*

All through the controversy Dr. Flint, Jr., played the part of a skillful politician, but eventually lost.

At the next meeting Dr. Adams presented a protest on the last action on grounds of five rules of parliamentary procedure violated in the action. His protest was laid on the table.

The whole thing was a miserable, unfortunate affair, but it established, for all time, the Academy's position as an organization devoted to scientific matters, aloof from all standards of ethics, except as affecting its own organization. It was perhaps worth while.

In November the normal course of events was resumed, after six months of futile strife.

The Academy was in serious difficulties financially. A Committee of the Council was appointed to consult with a similar Committee of the Trustees as to ways and means of cutting expenses. It was decided to stop payment for special notices and postage for the Section meetings; to dismiss the "hall boy," as the Janitor and "Tommy" could answer the door; to exercise economy in use of gas; and to consider raising the tariff for meeting rooms, benevolent societies to be charged one half the usual rates. To meet the emergency, a temporary loan was made by members of the Council, and three Fellows loaned $500 to pay in advance for journals for the next year. The Academy then, for the first time, voted an assessment on each Fellow of $3.00.

As was inevitable, the papers were few this year. Eight were presented before the controversy and few thereafter.

Publication of *Transactions* was ordered resumed after an interval of seven years.

After the turmoil of the last year, things started peacefully again. Resolutions were passed approving the Society for Instruction in First Aid to the Injured (which was giving a series of lectures on the subject) and urging the acquisition of more land for parks in the city. The latter resolution was sent to the Governor.

Scientific papers were read with the utmost regularity, eighteen in all, and they were all creditable.

A committee was appointed to devise means of paying off the mortgage, now reduced to $7,000.

In June, Dr. Barker spoke feelingly of the deaths of Dr. Willard Parker and Dr. S. D. Gross of Philadelphia. He paid a fine tribute to them as physicians and citizens.

When the Academy reconvened in October, after presentation of a bust of Dr. J. Marion Sims, Dr. Agnew described a new local anaesthetic, hydrochloride of cocaine, and demonstrated its action on two subjects. He was unable to say whether it would work on tissues other than the conjunctiva.

At the last meeting in December, Dr. Barker, after the minutes had been read, turned the chair over to Dr. R. F. Weir, first Vice President, and the Academy heard the report of the Committee on Ethics on charges brought against a Fellow—Dr. Fordyce Barker. Attempts were made to go into executive session, in order to exclude the daily press, and avoid "washing its dirty linen in public." But it was urged that the side of the accusers already "in some mysterious way," perhaps not so mysterious after all, had found publication in some of the daily papers, and now *all the proceedings* should be open and above board.

The charge was that Dr. Barker had committed an "act which unfavorably affects the character of the medical profession" to wit:

1) He had signed, with his own hand, the signature book of the Academy, stating he was a graduate in medicine of Paris, 1844, whereas he was not a graduate of that date or any subsequent date;
2) that he signed the register in the County Clerk's Office in 1880, making the same statement;
3) that he had practiced in New York State in violation of the law

of 1880, because his statement of graduation from Paris was false;

4) that false statement rendered him liable to punishment for perjury.

The charges were signed by E. S. F. Arnold, Nathan Bozeman, *Austin Flint Jr., S. S. Purple*, C. S. Wood, and William Young.

Dr. Flint, Jr., who was the prime mover in this matter, had taken infinite pains to verify these charges; copies of the registration in the County Clerk's Office, with affidavit of its correctness; a statement from the office of the Minister of Public Education and from the Faculty of Medicine in Paris stating Dr. Barker's name was not on their lists and that there was no record of Dr. Barker's ever defending a thesis before the Faculty of Paris, a proceeding necessary to secure a degree.

Dr. Barker's defense was that he had been granted a diploma from Paris, dated 1844, though he did not take the final examinations or defend a thesis, being called home on account of the illness of Mrs. Barker's mother; he had informed Professor Orfila, Dean of the Faculty, of his return home; that in 1861, when in Paris, he had received through Dr. Trousseau, his diploma from the Minister of Public Instruction, in which office it had lain since it was signed in 1845.

He showed it, with other interesting documents to several medical friends on his return, but it was lost soon after when he moved. Drs. E. H. Davis and R. O. Doremus were two of those friends, and they wrote confirmation of everything Dr. Barker said, even the date when he showed them the diploma, by undeniable associated events, and both remembered Orfila's signature being attached to the diploma because they knew of his work.

The Committee on Ethics unanimously reported the charges unsustained, without foundation and absolutely untrue. The lay press tells us the report was "received with immense applause, and was accepted and adopted without a dissenting voice." The report stated that the entry after Dr. Barker's signature in the book of signers of the Constitution had been tampered with and the Academy voted it be investigated, employing handwriting experts if necessary.

Dr. J. C. Peters stated that the accusers had not complied with the By Laws, in not informing Dr. Barker of the charges, and thus providing for a *cour médicale.* He moved a vote of censure for the accusers, for failing to observe the rules of professional courtesy of the State Society.

Dr. Roosa moved, as an amendment, that they be asked to resign. Dr. Jacobi approved of the proposed censure, but was unwilling to vote for the resignations, which was practically expulsion. Dr. Pooley moved to amend, that they be expelled, which was vigorously supported by Dr. Henry. Dr. Dalton thought the Committee's report was just what the Academy wanted, and moved to table all resolutions. Dr. Barker was allowed to say he agreed with Dr. Dalton, was perfectly satisfied with the Academy's action, and that it would be injurious to go farther.

The motion and amendments were withdrawn, and the President, resuming the chair remarked, "Here endeth the second lesson. The Academy will now resume its scientific work, which has been continued harmoniously for thirteen months, until interrupted by this supreme effort to elevate the character of the medical profession."

Dr. Griswold, who was to read on "Electricity as a Cardiac and Respiratory Stimulant" evidently did not think this an opportune time, so he asked for postponement till a later date.

After voting to discuss the proposed bill to form a State Board of Examiners at the next meeting, the Academy adjourned. "An ovation to Dr. Barker followed, and he was overwhelmed with expressions of sympathy and congratulations. Dr. S. S. Purple sat very still in his seat."

This was the direct result of Dr. Barker's efforts to divorce the Academy from medical politics. The lay and medical press reported the proceedings in great detail and editorially, and the accusers were condemned in no measured terms. They felt it necessary to publish a full and detailed statement of the affair, with reproductions of all the documents submitted.

A "card" from Dr. Barker appeared subsequently in the *Medical Record* acknowledging the receipt of over 200 letters from members of the profession in New York and Brooklyn, and many letters and telegrams from other places.

The whole controversy had far-reaching effects. Dr. Purple was a broken man. He had worked hard for the Academy, but his loyalty to the Code overshadowed everything else. In January, 1885, a letter from Dr. G. M. Smith, asking him to contribute to the Library fund, brought this response:

36 West 22nd Street
New York January 9th 1885

My dear Doctor:

I have delayed answering your very cordial note of the 31st ult till now hoping to be able to bring my convictions of duty to a point in accord with your request. It is now nearly twenty years since a small number of the Original Fellows of the N.Y. Academy of Medicine made a decisive step which resulted in the Academy's present home. No substantial progress was made until the movers themselves subscribed liberally—yes, more than liberaly [sic], of their moderate means, in order to lead the movement on to success.

An arrangement was early entered into among the movers to leave bequests in perpetuity of the object. And a quiet and unobtrusive method was instituted to interest members of the profession not Fellows of the Academy in our object and purpose. With what result the development of the past speaks for itself.

Within the past two or three years an element of discord directed against the Constitution and by laws of the Academy, and which has been abbetted by a temporizing policy, has signally alienated the confidence of our best pecuniary friends—original Fellows and Benefactors, to that degree that at least Seventy thousand dollars have actually been withheld from the Academy, and thus the best work of Drs. Hubbard, Adams, myself, and others has been thwarted and brought to nought, and the healthy growth of the Library impeded.

I speak of these unfortunate results in feelings of warmth—but in all charity, and with the kindest of intentions.

In our labor to bring success to, and command respect for the Institution, Dr. Hubbard, Adams and myself made investments and purchases for the Academy which have never been made known nor presented to the financial department for payment—the amount of my own contributions of this kind is over six hundred dollars.

As the seed which has thus been sown may yet bear fruit—and as present circumstances do not encourage further investments I shall have to kindly decline your request.

My dear Doctor you are at liberty to show this letter to your confreres of the Committee and to say to them that I entertain no unkind feelings toward any one and in the words of a noble martyr to liberty and human progress, "With malice toward none and charity for all" I wait patiently for better and happier results.

Be pleased to Ever believe me Dear Doctor

Your friend truly

Samuel S. Purple

After the action in 1884, Dr. Dubois ceased to contribute to the Library. He had intended to leave a large sum to it in his will, but as a result of this action he changed his will and left it all to the New York Eye and Ear Infirmary. If Dr. Adams had intended to leave a legacy he also changed his mind. He died en route to England in 1884.

Dr. Purple is only heard of again in Academy affairs twice. In 1889 at the laying of the cornerstone of the new building, he and Dr. Barker were both on the platform, and again in 1897 at the Semi-Centennial, he made a short speech. He was then seventy-five years old.

Dr. Flint, Jr., resigned in 1885.

The elections for 1885 passed off quietly, and Dr. Jacobi was elected President. Almost everyone elected was a staunch supporter of Dr. Barker and his policies. When they voted, the names of candidates were written on the blackboard—thus saving the expense of printed ballots.

The Committee on Medical Education recommended it was inexpedient to take any action in regard to a State Board of Examiners. Dr. Sturgis thought otherwise, and moved that the Academy believed that the interest of the public and the medical profession would be served by the establishment of a State Board of Examiners, whose certificate after examination would be the sole license to practice medicine in New York State. Action was deferred til the next meeting, but the motion was eventually adopted.

In all the six years Dr. Barker failed to preside only eight times. Four of these absences were due to his being abroad to receive an honorary LL.D. from the University of Edinburgh, on its three hundredth anniversary in 1884.

Dr. Barker's amendments were very simple and entirely in accord with the recent actions of the Academy. They abolished the inactive Committee on Medical Education and the Committee on Ethics, giving its powers to the Council. It is strange in view of the position he had acquired that they were not passed. He was very much disappointed and told the Academy so. But Dr. Flint, Jr., had his following, and was able to postpone action. The amendments were adopted, however, in substance during the following year.

1885–1888

Abraham Jacobi

THE MEETING at which Dr. Barker retired and Dr. Jacobi became President was an occasion. On the platform sat Drs. Weir Mitchell and Theophilus Parvin of Philadelphia, John S. Billings of Washington, G. B. Shattuck and J. R. Chadwick of Boston, James Anderson and Alfred C. Post, ex-Presidents.

In his Valedictory Dr. Barker stated that in the six years 16,000 volumes had been added to the Library, four times as many papers were offered as could be found a place for, and many of those declined were valuable. The only reference to the discord of the last two years was this:

> The truth of history demands that the fact should be mentioned that, nearly two years ago, the Academy passed through the segment of a cyclone; but, like a good steamship driven over a sandbank near a lee shore, with its engines temporarily disabled, it escaped being hogged, its seams were not opened, its barnacles have been scraped off, its bottom has been cleaned, and it has since gone on its voyage with favoring winds and fine weather. All who are familiar with its past history, and who are unbiased by personal feeling or prejudice, must agree that the Academy has more nearly approached its avowed aims and its high purposes during the past year than in any former one since it was founded.

He called attention to the fact, however, that the Section on Obstetrics and Diseases of Women and Children was the only one that was functioning satisfactorily. Standing Committees had faithfully discharged their duties, except that of Medical Education which "had little to do, and it has done this and nothing more. It should be one of the most important committees of the Academy." He suggested the Regents of the State University might appoint this committee as a board of examiners for the city!

He summarized the needs of the Academy, for the future, as:

First. A large fire-proof building, with ample room for a library containing all the medical literature of the past and coming times, and including:

Second. A large hall for its meetings, and others for smaller societies and committees.

Third. A large room for a museum, illustrating physiological and pathological anthropology, and which should include a craniological series, a pathological series, and a series of sections and dissections illustrating topographical human anatomy, and a comparative anatomy series.

Fourth. An anthropometric laboratory, provided with the best means of measuring human bodies, the faculties, and everything cognate to these subjects, and which should include a set of psychometrical instruments and everything pertaining to the series.

Fifth. A lecture hall, connecting with the laboratory and fully equipped with apparatus for lectures and demonstrations of all kinds.

Sixth. It should also have a thoroughly educated and trained pathologist, who should, by means of an adequate salary paid by the Academy, be able to superintend all the scientific work and report on the specimens furnished to him; and also a first-class mechanic, skilled in brass and glass work; and a good practical photographer.

This is a broad scheme which will require a very large endowment, but it is my firm conviction that it only outlines the future of the Academy, even if it demands a million of dollars.

It certainly was a broad scheme!

Dr. Jacobi, in his inaugural, expressed his appreciation of Dr. Barker's services and his gratification that it was under his guidance that the Academy had triumphed over dangers and strifes such as he hoped would never occur again. He gave a most interesting account of the development of medicine in England, France, Germany, and America in recent years.

At its close, Dr. Chadwick presented a photograph of Oliver Wendell Holmes and read a letter from Holmes to Dr. Barker:

My Dear Dr. Barker:

You must allow me to join my best wishes to those of the friends who will surround you as you take leave of the office which you have filled so ably and happily.

I trust that you have not forgotten the day when you were with us at the opening of our Boston Medical Library. I know full well that we remember your presence, and how much it added to the pleasure of the occasion. Our Library Association, I hardly need tell you, has proved eminently successful—I want to say because you smiled upon its birth, but I dare not, for you have smiled upon a great many births, not every one of which, perhaps, has had the good fortune of the infant institution which you joined us in welcoming.

You may have learned some of our secrets during that visit, who knows? There are sparks of intelligence still left among us. At any rate, ever since you left Boston we have kept an eye upon you. As soon as it was learned that you had been spending some little time here, you were made President of the New York Academy of Medicine. As soon as you got back, for *some* reason, the Academy took a new start and has been flourishing ever since. All my informants agree about the fact, and they add that it is due to your own faithful administration and energetic efforts.

We of Boston congratulate our brethren of New York that they have had the great advantage of your services during these last eventful years. The gratitude of the medical profession will keep alive the memory of its benefactors. We must trust the future for its *vis a fronte,* but in the broadest and loftiest period of progress the leaders will look back to the days of up-hill work when you, our honored friend, lent all your vigor to that *vis a tergo* which they will feel pressing them forward to larger and higher achievements.

Pardon me for addressing this open letter to you. You can retire "to blush unseen" while some friend is reading it, if it is thought worthy of that honor.

Always faithfully yours,

Oliver Wendell Holmes

To Fordyce Barker, M.D.,
President of the New York Academy of Medicine

Dr. Abraham Jacobi, eighteenth President, was born in Hartum, Westphalia, of poor parents. He managed to go to the University and received his M.D. at Bonn in 1851. Because of his activities in the revolution in Germany in 1848, he was imprisoned for a year and a half at Cologne, convicted of *lèse majesté.* He was again imprisoned in 1853, but with the help of a sympathetic jailor made his escape and fled to America.

He had been the first full professor of pediatrics in this country, at the New York Medical College and for two years, starting in 1862, gave the first bedside clinics for his students. Always standing up for what he thought right, he sided with the new Code group and helped keep medical ethics disputes out of the Academy. He had written much, was a fine and fluent speaker, and had been very active in Academy meetings. He was fifty-five when elected president.

In April, Mrs. John Jacob Astor presented to the Academy, through Dr. T. M. Markoe, a fine portrait of Dr. Barker. Dr. Markoe spoke eloquently and strongly about Dr. Barker—his impartial, just and sympathetic handling of the bitter struggle over the Code, and his calm, unimpassioned, and complete refutation of the charges of deliberate falsification at the end of his presidency. After formally presenting the portrait to be added to the collection, he ended, ". . . as our children or grandchildren . . . ask who was this, and who was that, some white-haired relic of this present assembly may say, 'This is the portrait of one of our most eminent and our best beloved presidents, *Dr. Fordyce Barker.*' "

The *Medical Record* states: "The chaste, kind, expressive, and yet uncompromising language of the presentation address was listened to with that profound silence which comes only with deep, heartfelt interest in the welfare of a tried friend and brother, and which bursts into spontaneous applause when the spell is broken."

In April, Dr. Jacobi was asked by the Council to read the By Law in regard to publication of papers, and to announce the forthcoming appearance of the *Transactions.* He then delivered an address, prefacing his remarks with this statement: "When you elect a President you not only mean to confer a great honor upon him and give him great powers, but also grave responsibilities and urgent duties." He considered one of those duties was to remind the Fellows that membership imposed certain obligations "which no gentleman among us can possibly forego." He alluded to newspaper notoriety. "The rules of the Code of the American Medical Association forbid any form or manner of advertising through other than strictly professional channels. That it has not succeeded in creating gentlemen out of men who have nothing but a diploma, a shingle, a carriage, and plenty of self-assertion, we all know." He then went on to deplore the sensational articles regarding operations and other medical matters that were constantly appearing in the papers, many of them in spite of the operator, and urged Fellows to be very careful of their reputation *within* the profession. Feeling as he did, he claimed the privilege, as President of the Academy, of proclaiming his convictions, which he had felt all his life to be those of the American medical profession.

Dr. Jacobi throughout his Presidency spoke out, and told the Academy what he thought.

It was voted to omit the September meeting, and when the Academy convened in October, the President made a long report on the International Congress at Copenhagen, which he had attended. He explained the reason for forming the "International Committee for Collective Investigation of Disease" and defended it against its critics. He was Secretary of the American Committee and asked the Academy and the profession to give the International Congress their interested attention, referring to the hesitation of the Congress to meet next time in America.

After describing the action of the A.M.A. in interpreting the Code's restrictions as to consultations, Dr. Jacobi outlined the changes he thought should be made in the Constitution and set forth his plans for increasing the activities of the Sections. It was a long address, attentively received.

The President announced that the Academy was out of debt, the last of the mortgage having been paid off. He presented from Dr. S. W. Francis of Newport a thermometer used by Dr. J. W. Francis in 1830, when thermometers were new gadgets.

It was decided to appoint a committee to revise the Constitution, the committee to include the President, Recording Secretary, Chairmen of the Sections and others the President thought necessary.

The Academy unanimously passed resolutions urging that proposed reductions in the Health Department Budget be not made at the cost of services of important physicians long in its employ, which were essential to its efficiency.

The Anniversary Address, after a lapse of five years, was resumed. It was delivered by Dr. H. D. Noyes on "Pathfinding in Medicine."

The Academy wound up the year with $880.58 in the Treasury, and $647.12 in the Trustees' Treasury.

In January, 1886, the Constitution and By Laws were amended according to the recommendations of the committee previously appointed. The Academy now had only *one* object: "The promotion of the Science and Art of Medicine."

The Committees on Ethics and Medical Education were eliminated and the Council was required, on a written statement signed by a complainant and duly forwarded through the Recording Secretary, to take cognizance of any complaint against a Fellow. It might, after investigation, discuss the complaint, or transmit its findings thereon to the Academy for further action. All this had been recommended by Dr. Barker in amendments that failed to pass at the time. To these had been added: "The Academy may suspend or expel a Fellow for violation of its regulations or the commission of any act which unfavorably affects the character of the medical profession or the interests of the Academy."

The Library was ordered open from 10 A.M. to 10 P.M. The summer recess was lengthened to cover the whole months of July, August, and September, and the Sections were only required to furnish *one* paper *or* prepare *one* discussion for a stated meeting instead of doing *both twice* each year.

At the April meeting, biographical memoirs of three Fellows were read: on Dr. Vander Poel by Dr. Vander Veer, Dr. Post by Dr. Stephen Smith, and Dr. Flint by Dr. Jacobi. Dr. Vander Poel had been Health Officer of the Port, and an excellent one. He had played an important part in the Academy's early history. Dr. Post, former President, was a busy and devoted Fellow all his life. Resigning in 1885, he was made an Honorary Fellow, and continued his regular attendance to the end. In April, 1885, he described an original operation for ruptured perineum, and one month before his death had discussed a paper. He was eighty years old.

Of Dr. Jacobi's tribute to Dr. Flint, the *New York Medical Journal* said: "In the performance of this work he was most felicitous, as everybody knew would be the case; without in the slightest degree sacrificing strict justice in obedience to the behest *de mortuis nil nisi bonum,* he wove such a fabric of eulogy as has been offered in tribute to the memory of few men, whether in the medical profession or in more public callings."

Dr. Jacobi's first term of office was noted for the receipt of the first large money gift to the Academy, and he was responsible for it. Mrs. Anna Woerishoffer, in memory of her husband Mr. Charles F. Woerishoffer, gave $25,000 to be used for increasing its facilities for the diffusion of medical science. The two Woerishoffers were both promptly elected Benefactors.

The Academy also received $5,000 from the estate of Dr. E. L. Beadle, a Founder. A group of physicians and laymen, of whom Dr. Jacobi was one, donated $1,155 to establish the Ernst Krackowizer Prize Fund, the income to be awarded every three years for the best essay on a medical subject. There was always difficulty in securing an essay, and some years later, Dr. Jacobi, as the last surviving member of the group, authorized the Academy to devote its income to the Library, as the Ernst Krackowizer Library Fund. Dr. Krackowizer had been an active and valuable early member of the Academy. He, like Dr. Jacobi, had been driven out of Austria by the government.

The Council had decided to beautify the "Parlor" with a "handsome ornamental fireplace," and the William H. Jackson Company built it at a cost "with fittings" of $136 and then presented it to the Academy.

The Anniversary Oration was carefully prepared for. Fellows were requested to send to Mr. Brownne, the resident Librarian, the names of friends whom they wished to be present, and Mr. Brownne would mail out special cards of invitation.

Dr. Jacobi made an introductory address in which he stated the Academy's foundation was contemporary with the introduction of anaesthesia in America and the origin of Virchow's Cellular Pathology in Germany. The Academy had not only followed the steady progress and advances in medical knowledge but had contributed much to it. He mentioned with pride that this anniversary meeting was for the first time open to the public according to the By Laws, and he was much impressed by the response of the laity to the invitation.

Dr. W. H. Draper, an eloquent and finished speaker, delivered an interesting address. He analyzed what the problems before the profession were, owing to the discoveries of the last twenty-five years. It is of interest today as showing what was thought sixty years ago.

. . . It is not possible for me to consider the present aspect of the germ theory in its relation to the many diseases to which it has been applied. It is sufficient to remark that it is continually invading the domain of pathology in new and unexpected directions. Not only all septic processes, but even inflammation itself; not only eruptive fevers, including syphilis, but even malarial and rheumatic fevers; not only phthisis and pneumonia, but even common colds; not only diphtheria, but ulcerative endocarditis; not only leprosy, but even the malignant infectious tumors—all of these general and local affections have been more or less reasonably suspected of hiding the secret of their origin in a specific germ. Admitting that the microbe etiology of many diseases is as yet only a theory, it has surely given a new and definite aim to therapeutics, through which it has achieved in certain directions marvellous results. It has revolutionized the art of surgery by converting what were formerly regarded as most formidable operations into safe and simple procedures. It may be said to have conferred an almost dangerous facility upon certain surgical undertakings and to have tempted the modern surgeon to enter upon paths which the angelic prudence of his predecessors made them fear to tread. . . .

. . . To the sanitarian it is the revelation of a new gospel. It gives a pith to the principle of cleanliness, which commands a respect that has never been secured by its supposed contiguity to godliness. It has so formulated the protective measures against the spreading of infection in hospitals and private houses that it must in this way largely diminish the ravages of disease. But when we come to the object which the germ theory holds out to art, to antagonize the morbid processes which germs set up in the living body, either by destroying the germs or by neutralizing their effects we are met by what seem to be insuperable difficulties. . . .

There are two directions in which the study of germ diseases seems likely to affect their preventative treatment. The first is prophylaxis by inoculation with a virus modified by attenuation of the constitutional conditions which favor the growth of the various specific germs.

After the address the guests were invited to inspect the Library and the hall. We do not hear they were invited to partake of the Loving Cup.

At the annual election there were three candidates for President, Dr. Agnew having declined nomination. Dr. Jacobi was reelected for a second term.

The great event of the year was the receipt of the bequest of $70,000 from the estate of Celine B. Hosack, to be used for the erection of a new building for the Academy or an auditorium in such a building. The executor and residuary legatee had held this fund for nearly a year, as entitled to by the will, in order to collect the interest, so the Academy knew that it was coming and had appointed, to investigate "eligible sites," a committee consisting of Drs. Jacobi, G. A. Peters, and F. A. Castle.

The Hosack bequest was the result of Dr. Purple's former efforts, and it was probably this $70,000 which he said was "lost" in his letter to Dr. G. M. Smith, previously quoted. Dr. Jacobi may have been responsible for its being "found" again. Mrs. Hosack was promptly enrolled as a Benefactor. Later in the year Dr. Purple "on account of past services and donations" was also made a Benefactor, which was just.

Another bequest of $10,000 was made by the Hosack will to Roosevelt Hospital to establish an endowed bed, the occupant to be designated by the "President and Trustees for the time being" (of the Academy). The terms of this bequest were printed as a note in the Academy's publications for many years and appears in the Annual Reports to the present day.

With $70,000 available for a new building, the Academy empowered the Trustees and Council "to purchase a site or building or to erect a new building for the Academy when such a course shall be considered expedient." A committee of thirty was appointed and began its drive of eight long years for a suitable new home. The Trustees promptly established a "Building Fund."

Things ran very smoothly all through 1887, as they had in 1886. The Sections were accepting their responsibility of arranging discussions. In March, Dr. Gerster opened one on the "Proper Selection of Chloroform or Ether as an Anaesthetic." Dr. Jacobi spoke of this later as "a question the merits of which have often been curtly, if not correctly decided by a coroner and his jury, guided by accumulated ignorance."

At another Section discussion, on the "Practical Value of Present Methods of Treating the Upper Air Passages," three papers were read.

In May the "Treatment of Empyema in Children" was discussed in papers by Drs. Holt, Huber, and Abbe.

In June a particularly interesting and important discussion was held on "Intubation of the Larynx." Dr. Jacobi had announced this forthcoming discussion in order to secure a large participatory attendance, "in order to enlighten the profession of Europe, who do not take kindly to intubation." Dr. Francis Huber gave a summary of forty-seven cases. Dr. Joseph O'Dwyer, the originator of intubation, exhibited anatomical specimens showing the tube *in situ*, and a number of tubes, old and new, including two made of hard rubber, as to the value of which he was not yet prepared to give an opinion. Dr. O'Dwyer's collection, augmented by much additional material on the development of intubation and including a large photograph of Dr. O'Dwyer, is a permanent framed exhibit in the Academy.

Dr. Dillon Brown gave the statistics, and Dr. Northrup described the pathological anatomy of the respiratory tract in fatal cases of laryngeal diphtheria, after intubation. Dr. Hanks recounted a case where laryngotomy was required after intubation.

All through his Presidency Dr. Jacobi stimulated the development of the Sections. He was constantly prodding them. He said that good abstract reports of their meetings were not only interesting, but were required by the By Laws, and he desired the officers of the Sections to report personally.

Volume VI of the *Transactions*, dated 1890, lists all the papers read at the Stated and Section Meetings from January, 1886, to December, 1889. It is a most interesting and creditable series of papers.

At the Anniversary meeting in 1887, all business was omitted except the announcement of gifts and the addresses. Drs. J. S. Billings, "National Medical Library, Washington," Barker, C. C. Lee, Vice President, and Dr. W. H. Draper, the Orator of the previous year, were invited to sit on the platform.

"It being a public meeting to which the public had been invited by special invitation, many ladies and gentlemen were present on the occasion, in addition to numerous professional friends and Fellows of the Academy." At the request of the Council Dr. Jacobi discussed "the status of the medical profession, and the present condition and future requirements of the Academy, with an appeal to the general public for funds for a suitable, fire-proof building."

The Academy had 511 names on its roll. The Library Fund amounted to $10,000, but $100,000 was needed to provide the "intellectual food" required. Dr. Jacobi read a long circular about to be sent out by the Committee of Thirty.

Dr. A. H. Smith, the Orator, spoke on "The Family Physician in the Future." He emphasized among other things the great importance of at least an *annual physical examination* of children, with a *permanent* record of their development, illnesses, vaccinations, and so on. That was in 1887.

At the annual election, while the Tellers were counting the vote, the Academy was entertained by memorials of four former Fellows, Dr. Alonzo Clark, who played a large part in the Academy's early history, by Dr. Francis Delafield; Dr. T. R. Varick of whose activities in the Academy's history we know little, by Dr. J. L. Corning; Dr. Jared Linsly, one of New York's great medical men, by Dr.

S. T. Hubbard; and Dr. Middleton Goldsmith, of Rutland, who left his library to the Academy, by Dr. J. C. Peters.

The vote being announced, there was no election for the member of the Committee on Library or the Committee on Admissions. Another vote was taken, and during the count the Academy took a recess to partake of a collation, at the invitation of the President. At ten P.M. when it reconvened there was still no election for the Committee on Library, and another vote was taken, without further adjournment. This was the first time there had been such competition in a number of years.

In January, 1888, Dr. J. D. Bryant, Health Commissioner, read a paper on "How the Profession Could Aid the Board of Health" and at his request a committee of five, Drs. Agnew, Janeway, R. H. Derby, Stephen Smith, and Jacobi were appointed to look into the matter. In June the committee presented a report on the Quarantine Station, New York Harbor, which had been drawn up by Dr. Agnew, its chairman. "The President referred to the great interest Dr. Agnew had taken in the matter and the success of the Committee in obtaining from the Legislature an appropriation for the improvement of the New York Quarantine Station."

The *Medical Record* commented editorially most enthusiastically on this report:

We are informed . . . the supply of water is insufficient, and warm water is almost entirely wanting. For a population now there [at Quarantine] of more than 500 persons, there are only about four water-closets, each closet having three or four hoppers, some of which are not flushed at all! The cleansing and disinfecting plant is entirely inadequate, making it impossible either to cleanse the clothes or the persons of the quarantined, or to keep them clean. . . .

That it should be considered necessary to recommend a proper flushing-tank for the sewers, and that "no sewage should be allowed to pass into the bay without being subjected to chemical treatment" needs no comment upon the necessity for the inspections made. . . .

We doubt not that the voice of the committee will now be heard, that the public will be satisfied that a radical reform of the whole system is called for at once, and that the time for political dickering has passed.

Thus was begun the Academy's long struggle that resulted finally in the establishment of nation-wide Federal control of Quarantine.

In 1888 the Academy lost two of its most valued Fellows. Dr. C. R. Agnew, a Trustee since 1884, was a most devoted worker in its interests. He died of peritonitis following appendicitis. The meeting at which his death was announced passed suitable resolutions and adjourned in honor of his memory. Dr. T. G. Thomas later read a most appreciative memorial of him and his work. Dr. Agnew had been especially helpful in securing exemption from taxes, which were constantly being reimposed. It was practically by his efforts alone that those imposed in 1885, 1886, and 1887, still unpaid, were annulled and judgment was promptly served on the tax officers and Comptroller. Dr. Agnew was such a prominent figure in New York that even the Tax Department listened to him. (Legal Counsel advised the Academy to keep a copy of the judgment "in case of further attempts to levy taxes.") In the Quarantine Investigation also he had been the most active figure. On recommenedation of the Council, in May, Dr. Agnew was enrolled as a Benefactor "in consideration of his faithful and valuable services and numerous gifts of money and books to the Academy."

Dr. Wesley M. Carpenter, the second loss, had been the efficient Corresponding Secretary since 1886. He took part in many meetings, and left the Academy $5,000, the income of which was to pay for an annual lecture, the "Wesley M. Carpenter Lecture," to be published immediately after delivery.

The Academy amended the Constitution, making physicians resident in New York State within a radius of one hundred miles eligible for Fellowship. As proposed by the Council, membership was not limited to New York State but the Academy preferred to so limit it.

In June, 1888, Dr. Loomis reported $11,000 had been promised for the new site for the Academy, and urged every Fellow to contribute at once and then take the circulars to his friends and interest them, "when it was confidently predicted the amount required would be easily and quickly raised"! In October it was unanimously resolved ". . . it is now expedient to take active steps to purchase a site and erect a new building for the Academy" and the Council and Trustees were instructed to so do.

The Trustees had not been idle in this matter. They held many special meetings discussing possible sites, but could not seem to agree. Drs. Jacobi and Loomis were most insistent that something should be done at once. Sites investigated on 59th Street and Sixth Avenue were objected to as too noisy on account of the Elevated Railroad and two car lines. Fifty-seventh Street near Broadway was favorably considered, and many sites in the lower West Forties were also contemplated. Finally, in December, all agreed to a site on the north side of 43d Street, between Fifth and Sixth Avenues, but voted to keep the matter secret until the deal was consummated!

The Anniversary Meeting was again quite an event: "According to custom, the public had been invited to the meeting by special invitation, and in response a large audience of ladies and gentlemen, lay and professional, were present. The By Laws were suspended to omit all business. Ex-President Fordyce Barker and the Vice Presidents, Henry D. Noyes, William H. Draper, and Andrew H. Smith, occupied seats upon the platform."

Dr. Jacobi spoke most interestingly of this one meeting each year to which the public was invited, in order that the community at large might better understand the aims and objects of the Academy. He sketched the needs for such an organization, as instanced by legislation in regard to pauper insane, passed without consulting medical experience; the requirement that the *President of the Board of Health* of a city of one and a half million people must not be a medical man; the refusal to abolish the retaining of medical experts, not men with special knowledge, but employed by contestants all of which reminded us of past "semi-barbarism."

In introducing Dr. D. B. St. John Roosa, he stated: "Whatever he will say on his chosen subject . . . no one doubts two things, namely, that he knows exactly what he is going to say, and will exactly say what he knows or believes to be the truth, the whole truth, and nothing but the truth." Dr. Roosa spoke on "The Means of effecting the Unity of the Medical Profession."

Commenting on these annual addresses, the *Medical Record* stated: "The Academy ought to have better quarters, and to receive public guests in a less barren, white walled, inacoustic audience room. Distinguished laymen must find it hard to get *en rapport* with medicine while seeking sedentary comfort on a perforated board, dodging draughts, or sitting in a heated mixture of pulmonary exhalations and alleged atmospheric air." In 1879 the *Boston Medical and Surgical Journal* had lauded the acoustics and ventilation!

In December the By Laws were amended as recommended by the Council. Changes were made on the ever-present and ever-troublesome matter of Fellows delinquent in their dues. Handling of this had always been in the hands of the Trustees, who had authority to delay action as long as they pleased. The duty and authority were now transferred to the Council. After one year's delinquency it was required to notify the offending Fellows by mail, and within eight months thereafter to report all still delinquent to the Academy, which by a majority vote of those present could annul the Fellowship. The Council was also wisely given authority to "remit yearly the dues of any Fellow who has paid ten or more annual dues and is in physical or financial distress."

The time for opening the polls at elections was also changed from "after the reading of the minutes" to "at eight o'clock."

At the December meeting nominations for the next year being called for, Dr. Jacobi "as a Fellow" promptly nominated for President Dr. A. L. Loomis. Being himself renominated, he declined and the nominations were promptly closed. Since Dr. Loomis, the only candidate, was a Trustee and his election would create a vacancy, it was proposed "to save time and expense" to nominate a Trustee now to fill his place. But that was not considered proper procedure, and the motion was withdrawn.

At the annual meeting, while the vote was being cast and counted, the Treasurer reported a balance of $262.62. The total fluid receipts had been $6,397.42, of which $2,283.16 had been expended for general expenses and $3,581.90 for the Library. The Treasurer of the Trustees reported $109,269.86 in the "General" and "Building" funds.

The Library asked for $5,060 for the next year, emphasizing the deplorable condition of unbound books, but "in view of the limited available income" only $4,000 was recommended by the Council and so voted.

No papers were scheduled for this meeting and, the Tellers not being ready to report, Dr. Jacobi called for case reports. Only one was forthcoming, so he announced the next order of business, without recess, would be a collation in the parlor. After the collation, the inspectors announced 134 Fellows had voted; there was no election for Corresponding Secretary to replace Dr. Carpenter, or for delegate to the State Medical Society. The polls were reopened. This time only forty-seven votes were cast, and the elections were completed promptly.

At the second meeting in January, 1889, the Council recommended that the amended By Laws' requirement that non-Resident Fellows pay $3.00 dues be enforced only for those *elected* after the date of adoption. The Academy considered this recommendation out of order, and rejected it.

These four years were the most peaceful, active, and prosperous years in the Academy's history. The Council had to investigate only three complaints against Fellows. Two of these were on the ground of undue newspaper notoriety in connection with operations; in both cases the Council reported that the responsibility could not be laid on the accused Fellows. A third charge was for certifying to the value of a proprietary medicine, and the Council ruled the gentleman be informed his action "in commendation of the alleged remedy is objectionable."

The Library was enriched by $5,000 to form the Philippine Meyer-Ernst Jacobi fund, the interest thereof to be spent on new books.

Many autograph documents were presented, including a letter written by Virchow in 1856 and containing a biographical sketch of himself, and a manuscript account of "A Medical Inquiry into the Use of Cold Water in Malignant Fevers, Especially Yellow Fever," by Julien Bouvier, who practiced in New York and who had sent the account to Alexander Hamilton, Secretary of the Treasury.

A collection of 400 works on congenital malformations was presented by Dr. W. L. Estes of Bethlehem, Pennsylvania, and the library of the late Middleton Goldsmith, 1,200 volumes, was willed to the Academy. Several other small libraries were also received. In 1887 the Academy put a sign on the outside of its building announcing the Library was open to the public.

The Academy's art treasures were increased by a portrait in relief of Dr. Mott and oil portraits of Drs. Benjamin Rush, S. A. Purdy, a founder and early Recording Secretary, and T. A. McBride, a Fellow who died at the age of forty.

In addition to the influential report on the Quarantine, a very important report on infectious eye diseases in institutions was presented. A committee appointed to investigate made two very full reports. The Academy passed resolutions urging legislation to correct these conditions and memorialized the Legislature, in conjunction with several lay organizations, to pass a law regulating the methods of prevention; this was eventually passed. The Academy memorialized the Legislature in support of a bill for the better accommodation and care of pauper lunatics, and urged the Committee on Ways and Means of Congress and the New York Senators and Representatives, "in the cause of humanity" to remove all duties on medicines and all appliances used in the care of the sick.

Comparisons are odious, but there is no question that the Academy never had a more industrious, tactful, interested president than Dr. Jacobi. In all his four years he failed to preside at only two of seventy-three Stated Meetings. He attended Council and Trustees' meetings with great regularity. He was determined to build up the Section meetings, and read two papers himself before the Section on Medicine, and two at that of Materia Medica. He was particularly interested in the Section on Pediatrics, organized in 1888, read two papers before it and demonstrated cases twice.

He served on almost every committee of the Trustees, of which he was President by election. He settled many minor questions himself. The American Philosophical Society of Philadelphia wrote inviting the Academy to participate in an international convention to establish a universal scientific language, such as Volapuk. He replied

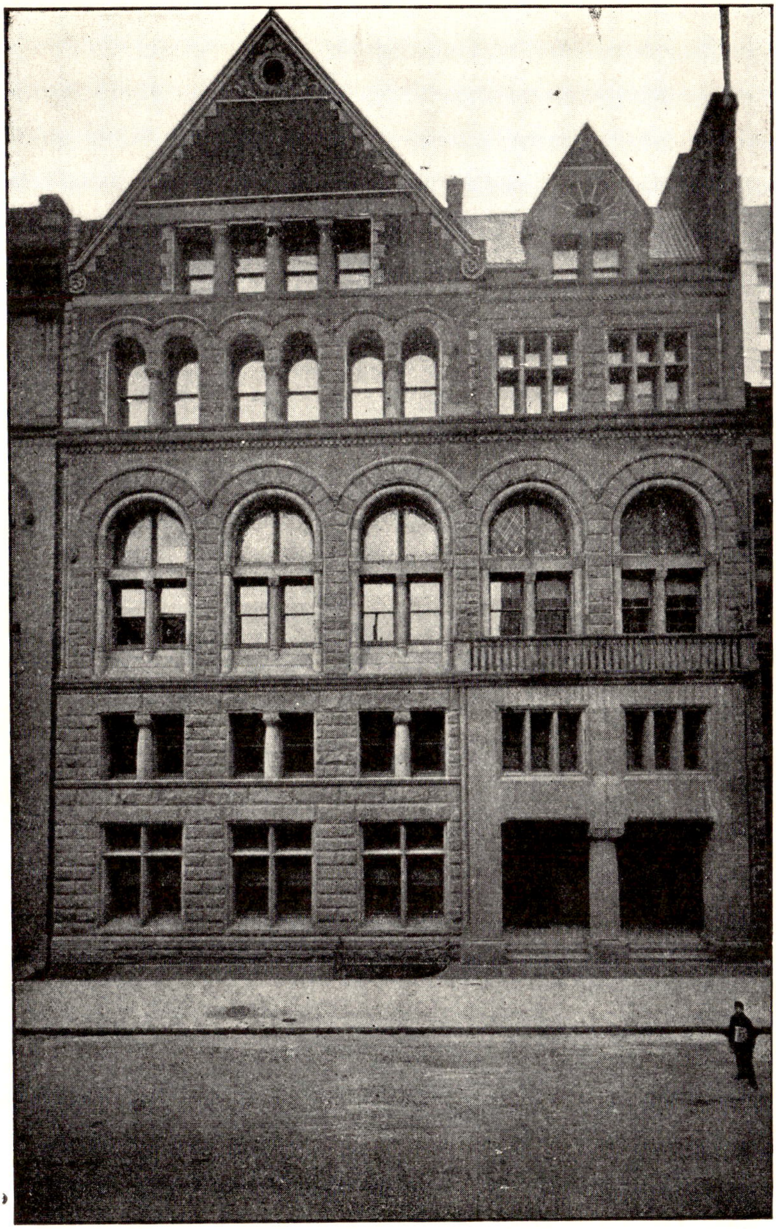

SECOND HOME OF THE ACADEMY, 17–21 WEST 43D STREET

Meetings Held Here from October 2, 1890, through November 16, 1926

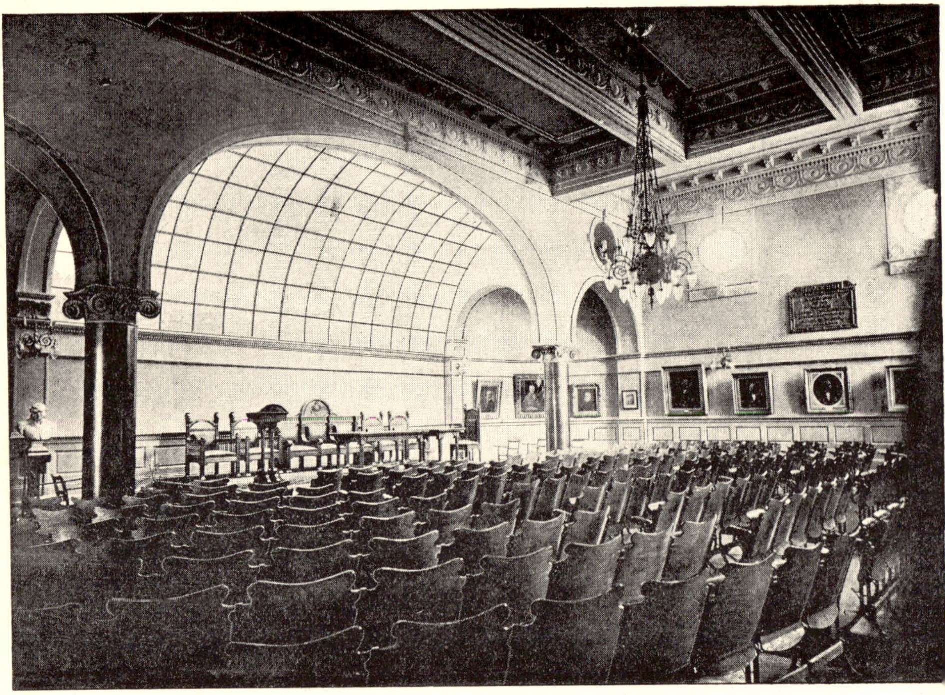

HOSACK HALL, 17–21 WEST 43D STREET

RIGHT, ABOVE: FELLOWS ROOM, 17–21 WEST 43D STREET
Smoking Room and Hosack Hall in the Background

RIGHT, BELOW: COLLATION ROOM, 17–21 WEST 43D STREET
Door of Elevator at the Right

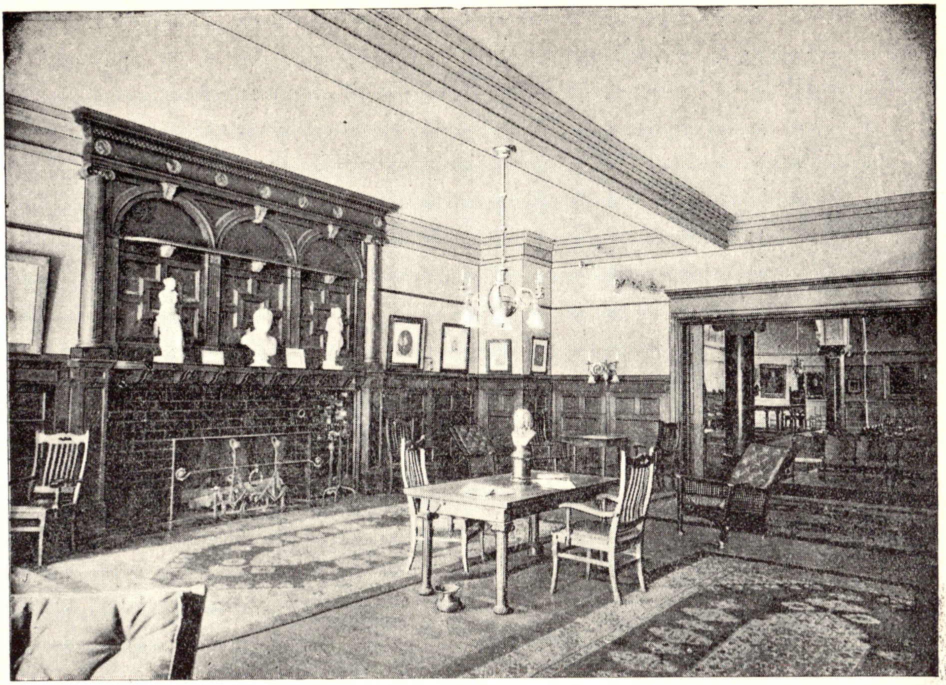

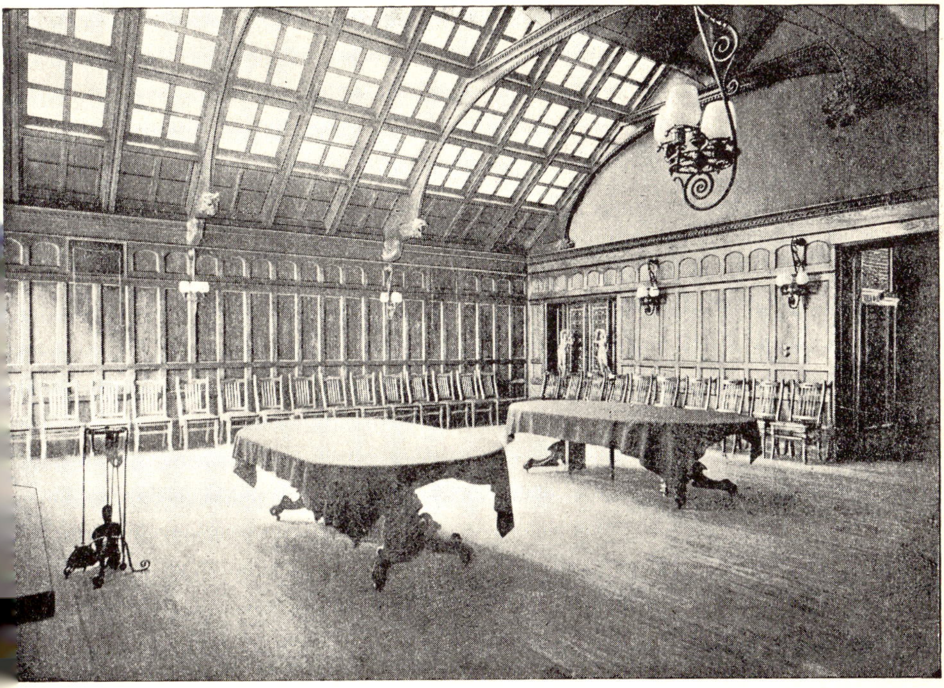

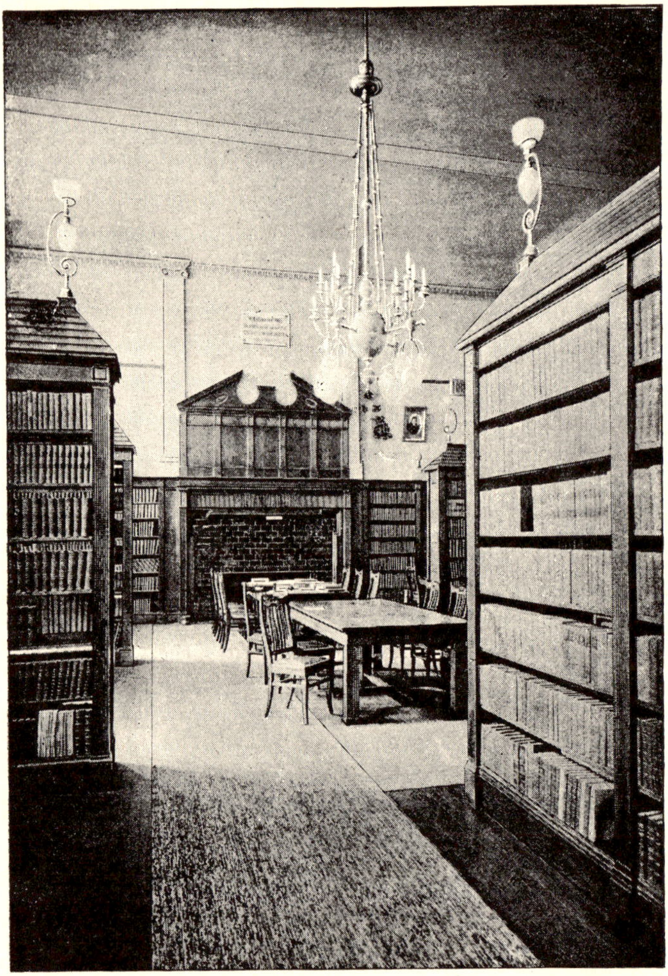

MAIN READING ROOM OF THE LIBRARY
17–21 WEST 43D STREET

that the "Academy was devoted simply to scientific medicine and was not likely to participate." The Council approved.

And his active interest did not cease when he retired. He was immediately elected a Trustee and served for seventeen years, with the exception of one year when, his term expiring at the same time as the President's, he was replaced by Dr. Janeway, as was customary. He was President of the Board from 1894 through 1911, excepting the one year mentioned.

1889–1892

Alfred L. Loomis

FEBRUARY 7, 1889, Dr. Jacobi delivered his Valedictory Address. He gave a very brief résumé of the four years' accomplishments and said the Council and the Committee on Site were unanimous in their views as to the need of a new site, that the delays were due to efforts to make no mistake as to site or as to the means available to complete the plan. He assured them of an early announcement that the matter was completed.

Dr. Loomis, after paying his compliments to Dr. Jacobi for the work he had done as President, spoke on "the Present Needs of Scientific Medicine in This City." He said the needs were great and urged making some special provision for scientific medicine instead of giving all money to found hospitals and dispensaries, with which we were already oversupplied. He also remarked on the overwhelming amount of medical literature which was uninformative, not new, and worthless.

Alfred Lebbeus Loomis was born at Bennington, Vermont, a graduate of Union College, and of P. and S. in 1853. With little money and poor health, he started practice in 1854. There had been much tuberculosis in his family, and he early gave much attention to diseases of the chest; the art of auscultation and percussion interested him strongly. He was associated with the New York University School of Medicine and procured for it $100,000 to build and endow the Loomis Laboratory. He was associated with Dr. Trudeau in organizing in the Adirondacks a hospital for poor tuberculous cases. He joined the Academy in 1863 and was elected a Trustee in 1885 and served as such till his election to the Presidency. He had also been the energetic chairman of the Section on Medicine. He was fifty-eight when elected President.

After his address Dr. Loomis expressed his pleasure at the presence of Dr. Barker, and invited him to address the Academy. Dr.

Barker commented upon the wonderful growth of the Academy in the past few years and moved a vote of thanks to the retiring president, Dr. Jacobi, for the devotion, zeal and perfection with which he had performed the duties of presiding officer. "These were unanimously carried and Dr. Loomis tendered the same to Dr. Jacobi in person."

At the next meeting Dr. Loomis announced that the Council had purchased a site on West 43d Street, near Fifth Avenue, 75 by 100 feet, at a cost of $90,000. Together with the Building Fund, the Hosack Fund of $70,000 and the sale of their present property would nearly pay for the new building, but from twenty-five to thirty thousand dollars more must be raised to ensure possession of the new building within a year free of debt. Every Fellow was urged to start earnestly and at once to raise money.

Dr. Loomis personally signed the deed of purchase, and in October he and Mrs. Loomis deeded it over to the Academy. Dr. Loomis and Dr. Jacobi also purchased twenty-five additional feet to the west of the property, in case the Academy should need it; but this was not announced.

Three firms of architects were invited to submit plans and by April that of R. H. Robertson had been selected. As originally suggested, only the Library was to be fire-proof. But an entirely fire-proof building was now decided upon, and it was estimated the cost would be $145,000, exclusive of architects' fees.

In June the architect exhibited and explained the plans before the Academy and its friends, and an informal reception and "collation" followed, all business being suspended.

All year the Council was busied with plans and the Trustees with financial problems connected with the building. A committee of five was appointed to arrange for the laying of the cornerstone and another of two to prepare a history to be deposited therein.

The President felt the Constitution and By Laws should be amended and the business procedures simplified before the Academy moved, and to this end a committee of three was appointed.

The cornerstone was finally laid on October 2, 1889, "in the presence of an audience composed of several hundred prominent ladies and gentlemen, both lay and professional." The *Medical Record* reported:

> The N.Y. Academy of Medicine laid the cornerstone of its new building at 17, 19 and 21 West 43rd Street, on Wednesday afternoon, October 2nd with the assistance of Bishop Potter, the Rev. Dr. John Hall, Grover Cleveland, Dr. A. Jacobi and A. L. Loomis. The medical profession turned out in force and filled every space within hearing distance of the speakers. The platform was occupied by officers and ex-officers of the Academy with the distinguished laymen who were invited to participate in the ceremonies. Among the medical gentlemen on the platform were Drs. Fordyce Barker and S. S. Purple, ex-Presidents of the Academy, Gouverneur M. Smith, George A. Peters, S. T. Hubbard, W. H. Draper, F. N. Otis, A. M. Jacobus, F. A. Castle, Alexander S. Hunter, C. A. Leale, and George F. Shrady.
>
> Bishop Potter opened the exercises with a prayer, and an address was delivered by Dr. A. Jacobi, an ex-President of the Academy and the Chairman of the Committee on Funds for the new building.

Dr. Jacobi outlined what the Academy had done for the profession and especially for the public. He emphasized its needs and suggested the lay public ought to meet them. Only $50,000 was needed to complete the structure. Mr. Cleveland congratulated the Academy and spoke of its splendid work as a part of the general spirit of citizenship of the whole country. Dr. Loomis laid the cornerstone, and the Rev. Dr. John Hall pronounced the benediction.

The Council had authorized the Committee on Arrangements to furnish carriages to convey Bishop Potter and Mr. Cleveland to and from the ceremony, and at the Stated Meeting the day after the celebration a vote of thanks was passed to "Bishop Potter and Honorable Grover Cleveland for the honor of their presence and their kind participation in the ceremonies of laying the cornerstone." No mention was made of the Rev. Dr. John Hall.

The final payment on the property had to be made in May, and although considerable sums had been contributed, the funds at hand were not sufficient. The Trustees were authorized to borrow from the Fifth Avenue Bank not more than $30,000 at 6 percent interest.

One of the contributions was from Dr. Jonathan Wright, who wrote that his father, the late Dr. Aaron, an original Fellow of the Academy, "left the city in 1857, was dropped from the roll for non-payment of dues in 1863?, and died in 1885." The amount enclosed represented his father's dues from 1857 to date. The Secretary was directed to instruct the Statistical Secretary to restore the name of Dr. Aaron Wright to the roll of deceased Fellows and make a note of the same in the book of signatures of the Academy.

Later in the year the President was authorized to appoint a committee of twenty to solicit subscriptions from all those who had not already subscribed to the Building Fund, to report on or before the second meeting in February, 1890.

In 1890 the Academy decided to issue bonds of $500 each at 5 percent interest to run for ten years, unless redeemed earlier, and subscriptions were solicited. Thirteen Fellows promptly subscribed $18,500, Drs. Loomis and Herman Knapp for $3,000 each, Drs. Jacobi, E. Herrick, and C. W. Stimson for $2,000 each. In order to increase the funds for retiring these bonds it was voted that all donations not otherwise provided for, the interest of the Permanent Fund, and one-half of the assessments for rooms be turned over to the Trustees for this purpose.

In 1889 Mrs. Horace P. Farnham offered to transfer a mortgage for $10,000 to the Academy in memory of her husband, who had been Treasurer, 1877–82, and Vice President, 1883–85. The income was to be used to pay the initiation fees of "poor but worthy young physicians desiring Fellowship in the Academy, the candidates to be nominated by the Council or Trustees."

The Trustees agreed to accept the trust, if the surplus each year be spent to pay the *dues* of impecunious Fellows; any sum still remaining was to go toward the support of the Library. Mrs. Farnham wisely changed her mind and left the whole amount to form a special Horace Putnam Farnham Library Fund. The Journal Room, which Mrs. Farnham later fitted up, was named the "Farnham Room."

In April, Dr. A. Caillé presented on behalf of twenty-nine Fellows a framed portrait of Dr. Jacobi and, in May, Dr. O. D.

Pomeroy, as Chairman of the Section on Ophthalmology and Otology, presented on behalf of forty-two members of the Section and other Fellows a portrait of Dr. C. R. Agnew by George H. Yewell. He gave a biographical sketch of Dr. Agnew, which was followed by brief eulogies by Drs. Barker, Jacobi, Noyes, and A. H. Smith.

In November the Treasurer reported unpaid bills of $373.58 and $248.99 in the Treasury with which to pay them. Dr. Loomis came to the rescue and loaned the Academy $1,000, which was promptly repaid the next year.

Dr. W. M. Polk delivered the Anniversary Address, "The Relation of Medicine to Some of the Questions of the Day." He emphasized the duty of physicians to teach the masses of the people, as part of their daily intercourse with them, the need to *keep* their bodies well in the struggle for existence, and *how* to do it. "The meeting being a public one, many prominent ladies and gentlemen of the city were present by special invitation."

The Academy had decided to send a set of its *Transactions* to the Paris Exposition of 1889, and the Exposition authorities granted it a diploma, which was duly received.

During the year seventy-five new Fellows signed the roll, "the largest number in a single year in the history of the Academy."

In February, 1890, the property at 12 West 31st Street was sold for $60,000. It was bought in 1875 for $28,000 and some $10,000 had been spent on the addition and improvements.

Newspaper notoriety had been a source of considerable concern. Dr. Jacobi reported that during the year without connivance on his part, the expected arrival of some of "Koch's lymph" had been featured in the daily press and also that without his authority he had been mentioned as approving "Seibert's Sterilizing Apparatus." Dr. Loomis stated that his son, Dr. Henry P. Loomis, had been reported as having an interview in which he praised the value of "Koch's lymph"; this was absolutely denied.

On the invitation of the Trustees of Columbia University, the Academy appointed Drs. Loomis, Jacobi, Roosa, A. H. Smith,

G. M. Smith, and E. Herrick to represent it at the inauguration of Seth Low as President.

The major part of the year was occupied in preparing to move to the new site. In April it was announced that after the 15th, the Library would not be open until further notice, but the Journal Room was ordered kept open to Fellows till May 8. The House Committee was instructed to arrange for a place to hold Stated Meetings in May and June, but they were held at the Academy Hall, as usual. The Sections were informed that no provision had been made for holding Section meetings after May 7. The Section meetings were held, however.

The moving began in May and was so far completed that on June 25 the Council instructed the Resident Librarian to have all the employees of the Academy on duty from 9 A.M. to 6 P.M., and also for him and the Assistant Librarian to begin immediately arranging the books on the shelves and the journals in Room 21, so that they could be used by the Fellows without further delay.

The question of assessment for rooms was taken up by the Trustees, and it was decided that the Society for the Relief of Widows and Orphans of Medical Men, the New York Physicians Mutual Aid Society, the Medical Boards of Hospitals (provided they met in the daytime), and all regular National Medical Associations be granted the use of rooms free, at the discretion of the House Committee.

For others it was voted that the tariff be raised 50 percent on rooms similar to those in the old building. Societies meeting twice a month were to receive 16⅔ percent reduction on rates. At a special meeting of the Trustees Dr. Jacobi reported the rates had caused much criticism and it was finally decided not to establish fixed rates, and Drs. Jacobi and Johnson were given authority to fix the rate in each case, medical societies to be informed that they could obtain the use of rooms "upon terms to be agreed upon." Also instead of a flat rate of $10 for the use of the kitchen and table furniture, the actual expense thereof should be charged.

The Secretary secured subscriptions from the Officers and Fellows of the Academy to the amount of $34.50, which he had expended for a white standard, 10 by 15 feet, with the initials of the Academy on it, and also an American flag 10 by 18 feet, which were to be presented to the Academy, the former to float daily in clear weather when the Academy should be open and to fly at half mast on the death of a Resident Fellow for the usual period, and the national flag to be used on public occasions or holidays.

A committee was appointed to attend to the furnishing of the Academy. One bill authorized for payment was to Lewis and Conger for twenty-three cuspidors at a cost of $15.50.

On October 2, 1890, the Academy met for the first time at its new home. The President made a few remarks on the unfinished condition of the building and announced that the formal opening would take place November 20, "Anniversary Day," by which time it would be completed. Dr. McBurney read the first paper in the new building on "Skin Grafting after the Method of Thiersch."

The Council appointed Drs. Starr, Laurence Johnson, F. A. Castle, W. H. Katzenbach, A. M. Jacobus, and the President ex officio, as a Committee on Arrangements, which was to have complete charge of everything pertaining to the official opening, including the selection of Committees on Invitation and Reception, securing funds for a collation, and so on.

Engraved invitations with admission cards were to be sent to the Fellows, the subscribers to the building fund, the press, prominent laymen and resident and non-resident physicians. All members of the societies composing the Congress of American Physicians and Surgeons, which met in 1888, were also to be invited to attend the reception.

The meeting was in Hosack Hall. Music preceded the exercises, the program of which was:

Invocation.	*Rev. Howard Crosby*, D.D.
Address by the President.	*Alfred L. Loomis*, M.D.
The Anniversary Oration. "The New York Academy of Medicine."	*Edward L. Keyes.*
Address. "Our Library."	*Abraham Jacobi.*
Music.	

Address. *Fordyce Barker.*

Addresses of Congratulation:

John S. Billings, LIBRARIAN, Surgeon General's Office, Washington, D.C.

S. Weir Mitchell, Philadelphia.

Reginald H. Fitz, Boston, Massachusetts.

Mr. D. Willis James was to have delivered an address on the "Influence of Scientific Associations upon great Cities," but sent a letter regretting his inability to be present owing to serious illness. His letter was really a brief address on the topic chosen by him and, after it was read by the President, it was placed on file in the Academy.

Many letters of regret were also received, the President reading those from President Grover Cleveland, Drs. Oliver Wendell Holmes and Henry I. Bowditch, of Boston; Nathan S. Davis, Sr., of Chicago; William H. Welch of Johns Hopkins University, Baltimore; and L. L. Seaman of the Academy.

Dr. Seaman's letter accompanied a piece of marble statuary, called Esmeralda, sculptured by Tagolini, of Rome, in 1867, and which is now on exhibition in the Reception Room of the Academy.

During the evening an orchestra rendered various musical selections and at the close of the exercises, the President invited the guests and Fellows to inspect the new building and partake of the substantial collation prepared.

There were in attendance during the evening at the meeting and the reception about 1,500 ladies and gentlemen of the laity and the medical profession.

All the expenses of this evening were paid for by voluntary subscriptions from the Fellows.

At a later meeting Dr. Keyes presented a check for $1,000 from an anonymous donor, which was directly due to the appeals made at the opening ceremonies of the new building.

No transactions of any kind had been published by the Academy since 1885. The finances would not permit. Dr. M. Allen Starr was appointed a committee to edit a volume or volumes to cover this period. He reported that 113 papers had been read before the Academy during four years, and 371 before the Sections. It would require four volumes of several hundred pages, costing nearly $1,800. It was therefore decided to publish one volume containing the Anniversary Addresses, Dr. Jacobi's and Dr. Loomis's Presidential Addresses and a list of all papers read before the Academy and its sections, with references to place of publication. It also was to include a record of the exercises at the laying of the cornerstone and a picture of the new building. This volume, dated 1890, consisted of 199 pages and cost the Academy $271.25.

The Constitution and By Laws were clarified and amended. There were no drastic changes, except that the "maintenance of a public medical library" was made the *second* objective.

At the annual meeting the Treasurer reported a balance of $555.44. During the year ninety-two applications for Resident membership had been received, and fifty-eight were recommended for election; one non-resident, one honorary, and one corresponding Fellow were also recommended. Only two were rejected and the rest were under consideration. The Library had secured a trained assistant at $800 and asked for $5,700 for the next year. It was only allowed $4,500.

Dr. Loomis was elected for a second term.

In spite of the moving, the two years had been busy ones professionally. A number of excellent papers were read: Dr. McBurney, "Radical Care of Inguinal Hernia"; Dr. Delafield, "Acute and Subacute Nephritis"; Dr. L. A. Stimson, "Gunshot Wounds of the Abdomen with Special Reference to Wounds of the Intestines."

Several meetings were given over to discussions of special subjects. Six papers were read on various phases of "the place of electricity in therapeutics"; four on the tubercle bacillus and its relation to the etiology, diagnosis and treatment of phthisis pulmonalis. Four papers were read on the prevailing influenza epidemic; three on the forms of pneumonia which complicate influenza (of these, two were by Drs. William Pepper of Philadelphia and F. C. Shattuck of Boston); five on the "Relation of Diseases of the Upper Air

Passages to Reflex Neuroses"; and three on the relation of peripheral irritation to disease. Another series of papers dealt with hydrophobia, one of which by Dr. H. M. Biggs was on "The Present Experimental Aspects of Pasteur's Prophylaxis for Rabies."

One meeting was given over to the report of the delegates to the Tenth International Medical Congress in Berlin. Dr. Jacobi read the general report and nine others reported on special branches of medicine.

The Academy was very busy with public health measures. An ordinance of the Board of Aldermen requiring ashes and garbage to be placed near the curb to await collection met with its disapproval. It was considered a "backward step in the cause of sanitary reform" and the Mayor was requested to use his full power to prevent its becoming a law.

Dr. Jacobi objected to a proposed change in the law regarding education preliminary to the study of medicine. His objections were adopted and ordered sent to each member of the Legislature.

There was a report that 2,800 nuisances existed in the Croton watershed; a committee of three was appointed to bring the matter before the proper authorities.

The Assembly passed a bill allowing Madison County to care for its own indigent insane, thus being relieved of the necessity of paying for state care. This was strongly objected to, as against the long fought-for principle that small communities could not adequately care for the insane. A large organization was needed. Considerable detail was gone into and it was voted to submit this opinion to the Legislature through a special committee.

At Dr. Jacobi's suggestion, Dr. Bryant, Commissioner of Health, was requested to read a paper on manure disposal.

The Section on Public Health proposed resolutions in regard to stamping out yellow fever epidemics. After considerable discussion this was referred to a committee of three, which reported: "the resolutions are in conflict with the Constitution of the United States, the present quarantine laws and the existing facts. Therefore the committee is not prepared to recommend said resolutions for consideration by the Academy."

The Academy was being embarrassed by a surplus of portraits, usually crayon drawings or large photographs, of deceased Fellows who had had little to do with its activities. It was decided that hereafter no portrait or photograph of a physician be accepted, until approved by the Council.

The new building was expensive to operate. The bills for light and heat were naturally greatly increased and the elevator was an additional expense. A night engineer was needed. And there was the interest on $28,500 bonded debt to pay. The Trustees were kept very busy.

Dr. Loomis, in his second inaugural (1891), painted a very rosy picture of the Academy's accomplishments. He urged that the *Transactions* or a *Bulletin* appear regularly. The contributions to medicine were of such value he felt that a regular periodical would be self-supporting. At his suggestion the Council had appointed a committee to solicit subscriptions for such a *Bulletin*, to be published at no expense to the Academy. Nothing had been heard from it.

Dr. Loomis was in favor of holding an extra meeting each month or reserving a part of one meeting for social intercourse. He paid a deserved tribute to Dr. F. A. Castle, retiring after seven years as Treasurer of the Trustees, "whose faithfulness to detail, as well as a comprehensive grasp of the whole work, whose patience and perseverance, whose indefatigable activity and hard work, have done more than anyone to make our house a home." The Academy promptly voted a committee of three to raise funds for and have charge of a social gathering each month, and referred to the Council the matter of publishing a *Bulletin.*

Dr. Jacobi was chairman of a committee to investigate and he promptly handed in this report.

The Stated Meetings of the Academy furnish annually twenty papers and discussions, and the Sections one monthly for ten meetings each. A paper averages 10,000 words, a discussion 5,000 words; total 15,000 words, which at 340 words per page makes 45 pages.

Lowest estimate for 1,000 copies of a page $1.25; for 45 pages $57.00

Lowest estimate for 5,000 copies of a page $2.50; for 45 pages	114.00
For 120 papers and discussions for 1,000 copies	7,000.00
Ditto for 5,000 copies	14,000.00
Expenses for stenographer $12. per night, for 120 papers and discussions	1,500.00
Editor	2,000.00
Required annually	17,500.00

It does not appear that the Academy can afford the expenses. Besides the members who have been interviewed decline limiting the privilege of the papers to the *Bulletin,* when they have the opportunity of publishing in journals of large circulation. If the Academy claim proprietorship of the papers, probably the best papers would not be presented before the Academy.

It was voted that the report be received, that the question be laid on the table, and that the Committee be discharged with thanks.

The Council appointed a House Committee, consisting of three members.

Dr. Loomis presented the Academy with the furniture for the platform in Hosack Hall and sent the receipted bill for $817 to the Trustees. A vote of thanks was given.

In May on recommendation of the Council, after long discussion, the Academy unanimously voted to assess each member $10 this year to meet the estimated deficit of $6,000 at the end of the year. There was considerable protest of this action afterwards, mostly in letters written to the journals.

At the end of May, Dr. Fordyce Barker died. There is no record of any action taken by the Academy at this time, but a letter was read later from Mrs. Barker:

To Alfred L. Loomis, M.D.
President of the New York Academy of Medicine:

The family of Fordyce Barker, M.D., LL.D. who held the position of President of the New York Academy of Medicine with honor, three successive terms, desire to express their deep appreciation of the noble act of you his successor, by which you and the Fellows of the Academy placed a laurel wreath upon his brow by so touchingly and impressively acting as his Guard of Honor on his last progress through the Avenue [Fifth] where once his form was so familiar to the eye. We knew that you mourned with us at St. Thomas' Church.

May we further ask you fittingly to express our thanks to the Fellows of the Academy?

With high regards

Elizabeth Lee Barker wife of Fordyce Barker and
Mr. and Mrs. Fordyce D. Barker

24 East 38th Street, N.Y., June 19, 1891.

A memorial address was delivered by Dr. William T. Lusk, one of his closest friends, in November. Dr. Barker left to the Academy all his library dealing with obstetrics and gynecology and at the same time his son donated the rest of his father's medical collection, 1,800 volumes in all.

At the same meeting a memorial of Dr. Abram Dubois was read by Dr. Ball.

A committee of forty was appointed to raise funds to liquidate the bonded debt of the Academy.

The Committee on Admissions reported to the Council that a suit had been brought against Dr. A. S. Hunter, a former member of the Committee, by a Dr. Gould, who apparently was aggrieved at his failure to be recommended for Fellowship and laid the responsibility therefor on Dr. Hunter. The Committee had been ordered to produce its minutes in Court. The Chairman was instructed to obtain possession of the minute book and papers of the Committee at once and place them in the custody of the Academy. Dr. Hunter won his case, and was awarded costs of $400. His attorney's fees were, however, $650, and the Academy voted to reimburse Dr. Hunter. This is the only instance in the records of such suit being brought against the Academy.

The question of raising the dues from $10 to $20 was brought up and caused much discussion. Dr. Jacobi thought $15 was enough. Others thought an assessment was preferable, in case of a deficit. It was finally voted to increase the dues to $20. This met with considerable criticism in the medical press, but most of the Fellows realized the necessity.

The Anniversary Address was delivered by Prof. C. F. Chandler, on "Arsenic in Common Life." Dr. Chandler did not submit his paper for publication. "After the address the Fellows and guests were invited to a collation."

A Resident Fellow's new overcoat was stolen from the coatroom at this meeting and he made claim for $65. The Council paid it.

A very complete volume of *Transactions*, covering the year 1890, was published. The editor, Dr. George T. Jackson, did a very creditable and difficult piece of work. Almost every paper read was included, together with a list of the papers read at each Section meeting and the discussions, and a reference to publication elsewhere. They occupy 393 pages, and cost $676.75 to print 900 copies. A vote of thanks was given Dr. Jackson, and he was continued as editor for the second year.

Thanks to the assessment, the Academy finished the year with a balance of $895.53. House expenses amounted to $7,431; library expenses $5,339.

Dr. A. M. Jacobus, at his own request, retired after nine years' service as Assistant and Recording Secretary. He acted also as Secretary of the Council, and kept excellent minutes. His last report of the Council is followed by this note, "Thank the Lord that it is all over, and that I am now ex-Secretary. A. M. J." A vote of thanks for his services was given.

During the year Dr. R. W. Taylor contributed $100 to complete the furnishing of the smoking room and also gave a set of fire irons for it. Mrs. Woerishoffer gave a tablet for Woerishoffer Hall; Dr. Herrick, fire irons for the dining room, and Mrs. Herrick a clock for the dining room.

Dr. Loomis's second term was a very uneventful one. The most important event was the obtaining of "subscriptions" to the amount of $20,000 to retire bonds. We have no actual information on this, but there is very good reason to believe that most of the "subscriptions" were from the holders of the bonds themselves.

The Stated Meetings ran very smoothly. Dr. Loomis arranged for the Sections to be responsible for the second meeting each month. Usually only one paper was read at such meetings. There were many evenings when several papers were read on a special subject. One such meeting was devoted to observations on the use of Koch's tuberculin in the treatment of tuberculosis, with reports from St. Luke's, Bellevue, Mt. Sinai, and the Adirondack Sanitorium. Another was on epilepsy, and a third on tuberculosis, its prevalence, spread, and prevention.

At all these meetings well-known physicians were announced, beforehand, as discussants. Complaints were made, chiefly in the medical press, that the younger men were neglected. In reply to these criticisms Dr. Loomis, in opening the discussion on tuberculosis, stated that during his occupation of the chair, on but one occasion was the discussion limited to the announced list of speakers and then only because of the lateness of the hour. The reason for the selection of participants in the discussion was in order to make the discussion pertinent, pointed, and instructive. Every member present had a right to be heard and that right was secured to him.

In the field of public health, "Public Baths for the Poor" was discussed by Dr. Baruch, and it was voted that "the Academy approve of the construction of free public baths in the city as a sanitary measure of the highest importance."

Dr. W. H. Draper presented a preamble and resolutions of approval of the report of the Advisory Committee to the Mayor on the condition of the streets of the city and on the methods of the Department of Street Cleaning, and urging the Mayor to use his influence in carrying out the suggestions of the said committee in the matter. The resolutions were unanimously adopted and the Recording Secretary was directed to have a copy, properly authenticated by the President and Recording Secretary, sent to the Mayor, to the Commissioner of the Department of Street Cleaning, and to each of the five members of the Advisory Committee. The Mayor's Secretary acknowledged its receipt.

A special meeting was held in September, 1892, to consider the vexing question of quarantine, and a committee was appointed to consider the feasibility of urging legislation in favor of a National Quarantine. This committee was heard from later.

At the Anniversary Meeting, Dr. Lewis A. Stimson read or

"Pasteur's Life and Work in Relation to the Advancement of Medical Science." It was a very interesting account, and the *Medical Record* commenting on it said: "Even the doctors present, whose practice has been so largely modified by the discoveries of Pasteur in relation to the part played by germs in the production of fermentation and disease, and the correlated fact of prevention by inoculation, were led to a clearer understanding of the Chemist's work, and made to feel more deeply their obligations for his pains-taking and conscientious industry."

A special meeting, November 22, 1892, was called by the Council to hear Dr. J. J. Kinyoun of the Marine Hospital Service, Washington, D.C., deliver the first Wesley M. Carpenter Lecture: "Modern Treatment of the Infected Vessel."

The Library was very active. Through the efforts of Mr. Brownne two lists of periodicals in the Library, one, "English Journals" and the other, "Foreign Journals," were published. The Academy was very proud of those lists. Mrs. L. E. Smith was engaged as Assistant Librarian, to be on duty daily from 9 A.M. to 5 P.M. The older Fellows of the Academy will remember the always efficient Mrs. Smith. She served loyally until October, 1929, when after thirty-eight years, she was retired on pension.

Dr. A. L. Northrop, D.D.S., contributed 517 volumes, 50 pamphlets, and 18,000 numbers of dental periodicals. From this, "475 volumes were added to the reference library, making it one of the most valuable dental libraries in the United States." Dr. Northrop later announced his intention of continuing his subscriptions to the journals and paying for their binding during his lifetime. On Dr. Northrop's death the First District Dental Society sent $250 to start an A. L. Northrop D.D.S. Dental Library Fund. This fund was never increased.

A "want book" was placed in the Library, in which anyone wanting a book not on the shelves could enter the title which was then considered by the Committee. Notices were also sent to each Section asking for suggestions for new books to be added.

In 1891 readers signing the register numbered 3,888, and in 1892, 7,752.

The Library Committee already was asking for more shelf room, and asked for $3,600 to provide it.

The Academy closed the year with a balance of $1,124.09. Maintenance cost $8,931.33, and Library expenses, outside of salaries, $2,829.99. Fellows were in arrears for dues of $1,783.

At the annual election, Dr. Loomis declined to serve again as President, and also declined the nomination for Trustee. He was in poor health. Dr. D. B. St. John Roosa was elected President.

Dr. Loomis was a fine president, generous of himself and his money. He failed to preside at only five meetings during the four years of his service, and was very regular at the meetings of the Council and Trustees. At the last meeting of the Council for the year it was:

Resolved, That the Council wishes to make record of its appreciation of the courtesy, enthusiasm and efficiency of its presiding officer during his administration of the affairs of the Academy.

Resolved, That during his occupancy of the Presidential Chair, the Academy has conspicuously carried out the various objects for which the association was founded and the establishment of the Academy in its present edifice, and the reduction of its debt, has marked an epoch in the history of the society, which is in a very large measure attributable to his indefatigable zeal.

Resolved, That the Council feels assured that, while declining to accept the nominations which had been tendered to him, Dr. Loomis has his heart still as cordially interested in the welfare of the Academy as in the past and that he will continue in the future to labor as faithfully in its behalf.

Resolved, That a copy of these preambles and resolutions be engrossed upon the minutes of this meeting, and a copy of the same be transmitted to Dr. Loomis by the Secretary.

1893–1894

D. B. St. John Roosa

In his Valedictory Address, Dr. Loomis summarized the splendid advances and accomplishments of the previous four years, closing with a few words of appreciation of three Fellows who had died—Drs. Dubois, Barker and Leaming. He said the Academy did not " 'mourn their loss.' . . . They did their part in life with faithful zeal until their powers gave way . . . and when at last their summons came, the best of all they had—the essence of the man, his quality—they left with us."

Dr. Roosa delivered an eloquent address in which he emphasized the necessity of the Academy making widely known its opinions and plans to improve the health of the community and the country, referring especially to the question of quarantine reform, the obsolete and inefficient coroner situation, and the presidency of the Board of Health which could not be filled by a medical man. He also urged the establishment within the Academy of a *club* feature.

Dr. Roosa, twentieth President, was fifty-five, a fine talker and well thought of by the profession. Confining his practice to ophthalmology and otology, he had been professor in those subjects at New York University Medical College, and had been Surgeon to the Manhattan Eye and Ear Hospital, and the Eye and Ear Infirmary. He had also been president of the American, New York, and International Otological Societies and Medical Society of the State of New York. He was one of the most ardent advocates of the new Code of Ethics. During Dr. Roosa's administration the Academy gave much time to public health matters.

The first action was to hold a special meeting to hear the report of a Committee on Quarantine appointed in September, 1892. It had acted in an advisory capacity to a Committee of the Chamber of Commerce, which financed it. The city had been afflicted with cholera the previous summer and now the Committee, "looking forward with the gravest apprehension to the advance of the Asiatic Cholera to our shores in the season that is now almost at hand, recommend the New York Academy of Medicine to memorialize Congress to give us the only relief that seems to us possible, namely, a National Quarantine that is paramount to all others."

As a result, a committee of twenty-one was appointed to go to Washington and offer a formal protest to the pending, and inadequate, Harris National Quarantine Bill; to draft and support a suitable substitute bill; and to appeal to the profession in Boston, Philadelphia, Baltimore, and Chicago for cooperation, as well as to the State Society and various medical societies of the country.

The Committee sent a strong memorial to Congress, which was acknowledged by the President of the United States and the Speaker of the House. But in spite of these protests Congress passed the bill. When the Committee reported the fact to the Academy on February 16 it was thanked for its efforts and discharged. The *Medical Record* commented:

> While the action of the Academy was altogether commendable, the delay in taking that action rendered its effort useless. We have often expressed the regret that the Academy usually remained so indifferent to great public questions which fall within the scope of its legitimate work. It has a power for usefulness in the fields of social, sanitary and political science, unequalled by any other body. . . . It should be prepared to take the lead, rather than follow in the wake, of public opinion, as in this instance.

This was headed "The Useless Work of the Academy." Several letters were also published, some condemning the Committee, others supporting it.

Eight days later a special meeting was called to reconsider the action of dismissing the Committee. Dr. Jacobi opened the matter, feeling that the work was unfinished. The Committee had established relations with committees in other localities; moreover, the daily press had interpreted its discharge as a rebuke. Dr. Loomis was opposed to reconsideration: the Committee had done what it was appointed for, and the County Society was the proper channel through which to influence legislation. The Academy was no place for discussions of a political nature. Up till a few weeks before it had been a purely scientific body, and he hoped it would return to that role. Dr. Derby then reminded Dr. Loomis of his activity, during his administration, in the matter of dirty streets. It was finally voted 77 to 67 to reappoint the Committee, and Dr. Roosa stated his intention to continue on the lines laid down in his inaugural.

Reports of this meeting called forth more letters and editorials on both sides. The Public Health Section was a little disgruntled, and one of its members complained at the lack of interest in its work on the part of the general Fellowship.

In June another special meeting was called and the National Quarantine Committee asked its powers be enlarged so that it could investigate and agitate the establishment of a National Bureau of Health. The Academy unanimously granted it the powers to do so.

In March, 1893, the subject of the Croton watershed was taken up. Dr. Cheesman read a report on an inspection of one sector of the area, with numerous photographs of the pollution of the waters, and Dr. Chapin read an abstract of the laws concerning watersheds. There was a bill before the Legislature to buy up the Croton watershed, and the Academy appointed a committee to go to Albany and oppose it on the ground it was an unnecessary expense and would not protect the area. The Committee went and also presented a substitute bill creating a Croton water commission. The *Medical Record* commented: "The committee was defeated in its object, the interests of the opposition being too strong. It has, however, the consolation of knowing that its position was right and its recommendations wise. In fact no arguments worthy of the name were brought against the bill. The views expressed have the support of the profession and of unbiased sanitary experts."

An amendment to the recently passed law was offered by the Academy and brought endorsement from the *Medical Record*, but of course, failed to pass. The Committee, without definite permission of the Council, ran up a bill of $369.34 for legal services, which after much protest was eventually paid.

Another activity of the year was action on the bill proposed by the Public Health Section on a change in the coroner system. Resolutions were passed condemning the present system of a layman as coroner and urging the position be filled by a physician trained and qualified as a medico-legal expert.

Dr. Roosa was very insistent that the Academy provide facilities for Fellows working in the Library to obtain light refreshments in the building, thus "saving much time in searching for a place to obtain a meal"!. Several requests for it had been made. Legal Counsel was of the opinion that the sale of beer, cigars, crackers, and cheese at cost could not be regarded as "a means for the promotion of medical science," nor was it a necessary or usual function of a public library. The effect on tax exemption was taken up with the Comptroller, who ruled that it was proper for the Academy to serve a meal at cost, but the sale of beer was for the Board of Excise to decide. The Board of Excise was then consulted and it stated that the serving of beer would not have to be licensed any more than in a club or a home.

The President now strongly urged the establishment of "Club Features." The Council then renamed the House Committee the "Executive Committee," and authorized the President to appoint a House Committee of three, which he promptly did, and it was instructed to report a plan for the "Club" features and probable costs. It reported in June:

1. The House Committee shall provide for serving in the Dining Hall of the Academy, from 12 noon, until 11.30 at night, refreshments consisting of cold meats, bread and butter, Lager beer, Bass Ale, Ginger Ale, Mineral Waters, Cigars, and so forth, to Fellows of the Academy and their guests, only.

2. They shall not allow those not Fellows of the Academy invited to the rooms to order or pay for refreshments. No credit shall be allowed.

3. No spirituous liquors or wines shall be served unless on special occasions by order of the Council.

4. If the various societies meeting in the Academy and serving refreshments so desire, the House Committee may, at their discretion, arrange to provide these refreshments, the profits, if any, to be applied to the expense account of the refreshment rooms of the Academy.

5. The House Committee shall have full charge of the caterer, servants, and the service in these rooms, and have power to maintain order.

6. The House Committee shall endeavor to adjust the expenses so that no loss may be incurred by the Academy.

7. The House Committee shall report to the Council at each of its regular monthly meetings.

8. The arrangement of the refreshment and smoking rooms shall be begun at such time in October of this year as the House Committee may suggest.

9. Notice of the opening of the refreshment rooms shall be given to each Fellow by a circular signed by the House Committee and mailed with the notices for the first meeting of the Academy in October.

The cost of installation "for furnishing refrigerator, crockery and glass, linen, knives and forks, tables, shelves, window curtains, chafing dishes, etc," was estimated at $200. "The above sum of $200 will, in the opinion of your committee, be sufficient to enable the buffet to be opened. It is the purpose of the House Committee to make the venture self-supporting in a short time." The $200 was appropriated.

In October the buffet was announced as opened, and the President informed the Council he would guarantee all deficit up to January 1, 1894. By the following March the disbursements for the grill room had exceeded receipts by $461.39 and it was discontinued. Dr. Roosa paid $143.58 of the deficit.

Dr. John A. Wyeth called the attention of the Academy to a recent occurrence at the New York Infant Asylum. The Board of Managers had refused to reappoint one of the Attending Staff for the ensuing year. The Medical Board protested and demanded that nominations to the Staff should be made by it. As other rules governing such matters had been in force for several years, the Managers refused to alter them, and the Medical Board then resigned. Dr. Wyeth wished the Academy to back up the Medical Board, approve its action, and condemn the Managers. He offered resolutions to that effect. After much discussion, the matter was wisely laid on the table and was not taken up again.

The Library Staff was small and its hours were long. It was voted to close on Saturdays at 6 P.M.; that no one but Fellows should use it after 6 P.M. on other days, unless provided with a card from a Fellow; and that, to protect the books, electric light should be used instead of gas. It was also decided to close the Library at 6 P.M. from June to September 15, and to suspend its functions for two weeks in August for cleaning.

In the fall, the Treasurer announced that there was a large arrearage of dues and therefore he had not enough cash to pay bills. He requested the Treasurer of the Trustees to pay back some $1,700 "loaned" to him in 1891, and with interest at 3 percent! The Trustees transferred $1,500 of the income from their funds, but without the interest.

The Wesley M. Carpenter lecture was delivered by Dr. Robert Abbe, on "The Surgery of the Hand," and Dr. W. H. Thomson gave the Anniversary Address at a special meeting, speaking on "Modern Experimental Medicine." The audience was said to have completely filled Hosack Hall, and guests were afterwards invited to inspect the building.

In October, 1890, Dr. Jacobi had urged the establishment of a "Bureau of Nurses" and asked favorable action at some future meeting. In April, 1891, the President was authorized to appoint a committee of three (he to be one) to consider the matter. Legal Counsel was consulted and he considered it was not the function of the Academy to do so. The plan lay dormant, though Dr. Jacobi was very anxious to have it carried out. In the meantime the County Society was considering establishing such a bureau, and a Conference Committee was appointed, which reported back that the County Society preferred to have the Academy do it.

In December, 1893, a committee of five was appointed to establish such a bureau in the Academy building. It was opened in February, 1894, with a trained nurse in charge, and was to function, at first, from 8 A.M. to 10 P.M. Nurses were to be charged $2.00 a year for registration, and each must have an endorsement from two "reputable physicians," who were to be asked for a confidential statement as to her character and capacity as a nurse. Patients provided with nurses were to pay $2.00, and when a case was terminated the physician was to be questioned as to the handling of it. A night a list of names was to be left "with someone around the building" (the night engineer?). When fully established, twenty-four hour service was planned. This was based upon the experience of similar bureaus in Boston and Philadelphia, the latter having cleared $2,700 in its eighth year.

A room was provided by the Academy and the Bureau was allowed $50 a month for expenses. A telephone was to be provided. In the first six weeks 275 nurses registered and fifty-four calls for nurses had been received. Night calls were reported promptly attended to. The Janitor's room was so far from the front door that the Executive Committee placed a cot in the Nurses' Bureau room to provide prompt response to the bell. This Bureau did good service for a number of years, more than paying its own way. It was discontinued in 1906, when the need no longer existed.

During 1894, the Academy continued its activities in promoting public health matters. A Constitutional Convention was held in Albany, to consider amendments, and a committee was appointed by the President to present the Academy's views on certain topics relating to public health. The Committee, consisting of Drs. Jacobi (who declined to serve), Daniel Lewis, and S. T. Armstrong, attended the Convention and reported it "was courteously received and granted all hearings requested. Taking into consideration the dislike which the legislator has to the scantiest meddling in lawmaking, we have been fairly successful."

The Committee recommended three things: first, to abolish the office of Coroner, substituting therefor a Medical Examiner. All this accomplished was that coroners were not "constitutional" officers. The second recommendation was to change the Regents' tenure of office from life to ten years. This failed. The third was to divide the Department of Charities and Correction into two departments. This also failed.

The National Quarantine Committee, which had been reappointed and authorized to agitate the establishment of a National Board of Health, had been very active and had done a tremendous job. The only mention of it in the minutes is, in December, 1894, when it reported "progress." The *Medical Record* tells us a great deal. On July 15, 1893, it published a first draft as submitted by the Committee to secure criticism and changes that all might agree on it. On August 19 it published a "completed text" of the bill, still in the first-draft stage, and again urged suggestions for improvement.

On November 4 the *Record* published the final bill to be submitted to Congress, with an editorial on the work of the Committee:

The Quarantine Committee of the Academy of Medicine has completed its draft of a Public Health Bill. . . . It is the outcome of an exhaustive examination of all the health laws heretofore introduced into Congress, of the laws at present in existence, and of the health laws of other countries. We may add that, as the Committee extensively circulated tentative drafts of the bill and invited criticisms and suggestions from the ablest sanitarians in this country, large numbers of whom responded, the bill embodies the best thought and experience of the practical laborers in the field of preventative medicine.

Again, December 2d,

We feel justified in saying, for the encouragement of those engaged in this most patriotic service, that indications of success are daily multiplying. The New York Chamber of Commerce has resolved to aid the Committee, and its example will bring the cooperation of the Boards of Trade throughout the country. Life Insurance Societies have indicated a desire to add the weight of their influence. We have reason also to believe that this measure will soon prove acceptable to the government.

And finally, March 10, 1894, it states editorially that the bill was now in proper shape for passage before both legislative branches at Washington. ". . . we congratulate the Committee on its eminently successful work, and bespeak for it a becomingly high appreciation of its arduous and unselfish labors in the cause of public health, and the consequent interests of public safety."

Unfortunately the bill failed to pass.

The Academy strongly opposed a rider to the Army Appropriations Bill, reducing the number of Surgeons by thirty-five, and sent the protest to the President, Presiding Officers of the House and Senate, and Chairmen of the Committees on Military Affairs. It also opposed again, a reduction of the appropriation for the Surgeon-

General's Library, from $10,000 to $7,000, and a memorial was sent to the "appropriate parties" in Washington.

Dr. Jacobi proposed the introduction of a bill forbidding the mailing of medical books, pamphlets and circulars "which are of a character not proper for general and indiscriminate perusal or circulation," unless enclosed in a sealed envelope and prepaid at letter rates, or unless addressed for delivery to, or in care of, physicians, surgeons, medical schools and colleges, or students in such colleges, or to dealers in medical publications. It was voted to send a copy of this proposal to the Chairman of the House Committee on Post Offices and Post Roads, and Dr. Jacobi was requested to present the subject to the Medical Society of the County of New York and kindred societies. The Chairman of the House Committee on Post Offices and Post Roads wrote asking what evils were proposed to be remedied by such a bill. Dr. Jacobi was requested to answer.

The *Medical Record* was against the proposal as limiting the distribution of medical literature. To this criticism Dr. Jacobi responded promptly, saying the *Record* had missed the point entirely. The *Record* published his reply and said it now gave the resolution its unqualified approval.

In April it was reported that a bill was before the Legislature increasing penalties for non-registration of births, deaths, and marriages, which would be ineffective and impose extra burdens on all concerned. A special committee was appointed to memorialize the Legislature and the Governor. In May the Committee reported the bill passed before it could take action, and all it had done was to urge the Governor to apply the veto.

The Academy passed resolutions offered by the Section on Public Health urging disposal of garbage by incineration instead of the unsanitary method in use.

Many excellent papers were read, some of them really important. Drs. McBurney and Starr read a "Contribution to Cerebral Surgery: Diagnosis, Localization and Operation for Removal of Three Tumors of the Brain." This was a real contribution. Dr. Northrup's on "Scorbutus in Infants" was valuable, and experience was submitted in writing by Drs. T. M. Rotch of Boston, F. Forchheimer of Cincinnati, A. D. Blackader, Montreal, W. F. Lockwood of Baltimore. Dr. Northrup was a pioneer in investigating the mysteries of infantile scurvy. It was still frequently not diagnosed.

Dr. W. B. Coley elaborated his ideas of the treatment of "Inoperable Malignant Tumors" with the toxins of erysipelas and bacillus prodigiosus.

Dr. H. W. Berg delivered a long discourse on "Diphtheria and Its Treatment," including the use of antitoxin, which was being tried out and offered hopes of success.

Dr. Abbe discussed the surgery of gallstone obstruction, Dr. A. B. Judson the importance and value of early treatment of infantile paralysis deformities, and Dr. J. B. Murphy of Chicago spoke on "Intestinal Approximation," stressing the use of the Murphy button.

At the Section meetings many very interesting cases were reported, and good papers were read.

At the Anniversary Meeting the President expressed his surprise that so few of the laity present knew what the Academy was, and told them. Dr. Dana's address was "On the New Uses of Some Older Sciences," after which the audience was invited to view the building "and see under what conditions medical research was carried on."

The Carpenter Lecture was delivered by Dr. Joseph D. Bryant: "Important Facts Relative to Malignant Disease."

Each year a volume of *Transactions* appeared. Dr. George T. Jackson was the Editor and did a fine job. Except one or two which were not in publishable form, every paper read in 1891 and 1892 appeared with a complete program of each Section meeting. The two volumes cost $646.

The Academy had only been in its building about four years. It was faced with many complaints, chiefly from the Library. First the gas used for illumination was spoiling the books and electricity was substituted; the ventilation was so bad it was hard on workers The Library was growing so fast the stackroom was getting crowded, and shelves were being added in the various rooms to the detriment of the rooms themselves and the administration of the Library. After being asked "for the third time," and after much study and worry, the Council and Trustees made extensive repairs. An addition to the stacks was built at a cost of $7,288, which was done during the summer season, and of course there was chaos during the work. Dr. Jacobi made all the arrangements and Dr. Jacobus supervised the whole proceeding.

Everyone complained of the poor ventilation in the meeting rooms, and the electric lighting, which had been introduced, worried the Trustees on account of the bills. In October, 1894, Dr. Jacobi reported a contract had been given for a complete plant—engine, dynamo, steam pipes, meters, wire connections, switchboard—for providing electricity for the Academy. The contract carried a guarantee to make all repairs from wear and tear for three years, to furnish an engineer to instruct in the running of the plant for one week, and to provide 16 candle-power Edison lamps at not more than 25 cents per lamp (!) Dr. Jacobi remarked that the electric bills had amounted to some twelve hundred-odd dollars each year, and that with the dynamo one half the yearly cost would be saved, making all allowance for interest on the cost, extra coal, lamp renewal, supplies, and wear and tear.

As usual, the Fellows were very slow in paying their dues. In October the Treasurer placed 134 bills for nearly $3,800 in the hands of a collecting agency, and in one month had collected $1,208 from twenty-nine of them. The rest, he felt, there was little chance of collecting immediately. He closed the year with a balance of $1,839.49, with bills for $2,274.12.

In Dr. Roosa's term the Academy took action which must have made its worthy Founders turn over in their graves. The Committee on Admissions asked the Council as to the eligibility of a candidate who was a graduate of the Hahnemann Medical College of Philadelphia. Dr. Herrick moved, with Dr. Jacobi seconding, "that he be recommended for election provided he make a statement in writing that he is not a sectarian practitioner nor connected with a sectarian institution." He was proposed and elected, the first graduate of a Homeopathic Medical School.

The Council was informed that a non-Resident Fellow, Dr. J. N. Merrill of Skowhegan, Maine, had advertised himself in the *Somerset Reporter* as a Fellow of the Academy. He was informed this was offensive to the Council and was requested to remove the Academy's name from the notice. When he wrote and said he had done so, the Council was "satisfied."

Dr. Allan McLane Hamilton complained that Dr. S. T. Armstrong, in a letter to a medical journal, had criticized an act of a committee of the Academy. The criticism was not in question; but he had signed himself "Chairman of the Section on Public Health." A committee of one waited on Dr. Armstrong and reported he insisted he had broken no By Law and was more critical of the Council for entertaining the complaint than regretful of his action. He was informed his act was incompatible with the dignity of his official position and he was to refrain in future from using his official title in any letter to a journal.

Dr. Everett Herrick, a Trustee who had served as President of the Board of Trustees since 1886, asked in January, 1894, to be relieved of that position, saying a younger man should be appointed. The Council then resolved, "Dr. Herrick objecting":

> WHEREAS, Dr. Everett Herrick has served as Chairman of the Trustees of the New York Academy of Medicine for a number of years and particularly during the trying period when the Academy was endeavoring to secure funds and plans for a new building, and during the erection of the same, and for several years since, and
>
> WHEREAS, During that long period, he has devoted his best energy and time as a Trustee in serving the Academy most faithfully and to the best of his ability,
>
> *Resolved*, That on his retiring from the Chair, the Trustees desire to place on record their appreciation of the valuable services rendered by Dr. Herrick and to tender to him a vote of thanks for the faithful manner in which he performed his duties as Chairman of the Trustees for the past eight years.

Dr. Jacobi took his place and began his long tenure of the office.

During Dr. Roosa's administration there was a latent, steadily increasing resentment and opposition to the powers of the Council and Trustees. It was proposed to have a House Committee not appointed by the Council but elected by the Academy, to consist of three members, one retiring each year. The Council disapproved, and the proposal was laid on the table.

The Treasurer's report for the year was the first to be printed and sent to the Fellows. The *New York Medical Journal*, summarizing the report, called attention to this fact and stated:

THE FINANCES OF THE ACADEMY OF MEDICINE

For the first time in many years, the report of the treasurer of the Academy of Medicine has been printed and sent to each of the fellows, who are the stockholders of the organization. This publication, we understand, was not accomplished without the vigorous opposition of some of the trustees, who are said to have taken the remarkable position that the fellows of the Academy should continue in ignorance regarding its financial status. Many of the fellows have desired a more detailed statement, but nobody has seemed willing to take the initiative toward requiring the trustees to print it. In fact, we have heard it stated that some of these officers seemed to think that the Academy was to submit to their dictation rather than they execute the will of the Academy. But the president, Dr. Roosa, urged that the fellows be made acquainted with the value of their property as well as with some of its needs, and a majority of the trustees have concurred in the sensible position and have published this report.

Dr. F. P. Foster, Editor of the *Journal*, was a Fellow of the Academy. The statement was very unfair. It roused the ire of the Trustees, who wrote a letter to the *Journal* and asked that it be published. The letter stated that while declining to notice the gratuitous insinuation of "dictation," there never was any difference of opinion on important points between the Trustees and the President; that a detailed report was read each year to the Fellows; that heretofore it had been considered unnecessary to print the report and send it to each Fellow, the expense being an important item, but that when this was suggested, there was "no objection, no unwillingness, no opposition, no discussion at all, but an instantaneous unanimous concurrence." They claimed the affairs of the Academy should not be the subject of unfounded reports. The *Journal* almost made an apology.

Matters came to a head over the annual election. Dr. F. R. Sturgis sent out the following circular letter:

Dear Doctor:

May I beg your kind attention to the candidacy of Dr. Thomas Addis Emmet for the Presidency of the New York Academy of Medicine, and of Dr. W. M. Polk for the Vice Presidency, and of Dr. George L. Peabody for Trustee of the same association. It is not necessary for me to eulogize these gentlemen. They are well known and their fitness for the positions to which they are nominated is unquestioned.

The opposition to the candidacy of Dr. Bryant is not based upon any personal feeling against him, but upon the fact that he is the nominee of the Trustees, who by thus taking an active political part in the nominations and elections of the Academy are establishing a bad precedent in seeking self-perpetuation of their numbers in office, and are bringing the Academy to the low political standard adopted at the last presidential election, when it was openly boasted that members were so pledged that the election was a dead open and shut thing. The same boast has been made this time. Information has been conveyed to Dr. Emmet that Dr. Bryant is certain of election and it has been suggested that he, Dr. Emmet, should withdraw from a contest in which he must be sacrificed. Surely it is time that such electioneering methods were put a stop to. This can be easily done if members of the Academy will take sufficient trouble to vote.

If they care so little about the Academy that they will not take the trouble to stamp out this disgraceful exhibition of politics then it may be reasonably feared that the association will become one in which decent members of the profession will take neither pot nor lot.

With many apologies for intruding upon your time, believe me to be

Very faithfully

F. R. Sturgis

Dr. Jacobus considered the charges were libelous against the Trustees as a whole and himself personally, as a Trustee. They had had nothing to do with the nominations and he considered the charges scandalous.

Dr. Jacobi said that as Chairman of the Trustees, he was in posi tion to say that the Board had not meddled in the least in the matter of nominations. He had also been President of the Academy for two terms and then knew what was going on. He said that the Trustees were careful to abstain from using any influence to direct any nomination. He characterized the letter as containing inventions from first to last, and were the charges not so serious they would be ridiculous.

Dr. Sturgis moved that a committee of three be appointed by the Chairman to hear what the writer of the paper complained of had to say in reply, which was done.

The Committee met and heard Dr. Sturgis's explanations. Every Trustee individually denied he had electioneered in any way for Dr. Bryant. Dr. Sturgis said he had made his charges in good faith, but was now satisfied he had been misinformed, withdrew the charges and regretted he had cast any reflections. This was deemed satisfactory by the Committee, which reported the matter to the Academy and deprecated any electioneering by circulars or letters containing reflections of a personal nature against a Fellow.

At the annual election Dr. Bryant was elected President. Of two candidates Dr. Polk was chosen as Vice President, and of three for Trustee, Dr. Peabody was elected. With one exception, this was the first time the retiring President was not named a Trustee since 1873. When the nominations were made in 1884, Dr. Barker was under charges before the Academy, which probably explains the one exception.

During the year Dr. S. T. Hubbard died. He had served the Academy faithfully and devotedly. A Founder in 1847, he had been Domestic Corresponding Secretary, 1853–1859, Trustee, 1859–1872, Vice President, 1873–1875, and Trustee again, 1876–1885. He had declined nomination as President. Resolutions were adopted and a memorial address was delivered.

Dr. Roosa was a very faithful President. He presided at every meeting in his two years, including six special meetings—forty in all. He was not very active in affairs after his Presidency, becoming interested in other organizations.

1895–1896

Joseph D. Bryant

Dr. Roosa in his Valedictory Address replied to the criticism of the Academy's participation in legislative measures. He thought the Academy should "stand between the community and the Government" in public health matters and that, if it did not, others "of less moral standing" would.

Dr. Joseph D. Bryant, twenty-first President, was fifty years old, the youngest man ever elected to the office. He had been Health Commissioner of the City and had been responsible for bringing the Department and the Academy into closer working relations. Actively interested in the work of the Academy, he had been Vice President a year when elected. He was on the Faculty of the Bellevue Hospital Medical College and an Attending Surgeon at Bellevue.

In his Inaugural Address he reminded the Academy that, while being a definite and well-established organization, differences of opinion were bound to occur and, after discussion and debate, the views of the majority must be accepted. "The endurance and thrift of every organization depend on the honesty, the harmony and the productiveness of the administration of its affairs." Without the energy and loyalty of the entire fellowship the Academy would "suffer from the dire effects of the unheeded influences of time, temper and tempest." He begged cooperation and support in all matters that were just and equitable and urged the increase of the Library Fund.

The Academy promptly authorized a committee of not more than twenty-five Fellows, with "possibly the addition of a few prominent interested laymen," to raise an endowment of $100,000 for the Academy. The "interested laymen," through the Chamber of Commerce, sent out the following letter:

To the Members of the Chamber of Commerce:

Gentlemen:

The New-York Academy of Medicine, organized in 1847 for the elevation of the standard of medical education; the cultivation and advancement of the science of medicine; the treatment of public health, and the maintenance of a free Library, has issued an appeal for contributions to the permanent fund established for the purpose of enlarging the free medical Library, maintained in its noble building erected at a cost of over $200,000. In order that the Library may be supplied with the current publications necessary to maintain its efficiency, it is estimated that a fund of $100,000 is required. Without this addition to the Library the younger members of the profession will not be able to keep up with the current developments in the line of their work, and the public will be deprived of the benefit of the latest scientific and therapeutical discoveries.

The medical profession, as represented in the Academy, are engaged in unremitting and gratuitous labor among the poor, and its members have also unselfishly and successfully exerted themselves to promote public health, and to protect the City against epidemics of contagious diseases, notably during the threatened cholera invasion in 1887, and again in 1893, when the Academy was called upon to investigate and reform the Quarantine establishment of this port, which had become dilapidated, and had, therefore, ceased to be a protection against the dangers of contagion with which we were menaced. All these services were rendered without compensation, and oftentimes at great personal sacrifice.

The Chamber of Commerce, on the 5th inst., requested the undersigned to bring these facts to the attention of the members of the Chamber, and to urge them to make a generous response to the appeal of the Academy for an object which is closely related to the health of the City, and upon which its business is largely dependent. Checks may be sent to Dr. William F. Cushman, Treasurer, No. 325 West Twenty-second Street, or to

Yours respectfully,

Alexander E. Orr

President

HONORARY COMMITTEE:

Hon. Roswell P. Flower, Hon. Abram S. Hewitt, Mr. D. Willis James, Gen. E. A. McAlpin, Mr. James Stillman.

The death of Dr. Loomis was announced in February, 1895, and a committee of three was appointed to take suitable action. In April it presented resolutions and recommended that a memorial meeting be held in May. At that meeting Dr. L. A. Stimson, his lifelong friend, read a fine tribute. Rev. Dr. Henry MacCracken, Chancellor of the University of the City of New York, to whose welfare and success Dr. Loomis had contributed so much, followed, and Abram S. Hewitt, ex-Mayor of the City, testified to his service to the city at all times. It was an impressive occasion, and all business was omitted.

Dr. Loomis left $10,000 to the Academy to form a fund to pay for a "collation" after stated meetings. His name was placed on the roster of Benefactors.

Dr. Bryant's administration was for the most part a quiet and peaceful one.

The Department of Charities and Correction was a cumbersome organization, having charge of two fundamentally unassociated activities—the care of dependents and of delinquents—which placed its hospitals at a very serious disadvantage. The Academy appointed a committee to study and report on the matter. The Committee report, signed by Drs. Jacobi, W. T. Lusk, E. G. Janeway, P. A. Morrow, and A. H. Smith, presented a long statement of facts, showing that this one Department, besides being incompetent, handled six prisons, a penitentiary, a workhouse, seven hospitals, an almshouse, four insane asylums, an infant hospital, a hospital for children and one for incurables, and asylums for the blind and for idiots—a total of twenty-five institutions.

It was "Resolved that the New York Academy of Medicine respectfully urge upon the Legislature now in session the passage of an act by which the existing Department of Charities and Correction in the City of New York shall be abolished and two separate and distinct Departments created, one of Charities, one of Correction."

It was in 1895 that appointments to the Attending Staffs of Bellevue and other city hospitals were placed in control of the three medical schools, with an "Open" Division at Bellevue. This caused

Doctors Who May Eat and Drink Forever

When the Academy of Medicine Moves to Its New Home on Fifth Avenue the Alfred Loomis Entertainment Fund, Jolliest of Legacies, Moves With It

By JOHN WALKER HARRINGTON

Drawings by W. Fletcher White

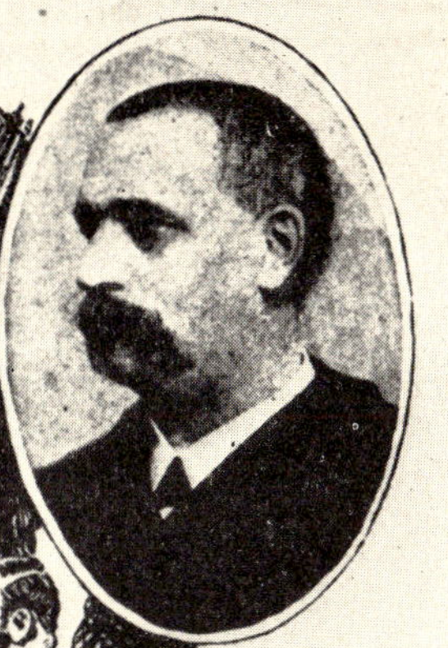

Doctor Loomis, patron of good cheer

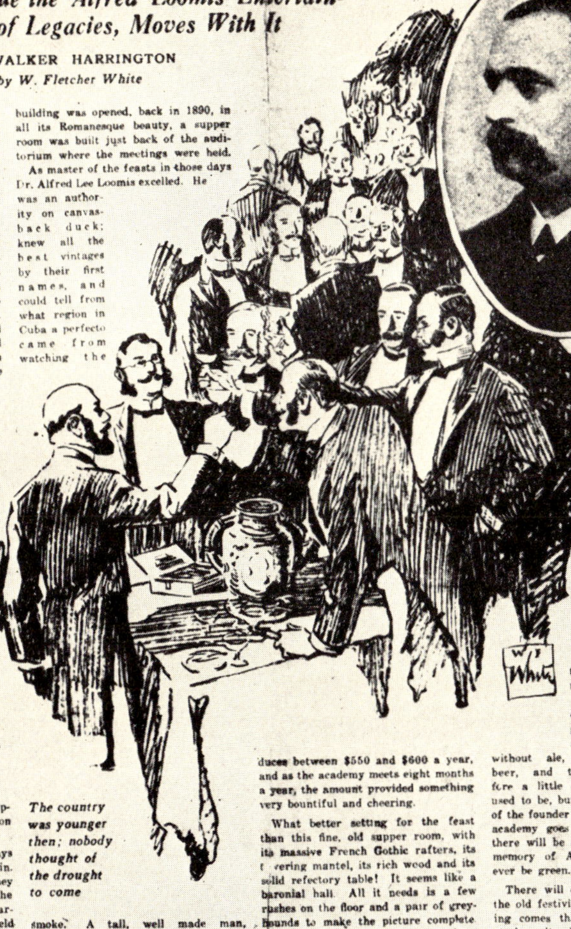

The country was younger then; nobody thought of the drought to come

DOCTORS are cherio folk, but happiest of all are the members of the New York Academy of Medicine. Without money and without price, every medical academician can be sure of having a good supper and a fine cigar after every monthly meeting.

Of course, it is well worth while to belong to that ancient and honorable institution for other reasons, for it is soon to have a new home in Fifth Avenue, which the Carnegie and Rockefeller foundations and hosts of grateful patients and its own means have provided millions to build and to endow. There it is going to take the second largest medical library in the United States, including vellum tomes with the mist of six centuries on them, rare relics of the healing art; time-mellowed old masters and a wealth of tradition. Just the same there is nothing it values more highly than the Alfred Lee Loomis Entertainment Fund, which enables all the members and all the good fellows to stand around the festal board and eat and drink in memory of one of the merriest souls that ever lived.

We laymen might never have known of it had mention of the odd bequest not been made in the formal application of the academy to the courts for permission to sell its present building at 17 West Forty-third Street. The officers were required to give a detailed account of their stewardship and to describe their various resources, so that the judge could be sure the academy could afford to branch out as it is about to do. So, naturally, he wanted to know whether the Loomis fund was used for motion pictures showing delightful appendicitis operations or for lectures on the latest in splints.

New York's physicians have always had a reputation as epicures to sustain. Ever since the city was founded they have had their supper clubs, and the present academy grew out of the yearly banquets of a relief association held in the Astor House in the '40s, when moralists were wondering if so luxurious a hotel, with all its Frenchified food, was good for the safety of the Republic.

The actual organization of the academy took place in 1847, when, as one of the chroniclers states, the doctors did not meet at the Astor House, as usual, "but at Peteler's, a fashionable restaurant in Broadway, near Prince Street." This, by the way, was quite near Niblo's Garden, where the great-grandmothers of the Follies girls used to be glorified. Year by year the academy grew in membership and influence, and it always made sure that its social life was not neglected. When the present building was opened, back in 1890, in all its Romanesque beauty, a supper room was built just back of the auditorium where the meetings were held.

As master of the feasts in those days Dr. Alfred Lee Loomis excelled. He was an authority on canvas-back duck; knew all the best vintages by their first names, and could tell from what region in Cuba a perfecto came from watching the smoke. A tall, well made man, with a roaring voice and a contagious laugh, was he. As chairman of the entertainment committee Dr. Loomis usually contributed half of the amount required for supper and asked Mr. John S. Brownne, who for the last forty-five years has been the librarian, to gather contributions from the other doctors to make up the balance of the bill.

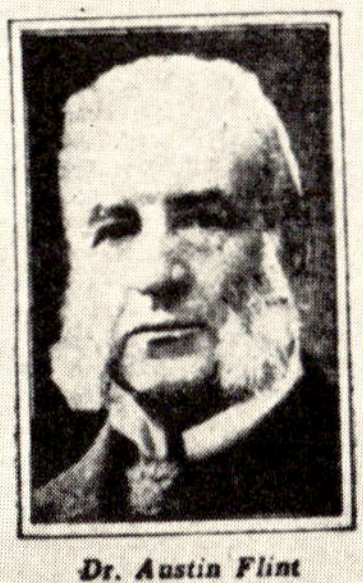

Dr. Austin Flint

"After I am gone, Brownne," said he one evening, "you won't have to do this at all. I have thought of an easier way."

When the jovial doctor went to the world beyond, his will revealed that he had left $10,000 to the academy as an entertainment fund to be used for the supper at the stated monthly meetings. This produces between $550 and $600 a year, and as the academy meets eight months a year, the amount provided something very bountiful and cheering.

What better setting for the feast than this fine, old supper room, with its massive French Gothic rafters, its towering mantel, its rich wood and its solid refectory table! It seems like a baronial hall. All it needs is a few rushes on the floor and a pair of greyhounds to make the picture complete. When this century was younger and nobody had ever thought of the drought which was to come upon the land there was brewed in a huge bowl a "high potency punch," said to have been an improvement on the dynamic mixture served by Mrs. Hicks Lord.

Dr. Loomis had bestowed much thought upon its formula. Under its influence, young doctors who were of modest demeanor usually talked to their elders in the bright spirit of all the ages. In one corner of the room could be found a keg or two of the best beer. There were heaping bowls of salads, sandwiches, not of the tea room sort, but enough to let a man know he had one; and there was ice cream in all the fanciful shapes known to the caterer's art. Urns of hot coffee gave forth a cheerful savor. The cigars were provided extra by various doctors, who individually took it upon themselves to crown the feast, and the rafters in time took on the tone of a meerschaum pipe.

Times and customs change and food prices go up to peaks. There are cakes these days without ale, and skittles without beer, and the supper is therefore a little different from what it used to be, but all the same the smile of the founder is over it all. When the academy goes to its larger quarters, there will be a supper room, and the memory of Alfred Lee Loomis will ever be green.

There will doubtless be so much of the old festivity when the housewarming comes that from its home in a steel vault will come forth the Astor loving cup, one of the society's most cherished links with oldtime New York. Often it appeared when noted visitors honored the academy and the day of grape juice had not dawned. And here is another gift with the rime of tradition upon it.

Back in the '80s, when the academy had moved from the lower city to a brownstone front of the Age of Innocence style, situated in West Thirty-first Street, there was much rejoicing. The president was Dr. Fordyce Barker, one of the handsomest and most impressive physicians of the period, who had assisted into this world most of the children

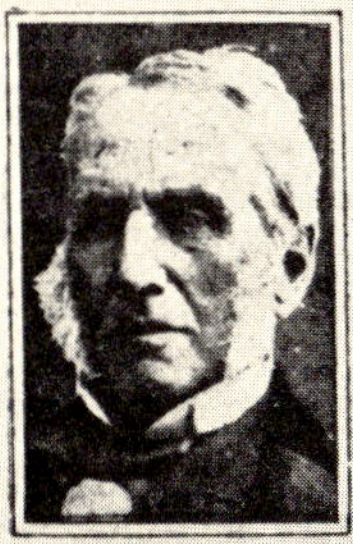

Dr. Willard Parker

Cont. on next page

FROM A FEATURE ARTICLE IN THE NEW YORK *Herald Tribune*, AUGUST 16, 1925

much discussion all over the city, and the opponents of the measure offered the following:

Resolved, That the New York Academy of Medicine deprecates the action of the Commissioners of Charities and Correction in abolishing the Consulting Board of Bellevue Hospital and the Consulting and Visiting Boards of the City, Harlem, Fordham, Gouverneur and Maternity Hospitals, the Hospital for Nervous Diseases, Almshouse, Workhouse, and Incurable Hospitals, and the Randall's Island Hospital.

Resolved, That the New York Academy of Medicine protests against the action of the Commissioners of Charities and Correction in placing the nominations, and practically the appointment, of the Consulting and Visiting Staffs of these Hospitals in the hands of the incorporated medical schools and the Fourth Division of Bellevue Hospital, (to all interests and purposes a monopoly), as contrary to the best interests of the institutions and of the medical profession.

Resolved, That a copy of these resolutions, signed by the President and Secretary of the New York Academy of Medicine, be forwarded to his Honor the Mayor and to the Commissioners of Charities and Correction.

This was such an important matter that a special meeting was called to discuss it but, after much exchange of opinion, the resolutions were not adopted.

The attention of the Academy was called to the fact that advertisements of Johann Hoff's Malt Extract were still appearing stating that it was endorsed by the Academy. This takes us back twenty-eight years to the trouble over that matter in 1867! On instructions, legal Counsel wrote the proprietors on behalf of the President of the Academy:

1. No report of any kind in favor of any such preparation was adopted by the Academy;

2. No report of any kind was made to the Academy by any of its committees, or by Dr. Bulkley or Dr. Griscom, in respect to the preparation advertised by you;

3. No report in language such as you profess to quote was made to the Academy by any of its committees, or by Dr. Bulkley or Dr. Griscom.

Under these conditions, the continuance of your publication must be at your own peril.

The Company replied "the officers had been misled into making the statements complained of under misapprehension of the true facts of the case"—and the circular was withdrawn.

The Carpenter Lecture in 1895 was delivered by Dr. H. M. Biggs, on "The Health of New York." His object was to discuss "the relative healthfulness of New York as compared with its past condition and with the past and present condition of other great cities of the world, and to point out where some of the gains have been made in the past and what we may hope to accomplish in the near future through improved hygienic conditions," prefacing his remarks with the statement "with certain limitations, the inhabitants of any city have it largely within their power to determine what degree of healthfulness their city shall have." It was a long and interesting talk.

The Anniversary Address was given by Dr. E. G. Janeway, on "The Progress of Medicine."

While other things ran smoothly, the Academy was in financial difficulties all the time. The trouble always appeared in the summer. What dues were paid voluntarily were paid early in the year. The Academy had expended considerable money on new stacks for the Library and the installation of its own electrical plant. Notes for $3,500, at 5 percent interest, were still unpaid. Instead of borrowing from the bank at 4 percent, the Treasurer of the Academy advanced the Treasurer of the Trustees the amount required to pay off the notes, "thus saving interest to outside parties." He was to be paid back "as soon as available funds would admit." By September, $1,500 had been paid back, but now the Treasurer of the Academy asked for the balance of $2,000, needed to pay the Academy's bills. There being no available money in the hands of the Trustees, at the moment, Dr. Bryant and Dr. Jacobi each loaned the Trustees $1,000 to pay back the loan.

At the end of December the Treasurer of the Academy reported he had "advanced a sufficient sum to pay the November bills, which sum has since been paid in, and we have a balance of $8. The bills offered for approval amount to $995.69. I will see that the salaries, $506.14 are paid, but recommend the other bills be held until the dues for next year be paid in sufficient amount to liquidate them." The Treasurer was advancing money to the Academy. Fellows were not the only ones derelict. The Treasurer reported that the Medico-Legal Society was in arrears for several months and that the officers did not seem to hold themselves responsible or care to pay. It was voted to put the bill in the hands of a collector, and inform the society that it could not use the rooms for meetings until the arrears were paid up.

In 1895 and 1896 volumes of *Transactions* appeared for 1893 and 1894. They were two years late, but contained a full and complete record of the papers read, and, again, a list of titles of papers read before the Sections. The Council authorized the publication for 1895 also.

The *American Medico-Surgical Bulletin* had offered to publish the *Transactions*. Dr. Peabody, appointed to investigate, reported the Company demanded the *Bulletin* be the official organ of the Academy, and have exclusive rights to publish all original papers. The offer was declined.

The scientific programs were arranged for one meeting each month by a Section, and very interesting papers were read at these meetings. One was given over to methods and results in amputations, five papers being read.

A meeting in 1895 was given over to diphtheria antitoxin, its production and usefulness. Another series of papers was presented in 1896 on its use, and the papers and discussion occupied two full meetings. Dr. Winters was opposed to it, but almost everyone else had had excellent results.

Another meeting was devoted to empyema in children.

Specialization was becoming more marked, and the Section on Obstetrics and Gynecology was divided into two Sections, one for each subject.

In 1896 the Carpenter Lecture was delivered by Dr. G. M. Sternberg, Surgeon General, U.S.A., on "The Etiology and Classification of Infectious Diseases," and the Anniversary Oration by Dr. George R. Fowler was "The Evolution of the Surgery of the 20th Century."

It would appear that the Section on Medicine was having some trouble in 1896, for its chairman reported it was in a deplorable condition, as regards interest and attendance. No provision was made by the Academy for sending postcard notices, which were absolutely necessary. The folder did not make any impression. The Fellows already were paying higher dues than "warranted by the privileges which we enjoy." The question was whether the Academy would pay, or whether it wished the Section chairman to bear the expense. The Secretary was instructed to inform Dr. R. W. Wilcox, the Chairman, that, in accordance with resolutions passed on previous occasions, the Council declined to attend to the private business of the Sections. Dr. Wilcox did not like this and the following January wrote: "You will oblige me by sending at once the exact minutes in regard to the Section notices, also the names of the Council who voted such minute. It is a very interesting matter to know what members are in the habit of voting that the Academy shall not pay its debts." The Secretary, as instructed, sent Dr. Wilcox the minute already sent him and added that the names of those voting for the resolution were not recorded, but he believed it was unanimous. Letters from Dr. Wilcox continued. In November, 1897, he was informed by the Council he had received all the information he was entitled to and it considered the matter closed.

The Library was flourishing, although constantly hampered by lack of funds. While it was usually acknowledged as the real backbone of the Academy, its budget, though carefully prepared, was never met by the appropriating authorities, for obvious reasons. By the end of the year the efforts of the Committee on Endowment had resulted in pledges of $30,000, contingent, however, on $20,000 more being secured. The Library contained 46,000 volumes at the end of 1896, of which 10,000 were duplicates. The journal room contained 680 different journals from twelve countries.

The Staff was small and little difficulties were constantly coming up. During an indisposition of Mr. Brownne, the librarian, an overcoat and two books were stolen. The Library Committee asked for a boy to act as page and *watcher*, and at the same time to be instructed in Library technique "so as to have an assistant librarian always in training." The Council did not see its way clear to this expense and suggested the person in charge of the Nurses' Bureau might serve. The Executive Committee deemed this "inexpedient."

Most surprising things were happening which kept the Council and Trustees busy. The Secretary reported that a Fellow had been using the reception room from one to three times a week for the last six months for the examination of patients! He had been told this could not continue, and the Trustees approved this action. The President reported that various national societies which had the free use of the Academy for meetings had let their rooms to exhibitors for a charge, and that on learning that the American Association of Rhinology and Laryngology had made similar arrangements, he had notified the Secretary of the Association that all applications for space must be approved by the Chairman of the Executive Committee and that the Academy declined to allow money to be received for the use of rooms provided gratis to the society which sublet them.

The Berkeley School, situated in 44th Street directly behind the Academy's building, suggested that the school be given the use of Hosack Hall every week-day morning from 9–9.30 for "exercises," and that a hole be cut in the north wall, at the School's expense, to avoid the boys' having to go on the streets to get there. Strangely enough this request was not granted.

There were constant complaints of the heating and ventilation of the Library and Section rooms. The Trustees purchased six electric fans for the Section rooms, and instructed the Secretary to find out the cost of a large suction pump to be placed over the doors of Hosack Hall. In his Valedictory Address Dr. Bryant said it needed no mention to remind the Fellows the heating and ventilation, "essentials of good health and personal comfort" were strikingly defective in the building, and the time was not far distant when radical measures must be adopted to correct them. "Certainly, it is hardly consistent in us to expose our friends or ourselves to contingencies of this nature while uttering learned disapprovals of their presence in other places."

In December, 1896, after having served seven years on the Board of Trustees, Dr. Jacobi resigned. A committee of one, appointed to see if the resignation was "final," reported that Dr. Jacobi's only reason was his feeling he was no longer needed. His resignation was not accepted.

Some strange gifts were presented to the Academy by its well wishers. Mention of the statue of "Esmeralda" has already been made. Dr. O. A. White presented a painting by his father-in-law, "one of South Carolina's greatest artists" (T. A. Thomas from Georgia), representing the "Fortuitous resuscitation from a state of trance at the entrance of grave robbers to despoil the body of valuable jewels." This hangs high up on the wall of the "museum" room of the Academy today.

Early in 1896, realizing that it had almost reached the half century mark, the Academy appointed Drs. Jacobi, A. M. Jacobus, and W. M. Polk a committee to report on the "advisability" of a until October to make up its mind, officially. It recommended the celebration should be held, limited to one evening, and that the semi-centennial celebration in January, 1897. It took the committee President appoint committees of arrangements, entertainment, and invitations.

These committees worked hard; that on entertainment raised by subscription $3,329 for its purposes, and sent out notices to all Fellows with an answer card reading:

I do ——— intend to be present at the semi-centennial of the Academy of Medicine.

I subscribe toward the expenses $———. Enclosed please find my check.

At the first meeting in 1897 officers for the ensuing year were elected. The question was raised when officers took office. The that except in emergencies, which did not now exist, the President should serve one term only. Dr. Janeway, the only candidate, was elected. The question was raised when officers took office. The President announced "at once." Dr. Janeway then moved that this year the President-elect take office at the first meeting in February. This was carried unanimously, and was a very gracious gesture on the part of Dr. Janeway so that Dr. Bryant could preside at the Semi-Centennial.

The celebration was held at Carnegie Music Hall, January 29, 1897. This elaborate engraved invitation on sheets of paper 8 by 11¾ inches was sent out:

THE PRESIDENT AND COUNCIL
REQUEST THE PLEASURE OF YOUR COMPANY
AT THE
SEMI-CENTENNIAL CELEBRATION
OF
THE NEW YORK ACADEMY OF MEDICINE
ON FRIDAY EVENING, JANUARY THE TWENTY-NINTH.

Joseph D. Bryant, M.D.
PRESIDENT

Reginald H. Sayre, M.D.
SECRETARY

Then follows the list of the Committee on Arrangements, Dr. W. M. Polk, chairman, with the eight other members; Committee on Invitations, Dr. J. H. Girdner, chairman, and four other members; and Committee on Entertainment, Dr. Daniel Lewis, chairman, and the six members of this committee.

Cards of admission were issued: engraved ones, for Mr. ——— and lady; small printed orange ones for admission to the balcony; and others for the Reception at the Academy building.

Dr. Bryant welcomed the large gathering and expressed the gratitude of the Fellows to the laity for its support in the past and his hopes for continuation of that support in the future. He emphasized the service of the profession to the public without remuneration, and the Academy's activities in improving the public welfare and the city's health. Of the original 184 Founders of the Academy, eight were still living and two were present and would speak.

Dr. S. S. Purple, now seventy-five, still true to his convictions on ethics, stressed the motives which led to the foundation of the Academy: "a barrier between quackery and medical integrity, the establishment of a stringent motive for ethical observance—a desire to stand well among one's fellows, and a determined step toward professional harmony." He hoped these motives would always be the same. He then spoke briefly of the Library, for the development of which he had done so much, and of its needs.

Dr. Lewis A. Sayre, seventy-seven, reminisced a little, and then Dr. Jacobi delivered the oration of the evening. It was a scholarly address, in which he spoke of what medicine had done for mankind in the past in spite of all obstacles, and of its future opportunities. He outlined the Academy's no small part in it. He asked for financial help for the Library, to make it self-supporting and he closed with these words:

> The rapidly increasing facilities of investigation have changed the methods and aspects of modern medicine to such an extent as to make me anxious to know what the orator of the next semi-centennial celebration will have to say to you. Part of it I know, and you will know it too when I beg you to consider with me during the last minute of my address the possibilities and the certainties of medicine. Its methods of investigation will never be changed, for they have become those of natural science, and these, because they are based on observation and experimentation, are unalterable. Indeed, medicine is a part of the natural sciences; the human organism, well and sick, physical and spiritual, is the subject of its scrutiny. Man's nature, both normal and abnormal, belongs to the domain of medical inquiry. Psychology has for some time past become a branch of physiology. The sound mind, its aberrations and freaks, the soul with its holiness or turpitude, no matter whether considered by the believing philosopher or the searching materialist, are topics of biological study. The explanation and relations of most intimate physical and psychical processes are sought for, will always be sought for, by the sanitarian, the teacher, the clergyman, the judge, the statesman. It is in medicine that they will find them. The time will soon come when the culture of a nation will be estimated according to the mutual relations of medicine and the people.

This makes interesting reading today.

Dr. Bryant, who was his personal physician, then introduced President Grover Cleveland: "It is now our distinguished honor to welcome a gentleman whose deep interest in the affairs of the

Academy of Medicine has caused him to lay aside for a brief time the duties of his great office, that he might join with us in the ceremonies of the occasion. It is my great pleasure to present to you one for whom sincere men have a profound respect, patriotic people a high esteem, and intimate friends an abiding affection."

Mr. Cleveland made an excellent address, appreciative of the efforts of the profession, and in high praise of the old country doctor. He urged the Academy never to forget its duty was not only, as highly intelligent members of the community, to develop the science of medicine, but to use its tremendous influence in the cause of true citizenship.

After the addresses the audience adjourned to the Academy building for a reception and collation, and were shown over the building.

Dr. Bryant was an excellent President. He was attentive to his duties and presided over all but three of the Stated Meetings.

1897–1898

Edward G. Janeway

Dr. Janeway, in his introductory address, outlined some of the important matters which might be handled by the Academy. He painted a dark picture of the status of expert medical testimony, and called for a careful study of the subject and suggestions for elevating its standards. Tuberculosis and its control were another challenge. Much was being done for the health of schoolchildren, but the profession was negligent of the health of those in medical colleges and in hospitals.

Portraits of three presidents, Drs. Cock, Post, and Austin Flint, and of an ardent worker in the Academy, as well as a great scientist, Alonzo Clark were absent from the Academy's walls.

Dr. Janeway mentioned the splendid and wise gift of a million dollars by J. P. Morgan to the Lying-In Hospital, not to found a *new* organization, but to develop an old one.

The Academy must face the expense of improving the heating and ventilation of its building, sources of great discomfort and complaint.

Dr. Edward Gamaliel Janeway was fifty-six years old when he became the twenty-second President. The son of a physician, he was not at all interested in studying medicine and it was not until 1862, in his second year at P. and S., when he became a Medical Cadet at the Army Hospital in Newark that he began to study in earnest. He received his M.D. from the College of Physicians and Surgeons in 1864, was on the interne staff at Bellevue for two years, and then became Curator of Bellevue Hospital for six years, devoting all his time to the Dead House. He had been Visiting Physician to the Charity Hospital, and by request became Chief of Staff and lived there, to the great improvement of the institution. He was Commissioner of Health, as a part-time job, 1875–1881, so the Academy had two successive presidents with that background. For a number of years he held various professional positions at Bellevue Hospital Medical College, succeeding Dr. Flint as Professor of Medicine, and was also on the Visiting Staff of Bellevue Hospital. An indefatigable worker, he did not maintain a private practice, but was one of the best-known consultants in New York.

One of the first things the Academy did was to appoint a committee of three to express to Mr. Morgan its appreciation of his "munificent donation." This is in contrast to the action of the County Society, which appointed one to wait on him to say it was unwise and contrary to the best interests of the profession.

The Section on Ophthalmology and Otology informed the Academy that reporters from the lay press were present at its meetings and had regular Academy folder notices which they said were sent to their offices. The Section asked whether these reporters should be allowed to attend. It was voted that the matter must be decided by the Sections themselves. A motion to send the folders regularly, in the future, was lost. The *Medical Record*, December 4, 1897, stated:

> The time to arrest an evil is at its inception, and for that reason we take occasion just now to utter a word of reproof to the officers of the New York Academy of Medicine. Through the negligence or the connivance of certain persons connected with this society, reports of the meetings of the general body and of individual sections have appeared in the daily papers with startling frequency and regularity this autumn. Reporters are not detailed to report medical meetings unless word is sent to the editors that the proceedings are to be of interest to the general public. The report of the annual meeting of the academy, with a full abstract of the anniversary address, is proper enough, for the occasion is intentionally made one of interest to the laity; but for reports of section meetings there can be no excuse whatever, except that of a desire to advertise boldly and badly. The latest offence has been committed by the section on neurology and psychiatry.

In January, 1897, a committee of eight was appointed to report on "tuberculosis in its relation to the public welfare and the measures which should be adopted to curtail its ravages and the ways in which the Academy may be useful in the attainment of the aims proposed." This Committee was enlarged to eleven later, of whom the President was one.

The Board of Health passed an ordinance making it mandatory to report cases of tuberculosis. Thereupon the Committee reported to the Academy:

1. In the opinion of this Committee, the Board of Health might wisely delay the enforcement of compulsory notification, but should adopt more stringent methods for the care of all sputum in factories, workshops, tenement houses, ferry boats, places of public assembly, and public conveyances.

2. In the opinion of this Committee the establishment and maintenance by the city of an hospital or hospitals, to which indigent tuberculous patients may be admitted, is advisable.

3. This Committee recommends the appointment by the Legislature of a commission for the establishment and management of sanitaria in healthy country districts in this state, for the care of indigent tuberculous patients in the early stages of the disease.

4. This Committee would commend to the State Board of Health the importance of careful regulation of the sanitary condition of hotels and sleeping cars throughout the state.

E. G. Janeway, CHAIRMAN
T. Mitchell Prudden, SECRETARY

The report was adopted and ordered sent to the Board and its Advisory Committee.

The Academy voted to appoint a committee of five or seven "to study and investigate the whole subject of expert medical testimony as now given in the courts of justice," as suggested by the President, and to make recommendations for improving its character, promote the ends of justice, and "redound to the honor and dignity of the medical profession." Dr. Jacobi seconded the motion.

During the summer the members of the Committee undertook to find out the methods employed in foreign countries.

The Committee reported it was necessary to establish some standard of excellence in those who wished to appear as experts; that experts should be appointed by the presiding justice of the court so that they should have a judicial function, should not become wit nesses for the plaintive or defendant, and should be free of all bias in their judgment. Fees should be fixed by the court. The Committee felt that it would be impossible to delegate to any County Society or even to the Academy the examination of candidates for the position of special expert. The Regents were the proper persons to handle the matter and they should require each person to register and present evidence of his qualifications, which would be similar in force to the qualifications for a commissioner in lunacy. Each candidate should:

1) Register what department of medicine he desires to appear in;
2) Have been in practice ten years and in the practice of his specialty for five years;
3) Have had special opportunities for research during three years, either in laboratory, dispensary, hospital or asylum practice; and
4) Present a certificate of good moral character.
5) Qualifications should be sworn to and endorsed by two officers of his County Medical Society.

The names of all applicants should be published by the Board of Regents in at least one medical and one legal journal for two months subsequent to the application, the Regents to be given power to refuse to grant the license on objections presented under oath.

The Committee had discussed the subject with Justices Barrett, Ingraham, Patterson, and Rumsey. It would be wise to have the appointment made by the Judge of the Court in which the case is to be tried upon the application of counsel for either plaintive or defendant, or in the wisdom of the court; if an expert was necessary, the court should appoint one, three, or more experts as judicial advisers, who were merely to give testimony by questions and cross-questions before the court.

In its discussion of a bill presented by Mr. Plessy for improving the procedure, the report admitted that the bill was a good one but did not go far enough, and recommended, at some length, amendments to the bill as introduced. It was voted that the committee be empowered to consult the legal counsel of the Academy in drafting a bill. This was a most cumbersome report, but represented a tremendous amount of creditable work done.

The Charter for the Greater City of New York was under consideration. Dr. Stephen Smith read a careful analysis of that part dealing with the Health Department, stating that the establishment of one Department for the whole area was "an event of transcendent importance in the history of Municipal or State Medicine," but that several aspects of the plan were subject to criticism, especially that the President of the Board of Health could not be a physician. The Health Commissioners of New York and Brooklyn and those of New Brighton, Port Richmond, and Clifton on Staten Island were all present and discussed the subject.

Dr. Grandin thought the exclusion of a physician from the Presidency of the Board was an insult and he believed it to be unconstitutional. Dr. Janeway left the Chair to take part in the discussion. He was strongly in favor of one lay member of the Board, but not necessarily its president. If the laity was represented on the Board, the public would pay more attention to its orders than if these were given by physicians only. Dr. Smith could not see that point.

The President was authorized to appoint a committee of five to consider the matter and report at the next meeting. It reported back that, while extraordinary powers were given to the Board of Health, these had already been in operation for thirty years. The Board had used them very charily,—and only in times of great emergency. It would doubtless continue to do so. Owing to the advanced state of the Charter, the Committee limited its suggestions to a few important changes: there should be three commissioners, two of them practicing physicians; the Health Officer of the Port and President of the Board of Police should also be members, ex officio; the President of the Board should be appointed by the Mayor; and the office of coroner should be abolished, substituting for it the "Massachusetts system."

The report was received, and then Dr. Piffard assailed the Code section authorizing the Board to require any physician to submit, within three hours after demand, an affidavit stating the name and address of any patient suffering from a pestilential, contagious, or infectious disease. Dr. Jacobi brought out that the next section made failure to comply a misdemeanor, and required every visiting, hospital, and consulting physician to report immediately any practitioner who was evading the rules, at risk of losing his position, and any other penalty the Board might impose. He objected to making physicians spies. It was "undignified, unworthy, and dangerous, and certainly ought to be stricken out. Moreover it was unconstitutional," for, while physicians were compelled to report a felony, this required them to report a misdemeanor, which was not in accord with the Constitution.

Dr. Janeway felt the law looked more aggressive than it was, for he knew of no case in the past—and the law had been on the books for eight years—in which it had been enforced. Dr. Jacobi replied that if the law was a dead letter it had better be stricken out; it could become very dangerous. In the end, the report was laid on the table, to be taken up later, when there was more time for discussion. At a later meeting the Committee's report was voted on, adopted, and recommended for communication to the Mayor and "if necessary to the government." This was another case of "wasted effort," for the Committee had been told there was little chance of any change now.

Dr. Baruch, an enthusiast on health and cleanliness, called the Academy's attention to the fact that although a law had been passed in 1895 providing for the establishment and maintenance of public baths for New York, "not one stone had been laid." He urged a committee to impress upon the city authorities the necessity of immediate action. This was done. The Committee found Mayor Strong sympathetic, and a city lot on Rivington Street was selected, plans were drawn, and bids advertised for.

Two years later, nothing further having been accomplished, the Committee waited upon Mayor Van Wyck, explained matters to him, and roused his interest. He promised to communicate at once with the Commissioner of Public Buildings and erect two moderately priced public baths on the East and West Sides of the City, in localities recommended by the Committee. The Committee was thanked and discharged.

In the fall of 1897, Dr. Jacobi called attention to an outbreak of yellow fever in the Southwest, during the summer. He offered a resolution which was unanimously carried:

> *Resolved,* That the New York Academy of Medicine authorize the President to call the committee appointed years ago, and never discharged, and direct it to resume its interrupted labors and to report to the Academy of Medicine, for presentation to the Congress of the United States for adoption, the old bill, or a new bill, or to support a proper bill offered by great medical or commercial bodies, contemplating the centralization under the National Government of the means to protect efficiently the health of the American people against the importation and dissemination of contagious diseases.

The report was made the next month and adopted, and the Committee was discharged with thanks. There is no copy of the report on file.

In December another committee was appointed

> to consider the question of public sanitation and hygiene in all its bearings, particularly in reference to the prevention and stamping out of widespread epidemic disease, to the collection of statistics calculated to benefit the public health, to the furnishing of public information both of a preventive and curative nature, and to the study of all those problems in connection with their solution, by the general Government; the said committee shall also prepare a bill or bills to be presented to the Congress of the United States by the New York Academy of Medicine, either independently or conjointly with other scientific or commercial bodies, with a view to finally establishing under the general Government a department or bureau of health.

The President appointed Drs. J. D. Bryant, A. Jacobi, T. M. Prudden, and T. G. Thomas.

This "Committee on National Public Health" reported, opposing the so-called Caffery Bill in the Senate in its original form or with the modifications. Passage of the bill would be a serious misfortune to the interests of the public health in the United States: it would tend to postpone the establishment of a genuine national health bureau, because the provisions disclosed a very narrow view of the real importance of public health organization and emphasized a single phase of health protection which science and practice had shown to be of entirely secondary importance.

The Committee endorsed another bill—practically that introduced by the Academy of Medicine a year before—and recommended its unqualified support.

It was then voted that

WHEREAS, The happiness and the physical wellbeing of a people and the business prosperity of a country depend on the wisdom, the force and the execution of the sanitary laws and

WHEREAS, A diversity of opinion and a division of responsibility without cooperation in sanitary measures cause confusion in the efforts, and defeat in the practice, of sanitary aims and

WHEREAS, The medical profession of a country are the proper custodians of its health, therefore be it

Resolved, That the Fellows of the New York Academy of Medicine do earnestly recommend the establishment of a bureau of health with the power to administer within the constitutional limits the sanitary needs of the United States;

Resolved, That copies of the foregoing be sent to the New York Chamber of Commerce and the New York Board of Trade and Transportation.

In 1898 a committee was appointed to confer with other societies attempting to secure a bill legalizing midwives in New York State. Conferences with committees from the County Medical Society, County Medical Association, King's County Medical Society and the Society of Medical Jurisprudence disclosed great divergence of opinion: some favored abolition of midwives; some favored restoration, registration, and regulation of their practice; others favored leaving things in *status quo,* because any legislation concerning midwives would give them a legal status, which was thought inadvisable. When the committee reported these facts and asked either to be discharged or to be instructed how to act, it was told to confer with the Chairman of the Section on Obstetrics and Gynecology as to a proper bill for the control of midwives. It did so and, at a meeting of the Section, resolutions were adopted strongly recommending the taking of immediate steps to secure the passage of a law providing for the supervision of all persons not legally qualified physicians now engaged in practicing midwifery and debarring from such practice all persons not proven to be competent and qualified, and also containing such provisions as, without conflicting with existing rights, would tend to confine the practice of midwifery to qualified medical practitioners.

The committee noted that these resolutions in effect provided for the gradual abolition of midwives. It asked for instructions as to how to proceed now. The report was laid on the table and the committee discharged.

The scientific programs were well arranged and many good papers were read. A few may be mentioned as showing the problems that interested the profession at that time: the prevention and spread of contagious diseases, tuberculous infection from dust, and "The Use of Climate" for the tuberculous; sunstroke and a report on 805 cases in 1896, by Dr. Alexander Lambert, occupying two meetings; intubation in various conditions, and the serum exanthemata after antitoxin; "The Use of Modified Milk in Health and Disease"—a "great advance"—by its advocate Dr. Rotch of Boston; "The Ultimate Results of Thyroid Treatment in Cretinism"; "Uterine Fibroids in Pregnancy, Their Pathology and Treatment"; "The Radical Treatment of Enlarged Prostate and Its Pathology"; "Experimental Observations on Uraemic Intoxications," by Dr. C. A. Herter; "The Successful Treatment of Hemophilia by Serum Injections"; and "The Sterilization of Urethral Instruments," by Dr. Edward Martin of Philadelphia. One meeting each month was under the direction of a Section.

During the year the Academy lost, by death, a number of Fellows who had played an important part in its history. Memorial addresses of gratitude and appreciation were given in honor of Dr. W. T. Lusk, a pioneer in aseptic obstetrics, by an early associate, Dr. A. A. Smith, and of Dr. J. Lewis Smith, pioneer pediatrician, by Ellsworth Eliot, Sr. The latter paper, well worth reading today, appeared in the *Transactions* (2d Ser., XIII, 220). The modest, retiring Joseph O'Dwyer, inventor of intubation, was eulogized by Dr. Northrup.

Dr. S. S. Purple, tireless, determined Secretary of the first building fund, President for two terms, Trustee, who was named by the Council "Founder" of the Library, also died in 1898. A firm believer in the necessity of a strict and detailed Code of Ethics, he was estranged by the Academy action thereon in 1884, but as time went on, and the Academy did not actually degenerate, he occasionally came back and gave a book to the Library from time to time. His eulogy was not delivered until the following year.

The Carpenter Lectures were given by Dr. Park, "Contributions of Bacteriology to Therapeutics," in 1897, and by Dr. C. A. Herter, "Modern Views of Certain Symptoms and Causes of Renal Disease," in 1898.

The Anniversary Addresses were by Dr. H. M. Biggs, "Sanitary Science, the Medical Profession and the Public" in 1897, and by Dr. W. H. Welch, "Landmarks in the History of Pathology" in 1898.

Portraits of Dr. Loomis and Dr. Roosa were presented to the Academy, the first by his family and the latter by a group of Fellows.

The Constitution and By Laws were amended and brought up to date, in a new edition. Except for slight details the changes were unimportant; the time for change in administration was set for the first meeting in January instead of in February.

On recommendation of the Council, the Academy elected the following Benefactors:

Hon. Grover Cleveland
Hon. Roswell P. Flower
James M. Brown
H. Holbrook Curtis, M.D.
James S. Cushman
W. E. Dodge
W. H. Draper, M.D.
E. P. Fowler, M.D.
Everett Herrick, M.D.
S. Inslee
A. Jacobi, M.D.
J. S. Kennedy
W. M. Polk, M.D.
D. O. Mills
M. Allen Starr, M.D.
F. W. Vanderbilt.

The *Transactions* for 1895 included all papers read and much of the discussion. This was the last complete record the Academy ever published. A volume appeared in 1903, which gave all papers read at the Semi-centennial, and a few of the memorials, Anniversary Addresses, and Carpenter Lectures for the period 1896–1901.

Financially the Academy was in difficulties. In October, 1897, there was a deficit of $863.07; the Treasurer reported 188 Fellows in arrears to the amount of $4,588.50 for dues. The Council voted to pay salaries and the gas bill, but to hold all other bills. Meanwhile the President and Treasurer were to send a letter to the Fellows stating the necessity for prompt payment of dues. If there was no response within a week, a collector was to be sent. By November, $1,300 had been received, but the deficit was $629.62.

At the end of 1898 the Treasurer was only $163 short, and Fellows only owed $2,744. The Council went into a committee of the whole and decided to cut all appropriations—the Academy must live within its income the next year.

In the main, the Library did very well. The Committee on Endowment handed in a check for $14,000, the fruit of its labors. Ex-Governor Flower had contributed $1,000 to found the Dr. Orville Ranney-Flower Fund; and another gift of $1,000 was to found the James S. Cushman Library Fund. In December, 1897, Mrs. Woerishoffer, who had contributed $25,000 in 1886, presented $15,000 to the Library Fund. In addition to the $14,000, considerable sums had been pledged conditional to the raising of $50,000. Dr. Jacobi persuaded Mrs. Woerishoffer to give her contribution outright and suggested to the Council others might influence their friends to do the same.

In 1897 the Library had 38,320 volumes, exclusive of duplicates. There were 8,582 names in the register of readers, who were already more than could be accommodated easily. The Committee felt a gallery would probably be soon needed for more space and for more stacks. The Library had overspent its budget by $512.

The year 1898 was a banner year. The Governors of the New York Hospital donated its library of 23,000 volumes. There were many duplicates, of course, and as the Governors wanted as many as possible to benefit by the gift, a number of books were given to twenty-one other libraries and institutions. The New York Hospital paid for the transfer and for a bronze tablet announcing the gift. About 1,500 new titles were added to the catalogue, making the library "without question" the largest medical library in the country next to the Surgeon General's. The Library Staff estimated it would take eighteen months to sort, catalogue and place these volumes, but the Library Committee took great pride in noting that the task was accomplished in four months.

Mrs. E. C. Seguin presented her late husband's special collection of monographs and pamphlets on the nervous system, bound, numbering some 367 items, which he had been thirty years collecting, and also a large number of other books. The collection included an oil painting of his late father, Dr. Edouard Seguin, a framed letter from Pope Pius IX commending the elder Dr. Seguin's work in ameliorating the condition of backward, imbecile children, a bronze medallion of Charcot given to him "by the Master himself," and the only extant large photograph of Brown-Séquard.

The widow of Dr. Mourraille, a former Fellow, presented his library of 232 volumes, mostly French works.

The Fellowship were asked to express themselves on the question of opening the Library on Sundays. Of the 815 Resident Fellows, 249 voted for it and 157 against. As it would increase the expenses by $600 a year, the plan was laid on the table.

The Library Committee stated that the stacks were practically full, and that more must be provided. A gallery around Woerishoffer Hall was suggested as the only solution; it would add 10,000 feet of shelf space. Another assistant librarian was also needed. The Trustees instructed its Committee on Investment to look into the desirability of purchasing the lot in the rear on 44th Street to increase its plot.

The Library Committee felt the Council were very short-sighted in keeping its appropriation down. It never got what it asked for, especially for binding books and pamphlets. In 1898 it was within its budget of $4,500, and took care to state it had been much handicapped in purchasing new books because of having to cut down expenses. In response to a request for $4,500, the Academy voted $3,500 for the Library and, on any surplus accumulating, an additional $1,000.

It is impossible to give any statistics for the Library for 1898, as the careful and detailed (typewritten) annual report of the Committee leaves blanks for every figure!

In 1899 there were approximately 70,000 volumes in the stacks and the Library Fund was yielding $2,218.46. All of this had to be spent for *new books*, however. The Council appointed Dr. Bryant and the Chairman of the Library Committee to look into the question of obtaining an appropriation from the City, as a "free circulating library." (Taking out of books was limited to Fellows only.)

Dr. Janeway was a splendid President. He only failed to preside at stated meetings once, and was very active at Council and Trustees' meetings.

1899–1904

W. H. Thomson · Robert F. Weir
Andrew H. Smith

1899–1900

THE NEXT six years were marked particularly by activity in the public health field, excellent scientific programs, financial difficulties and internal peace.

Dr. Janeway, in turning over the Chair to his successor, regretted the slowness in building up the Library Fund and the difficulties in improving expert medical testimony, the two chief obstacles being the constitutional right to trial by jury, and the attitude of the legal profession. He also still hoped the Academy would establish a laboratory.

Dr. W. H. Thomson, twenty-third President, the son of a missionary in Syria, was sixty-six years of age. A graduate of the Albany Medical College, he had joined the Academy in 1864. He had been Anniversary Orator in 1878 and 1893. He was a very dignified gentleman and was considered a great clinician. In his Inaugural he outlined some of the medical problems which confronted the profession and which might be cleared up by the Academy, and reiterated Dr. Janeway's hopes for a true research laboratory in the Academy. He mentioned no public health activities which should engage its attention.

The scientific sessions started off well, and throughout the two years were well planned and worked out. Three evenings were given over to ten papers on syphilis, its diagnosis, and early and late symptoms. One of them, a special meeting, was held to hear Dr. Adami of Montreal.

Malaria occupied two evenings, and anaesthesia, local and general, another. Three meetings were given over to discussion of cancer, and Drs. Park and Gaylord presented the results of their studies in Buffalo on its etiology.

Dr. Jacobi read a report on "Artificial Infant Feeding," which had been read at the Thirteenth International Congress, and the next meeting was given over to five papers on the subject, by Drs. Blackader of Montreal, Rotch of Boston, Crozer-Griffith of Philadelphia, Holt, and Northrup.

The Anniversary Address in 1899 was delivered by Dr. Lewis S. Pilcher, "The Development of the Surgery of the Kidney, with Some of the Lessons Connected Therewith"; and in 1900 by Dr. Robert Abbe, "The Problem of Appendicitis from the Medical and Surgical Points of View."

The Wesley M. Carpenter lectures were given by Dr. F. A. Packard of Philadelphia, on "Infection through the Tonsil, Especially in Connection with Acute Articular Rheumatism," and by Dr. James Ewing, "Conjugation in the Asexual Cycle of the Malarial Parasite."

In public health measures the activity of the Academy was carried on chiefly by Dr. Jacobi.

Dr. Nammack introduced resolutions, which were passed, calling attention to the fact that pulmonary tuberculosis, especially among the poor, caused more deaths in New York State than any other disease, and that treatment in special institutions had been proved advantageous. Because private endeavor was inadequate, however well directed, he urged that the Academy recommend the establishment of state and municipal sanatoria, for the treatment and prevention of dissemination of the disease.

Dr. W. W. Keen of Philadelphia, President of the American Medical Association, sent an appeal to the medical profession to oppose proposed legislation in the District of Columbia to outlaw vivisection. The Academy endorsed the appeal.

Dr. Jacobi introduced resolutions, which were passed, calling attention to the act, passed in 1898, laying a war tax on legacies to charitable, educational, and religious institutions. War taxes were unnecessarily large and needed to be reduced. Income to such institutions was seriously impaired and the Academy petitioned

Congress to relieve them. Every Fellow was requested to inform our representatives in both houses of Congress of the reasons for this petition.

Also at Dr. Jacobi's instigation, the Academy petitioned Congress to appropriate $9,000 for extra and much needed shelves for the Surgeon General's Library.

And, finally, the Academy passed this resolution offered by Dr. Jacobi and approved by the Council:

Resolved, That the committee appointed by the Academy be instructed to use its influence to have the municipal hospital constructed for cases in the early, and presumably curable, stage of phthisis;

Resolved, That while the proper designation for such a hospital would be for "curable cases," yet in view of the bad effect the refusal to be admitted would produce, the designation should be "Hospital for Incipient Cases";

Resolved, That the committee be instructed to use its influence to have the hospital placed in that locality which will be the most productive of good, and where there shall be such space that it will not be an injury to the neighborhood, which would be the case if it were placed in a populous locality;

Resolved, That the Committee be instructed to use its utmost endeavors to have such examinations for admission made by thoroughly competent physicians possessed of such moral stamina as shall prevent advanced and incurable cases from being sent to the hospital for incipient cases;

Resolved, That the committee be instructed to use its influence to have the rules and regulations of this hospital such that it shall not become an unnecessary burden upon the community.

An article appeared in the *New York Herald* frankly criticizing the Academy and quoting an interview with Dr. R. W. Wilcox (the gentleman who protested so vigorously because the Academy would not pay for postal announcements of Section meetings), and naming Dr. Allen Fitch as the reporter who had the interview. This was brought to the attention of the Council. Letters were exchanged, but the Council referred the whole correspondence to the Academy without recommendations.

Dr. Wilcox admitted the interview, but had prohibited the use of his name. Dr. Fitch (a Fellow) admitted he was employed by the *Herald*, but did not understand what it all meant and regretted the incident. The *Herald* had published his name contrary to agreement. A letter from the Sunday Editor was read, admitting Dr. Wilcox's name should not have been mentioned and expressing his regrets. The Academy decided the explanations were satisfactory.

Dr. Spreng had inserted advertisements in the *New York World* identifying himself as a former member of the Academy. The matter was submitted to the Council and Dr. Spreng was requested to withdraw his reference to the Academy or state that he had been expelled (1874) from it.

Financially, the going had not been smooth. The loan to pay off the bonds was repaid, "owing to the generous subscriptions of $2,000 from Fellows and the accumulation of initiation fees and other income withheld for that purpose."

In both years the Treasurer was in difficulties. At the end of 1899 the Academy was in debt for $834 for running expenses, with $3,163 unpaid dues. The next year his deficit was only $725, with unpaid dues amounting to $3,544. In both cases the Treasurer was instructed to pay salaries and to hold other bills until after the first of the year.

The Council had always been very slow in acting on delinquents, but, it must be admitted, less so than the Trustees whose responsibility it was. Dues were payable before February first. In June, 1899, thirty-five delinquents were reported owing from $20 to $90, not including dues for the current year. Nine were dropped and action on the rest was postponed.

The building had to be kept in repair, and Dr. Jacobi reported in 1900 "the lower or main hallway floor was beautifully laid in mosaic."

Dr. E. F. Brush, a Fellow, wrote that he had promised Dr. Loomis several years earlier to obtain a moosehead to hang in the banquet hall. He had finally secured a good head and offered it to the Academy. It was hung and the Council ordered a plate placed beneath it, saying it was the gift of Dr. Brush.

Dr. J. S. Billings, formerly of the Surgeon General's Library and now in charge of the Consolidated Public Library, agreed to cooperate with the Library Committee and extend his library's department of biology and other sciences allied to pure medicine, thus relieving the Academy from further expansion in that field.

At the end of 1900 the Library had 52,895 bound volumes on its shelves, not including duplicates (of which it had 36,105!). It was receiving 616 journals at a cost of $1,875. Readers signing the register numbered 11,520. The Committee warned that with the present increase the stacks would be full within five years. It also warned that the staff was insufficient and, while it was doing its best, with the increase of readers and books it would soon be utterly swamped. The deficiencies of the heating and ventilating plant were causing great damage to the books and bindings were fast disintegrating.

The Library Committee were not the only complainants. The *Medical Record* in 1900 comments editorially:

VENTILATION AT THE ACADEMY

The season's work is about to open in all its activity at the Academy of Medicine, with every prospect of success and interest we hope, but there is one point of which we should like to speak, though it seems almost an act of temerity to do so in connection with a temple partially devoted to the worship of Hygeia. The ventilation in the academy building, in the main hall, in the library, and in the section rooms is nothing less than abominable. After a meeting has been in session an hour, especially in the sections, the air becomes so foul that it is impossible to take a great amount of interest in the proceedings, and many become somnolent or seek relief in flight. Opening of windows gives some relief, but this is usually objected to by those who, from exigencies of space or for other reasons, sit near those openings. This matter is one which it ought not to be difficult to correct, and it seems almost an absurd anomaly that it should exist, but that it does exist will be made evident to any one who will sit through a moderately crowded section meeting, or attend one of the meetings in the main hall.

Several portraits were presented: of the late Dr. Flint, by his family; of Dr. Bryant by some of his friends; of the late Dr. E. L.

Beadle by bequest of his niece; and of Dr. J. T. Metcalfe. Drs. Beadle and Metcalfe had been prominent in Academy affairs in days gone by.

A portrait of Dr. John P. Gray, for forty years Medical Superintendent of the State Lunatic Asylum at Utica, was presented by Dr. Ordronaux. Dr. Gray had not been a member, and a few months later, the Trustees voted that no portrait should be accepted to hang in the Academy unless it were of an officer or official of the Academy, or someone prominently identified with its objects and interests.

There were a number of deaths of Fellows who had been very active in Academy affairs.

Dr. W. F. Cushman, a Fellow since 1880, had been Treasurer 1883–88, and Treasurer of the Trustees, 1891–98. He had rendered invaluable service to the Academy in troubled financial times. He had resigned at the end of the preceding year on account of ill health. He was sixty-five.

Dr. H. E. Crampton, Treasurer since 1898, died in 1899, at the age of sixty-two. He had been a Fellow since 1870.

Dr. Fessenden N. Otis, a Fellow for thirty-nine years, Assistant Secretary, 1862–63, had contributed many papers; he died at the age of seventy-five, leaving his library to the Academy. An oratorical memorial address was delivered by Dr. T. Gaillard Thomas.

Dr. Henry D. Noyes, a Fellow since 1862, a brilliant ophthalmologist, had read many valuable papers before the Academy. He was Orator in 1885 and Vice President, 1886–88. He was sixty-eight at the time of his death.

Dr. H. T. Hanks had served the Academy for many years. Elected in 1874, he had been Assistant Secretary, 1874–76, Recording Secretary, 1877–79, and Vice President, 1882–84. He was sixty-three years old.

The annual elections took place peacefully. Dr. Thomson had been renominated, but Dr. Weir was elected.

Dr. Thomson was not a very forceful President. He presided at every meeting his first year, and only missed two in the second. He left no impression, however.

1901–1902

Dr. Thomson's Valedictory was largely reminiscent. He had little to offer in the way of suggestion for the future.

Dr. Weir spoke of the yeoman service rendered by Dr. Barker and gave credit to Dr. Jacobi for the development of the Section work of the Academy. He mentioned the slow increase in membership and wondered if it was not owing to the heavy annual dues, which perhaps would have to be reduced.

Dr. Robert F. Weir, twenty-fourth President, was an outstanding surgeon, sixty-three years old. Graduating just before the outbreak of the Civil War, after serving as House Surgeon at New York, he became an Assistant Surgeon in the Army, and was on duty and in charge of the Army hospital at Frederick, Maryland, for several years. For his fine work he was cited by the Surgeon General.

He joined the Academy in 1866, but for some reason resigned in 1873 and devoted his attention to the New York Medical Journal Association, of which he was President in 1880 when it was absorbed by the Academy. He was readmitted a member at that time. He had been chairman of the Section on Surgery, and Vice President for six years.

After the reading of three papers on infectious or communicable ophthalmia by Drs. R. H. Derby, Carl Koller and Frank Van Fleet, Dr. Jacobi moved that a committee be appointed to make recommendations to the Board of Health for its control, but Dr. W. E. Lambert's amendment to refer the entire matter to Dr. R. H. Derby, Consulting Ophthalmologist of the Department, was carried.

In December, 1902, after a preamble relating the great mortality at previous excavations on the Isthmus of Panama and the results of the efforts of Major Reed and others to eliminate yellow fever by mosquito control, the following resolutions were presented:

Resolved, By the New York Academy of Medicine that in their judgment the amplest powers should be given to the medical officers in charge of the sanitation of the Canal, and that to attain this end, the medical officer should be a member of the Commission which the President of the United States is authorized to appoint to conduct the affairs of the proposed Canal. It is furthermore

Resolved, That the Secretary of the Academy be instructed to forward this preamble and resolutions, duly signed, to the President of the United States.

These were promptly passed, together with a resolution on the death of Major Walter Reed, Surgeon, United States Army. At the next meeting Dr. W. W. Keen of Philadelphia spoke briefly of a fund being raised for the family of Major Reed, who were in very straitened circumstances. As the movement was already under way, the Academy merely called the attention of its Fellows to the matter.

Dr. Dana called attention to a bill before both branches of the state Legislature removing the requirement that the President of the State Board of Lunacy must have had five years experience in the care and treatment of the insane, and presented a long preamble explaining the evils which would result. A resolution was passed urging the Legislature not to pass the bill, and a delegate was appointed to oppose it at the public hearing.

Senator Brackett was attempting to legalize the practice of osteopathy. Resolutions were passed disapproving the bill, to be sent to the proper Senate Committee, and a delegate was again appointed to attend the hearings.

In June, 1901, a Committee on Tuberculosis was announced, consisting of Drs. Jacobi, Peabody, Janeway, Alfred Meyer, and A. H. Smith. This Committee had been authorized on December 20, 1900.

Dr. Knopf introduced resolutions on the exclusion, by order of the Treasury Department, of non-pauper tuberculous persons entering the United States, which caused much discussion. It was voted to ask the Treasury Department the reason for this action, before proceeding further. The Department replied that the order was the result of a report of the Supervising Surgeon General of the United States Marine Service, which stated tuberculosis of the lungs was a "dangerous contagious disease," within the meaning of the law. On further discussion, Dr. C. E. Quimby thought it was unwise, without long and careful consideration, to accuse the government of acting upon ill-advised opinion and ignorance; that it was begging the question to say tuberculosis was not a dangerous contagious disease but a communicable one, and that the fifty or sixty members present could hardly represent the whole Fellowship.

Dr. Dana proposed that a special committee consider the matter before action was taken. Drs. Thomson, A. H. Smith, and Alfred Meyer were strong for immediate action, and the resolutions, slightly modified as follows, were adopted:

WHEREAS, The Treasury Department of the United States, upon recommendation of the Surgeon-General of the Marine Hospital Service, has recently decided to classify pulmonary tuberculosis with dangerous contagious diseases, be it

Resolved, That the New York Academy of Medicine deeply deplores this decision, which is not based either on clinical experience or on scientific experiments.

Resolved, That the Academy considers the exclusion of non-pauper tuberculous immigrants and consumptive aliens visiting our shores unwise, inhumane, and contrary to the dictates of justice.

Be it further Resolved, That, while the Academy upholds the fact of the communicability of tuberculosis and urges all possible precautions against the spread of the disease, occasioned by tuberculous sputum or food, the Academy is opposed to all measures by which additional hardship is imposed upon the consumptive individual, his family or his physician.

Copies were sent to the Treasury Department, the Surgeon General Marine Hospital Service and to the State Medical Society.

A Committee composed of Drs. H. P. Loomis, E. G. Janeway, and Alfred Meyer studied the question asked by Homer Folks, Commissioner of Charities, whether certain old buildings on Blackwell's Island were suitable for tuberculous cases, and it decided they were.

Dr. Bryant spoke on the care of the insane on Ward's Island, and offered the following, which was unanimously adopted:

WHEREAS, Lunacy Bill No. 368 recently passed by the Legislature, places about 4,000 insane male and female patients of Ward's Island under the medical supervision and executive care of a single superintendent, and

Whereas, In the opinion of the Fellows of the New York Academy of Medicine, the magnitude of such a burden as this is far too great to be wisely and safely borne by a single head, be it therefore

Resolved, That the Fellows of the New York Academy of Medicine hereby respectfully register their objections to such a course of action and earnestly petition His Honor the Governor of the State of New York that not less than two superintendents be placed in charge of said patients.

Resolved, That a copy of the preceding preambles and resolutions be provided by the Secretary of the Academy to his Honor the Governor at Albany, New York.

The programs of the scientific meetings were excellent, especially those arranged by the Sections. Fields of recent progress were discussed, and outstanding speakers from other cities participated in several series of papers. Three sessions were given over to the value of X-ray examinations, the use of X-ray in certain forms of cancer, and its value in the treatment of fractures of the lower end of the radius.

Gonorrheal infection occupied a session. Other discussions included backwardness in children and the causes thereof; cirrhosis of the liver, and operative treatment for ascites; the difference between human and bovine tuberculosis, and the role of cow's milk in tuberculosis; operations for the relief of paralytic deformities; and vertigo from various groups of causes. Two other meetings were given over to smallpox—one on the value of glycerinated virus as against dry points, and a second on the symptoms, early diagnosis, and treatment. This was occasioned by a large increase of reported cases of the disease.

"Contagious Ophthalmia," its prevalence, and the laws of the state in regard to it were also discussed. At a symposium on gallstones, Drs. W. J. Mayo of Rochester, Minnesota, and J. B. Murphy of Chicago took part. Dr. W. S. Halsted of Baltimore delivered an address on "The Harder Variety of Hodgkins Disease," and Dr. W. C. Gorgas reported on "The Disappearance of Yellow Fever from Havana." Dr. Osler addressed the Academy on "The Need of a Radical Reform in the Teaching of Medicine to Senior Students."

The Anniversary Addresses were delivered by Dr. R. H. Fitz of Boston on "Surgical Tendencies from a Medical Point of View" in 1901, and Dr. A. H. Smith on "Past, Present and Future of the New York Academy of Medicine," in 1902.

Dr. Jacobi's 1901 Carpenter Lecture was a classic, on "The History of American Pediatrics before 1800," and in 1902, Dr. J. H. Huddleston's was on "The Relation of Physical Chemistry to Medicine."

An appeal was made to the Academy for a fund of $300 to obtain a place in St. Luke's Home for the Aged for Mrs. Wesley M. Carpenter, widow of the founder of the Carpenter Lectures; Dr. Jacobi contributed the honorarium for his Carpenter Lecture for the purpose.

In this period there were several deaths of Fellows who had served the Academy well. Dr. W. H. Draper died at the age of seventy. He had become a Fellow in 1858 and had read a number of important papers. He was Orator in 1886, and Vice President 1887–89. He had done much for the Academy financially as well as in other ways and had been made a Benefactor in 1898. He was an outstanding citizen.

Dr. T. M. Markoe, one of the Founders, died at the age of eighty-one. He had been Treasurer in 1847, but resigned when re-elected. He was a very distinguished surgeon and a very busy man. He did not appear very often, but was selected to present, on behalf of Mrs. Astor, the portrait of Dr. Fordyce Barker.

Dr. F. A. Castle, elected in 1879, had been a most energetic and loyal worker for the Academy. Treasurer of the Trustees 1884–1889, he did yeoman service in raising money for the new building. He had been Trustee 1891–1895. He was only fifty-nine at the time of his death.

The Council was very anxious to resume publication of *Transactions* in a more complete form than the last volume. Negotiations were entered into by Dr. Gibson, editor of the last volume, with Lee Brothers, the publishers of the *American Journal of Medical*

Sciences, but the proposition submitted was considered "impracticable." Dr. Gibson resigned, and the Academy never again tried to assemble their *Transactions* for publication.

The Council's attention was called to an illustrated article concerning Dr. J. D. Quackenbos, which appeared in the *Evening Journal.* The Secretary, by instruction, wrote asking if the article was the result of an interview and whether it was published with consent; Dr. Quackenbos replied it was published without his "authority, consent, sanction or even knowledge." His reply was considered satisfactory.

Dr. W. T. Gibb presented charges against Dr. E. B. Cragin. The Council went to considerable trouble to investigate, the Secretary interviewing both doctors. The Council finally voted, unanimously, that when Dr. Cragin learned between October 20 and October 25, that the patient whom he had seen in his private office on October 7 was the one that Dr. Gibb had introduced to Dr. Cragin's Hospital about twelve days previously, he should have inquired from Dr. Gibb whether the relations between Dr. Gibb and his patient had been properly severed. The Secretary was directed to send these findings to both parties.

There had been in recent years a large number of resignations, and quite a few Fellows were dropped for non-payment of dues. December 19, 1901, eight resignations were accepted and seven Fellows were dropped. A "mortified Listener" wrote to the *Medical Record:*

Sir:

It is unfortunate that the last meeting of the New York Academy of Medicine, which was notable for an unusually large attendance, should have been marred by certain proceedings which were, to say the least, in very bad taste. The presentation of letters of resignation and the dropping of members in arrears of dues afforded an opportunity for certain playful allusions by members of the Council. If there had been nothing but humor, there would have been no occasion to trespass upon your space, for it would have served as a good setting for the excellent intellectual scientific treat which followed; but there was a serious side which seems to call for criticism.

When one member gave as his reason for his resignation that practically the same privileges were extended to outsiders as the members of the Academy, one of the trustees felt called upon to reply quite sharply to this simple, candid statement of a well-known fact. Certainly no one will deny that, aside from receiving the programmes and having a little more liberty in the use of the library, a member of the Academy has no privileges which may not be enjoyed by a non-member. It is true that one who is not a member is deprived of the honor that goes with the membership, but in these days when the medical profession is none too prosperous, I suspect that there are not a few who ask themselves, in the privacy of their homes, whether the honor of being a member of the Academy is a satisfactory equivalent for the twenty dollars a year paid in dues. . . . If the majority feel that they receive the just equivalent for their money, and that the present regulations regarding membership are what they should be, then let the majority accept the verdict; on the other hand, if there is any widespread dissatisfaction it is for the best interests of the Academy and of all concerned that it be made known. It seems to the writer not unduly mercenary for the members to insist that a substantial distinction should be made between the privileges of members and non-members.

This of course caught the eye of Dr. Jacobi, always alert to defend the Academy from unjust criticism, and he replied the next week to the "mortified listener," who "ventilates his grief at what occurred at a Stated Meeting." He quoted the By Laws requiring the action which was taken, and informed the "anonymous mortified moralist" who thought it "not unduly mercenary (what is duly mercenary, Mr. Editor?)" that the Academy was founded to be of benefit to the whole profession, and that the honor of belonging to it and helping to elevate the standards of medicine was worth much more than twenty dollars a year. A few other letters on both sides appeared, including a reply from the still anonymous ("for reasons that will be appreciated") Mortified Listener.

The Council was very careful before recommending a Fellow be dropped, and often leaned over backward to be just. Frequently, when a Fellow wrote frankly that he was hard up and couldn't pay now, the dues were remitted; this was authorized for Fellows of ten years' standing. In many other cases action was deferred for months.

But to many, including the President, dues of twenty dollars seemed too much. A Fellow sent direct to the Council the following proposal: "The initiation fee shall be $5.00 and the annual dues shall be $5.00 in the case of Resident Fellows who render recognized, gratuitous service six hours or more weekly in any laboratory or dispensary connected with a medical school. This reduction in dues shall be granted only during the years in which such gratuitous service is performed and shall in no case be granted to a fellow who has been a medical graduate more than eight years."

It was voted that if this proposed amendment came before the Academy the Council would state its disapproval. (The original motion was never presented to the Academy direct, by its proposer.)

The Secretary, Dr. Huddleston, moved a substitute amendment, that "during the first eight years after the date of diploma, shown on entrance to the Academy, the initiation fee shall be $5.00; the annual dues $5.00, and that, at the expiration of that time the annual dues shall be $20.00 and the difference in dues shall be a matter to be noted only by the Treasurer and shall not in any way affect the standing of the member." This was laid on the table.

Dr. Purple did not leave the remainder of his library to the Academy on his death. When it was learned that the collection was for sale, Dr. Bryant and Mr. Brownne examined it and made an offer of $500. Drs. Bryant and Jacobi were entrusted with the purchase. Dr. Jacobi advanced the money himself, and announced later that the books not needed had been sold to the Library of the Medical Society of the County of Kings for $250.

In some way in 1901 the Academy ended the year with a balance of $532. Dues must have been paid more satisfactorily, for those unpaid only amounted to $1,706. The Council extended its congratulations to the Treasurer, Dr. Collyer, on his management of the finances. But in December the salaries of Mr. Brownne and Mrs. Smith were raised, and the Treasurer had to face an additional $1,500 in expenses the next year. In January the Trustees voted, at the suggestion of Dr. Jacobi, that the Trustees pay for the coal bought in 1901 and that they do so each year in the future, or until otherwise ordered. This matter of two Treasurers, one for the Academy and one for the Trustees, was always causing complications.

In 1902, however, things did not run so well. Even Dr. Collyer was in difficulties. In October the Trustees authorized the negotiation of a private loan of $1,600 to pay salaries and urgent needs. The loan was obtained from Dr. Jacobi, who made it "without solicitation and without interest."

In November the Trustees voted that on and after January 1, 1903, with the approval of the Council (which was granted) the Trustees should pay out of their available income the salary of the Janitor.

The income from the Loomis entertainment fund was not sufficient to pay for a collation twice a month, and the Trustees voted that it be omitted in May and June each year.

As the Trustees were faced with continual complaints on the ventilation of the building, Dr. Jacobus and Dr. Sayre were appointed as a committee to obtain estimates for improvements. Dr. Jacobi was added later. The Committee reported, in May, 1902, in favor of: radiators and connecting pipes for using chiefly exhaust steam in the rear rooms and stack room of the Academy, at a cost of $746; a 30-inch suction fan, motor, and connecting pipe, and radiator to ventilate Hosack Hall at a cost of $468; renewing the piston rods and packing for the elevator, as ordered by insurance inspector, $112, with $16 for packing the piston; also a new doorway in the stack room wall, including an iron door into the Trustees' room, at a cost of $93. This was all authorized.

In April, 1901, Mrs. Sarah Barker Gibbs and Miss George Barker Gibbs presented $10,000 to establish "the Edward N. Gibbs Memorial Prize Fund," the income to be devoted and awarded triennially to the physicians of regular standing in the medical profession of the United States of America who shall present the best original essay upon the etiology, pathology and treatment of the diseases of the kidney. This fund caused no end of trouble.

A committee was appointed to announce the offer of the prize, to be awarded three years later. In 1904, Drs. A. A. Smith, Janeway, Prudden, and Bull were appointed to judge the two essays submitted. One was a printed book, which did not comply with the terms, and the other was not considered worth while. The prize was not awarded. It was decided that the income of $1,000, plus the accrued interest for the next three years, but not to exceed in all $2,000 be offered for an essay submitted before October 1, 1907.

The New York Hospital, wishing to dispose of its collection of "wet specimens," offered it to the Academy. A committee appointed to investigate declined the offer with thanks.

Perhaps the most amusing of all gifts ever offered the Academy is the following. The executor of the will of a former Fellow, Dr. John McNulty of Fort Dodge, Iowa, who was in frequent combat with the Academy, reported this legacy: "I give and bequeath to the New York Academy of Medicine my Military Badge as Medical Director of the Twelfth Army Corps, in trust, to be given to the Medical Officer of Volunteers who shall demonstrate the highest sanitary knowledge in the first war after my death, in which 100,000 or more volunteers are in the active service in the field one year or more. The Academy shall fix the standard of excellence and tests of examination of claimants." The trust was accepted. The Badge cannot be found now. It probably crumbled into dust.

A bust of Dr. Horace Green was presented by his family, and Dr. Roosa, in presenting it, gave a short, interesting account of Dr. Green's life.

At Dr. Purple's death the Council had ordered a suitable tablet; in May, 1901, it was unveiled, and Dr. Stephen Smith delivered an address.

Several portraits were presented: one of Dr. Thomson (Dr. Polk read a speech on the occasion of acceptance); one of Dr. J. A. Swett; and a portrait of Alexander Hosack and a bust of Dr. David Hosack, both given by Mrs. W. H. Draper.

The elections were mere formalities this year. For only one of the six places to be filled was there more than one nomination. Dr. Andrew H. Smith was elected to succeed Dr. Weir.

As a President Dr. Weir was not outstanding. He announced he was going around the world in the summer of 1901, and left after the second meeting in May. His return was delayed by "illness in the family" and he did not preside until March 6, 1902. Of the thirty-five meetings, he presided over only nineteen. He was not a very frequent attendant at the Council and Trustees meetings and he was not elected a Trustee on completion of his term of office.

1903–1904

Dr. Weir in retiring expressed his regret that the membership in two years had increased by only fifteen. He had hoped that dues could be reduced to allow more younger men to join, but the finances of the Academy had prevented it. He stated that only six surgeons, before himself, had been elected president, and gave a brief résumé of the lives of five of them. The sixth was still living.

Dr. Smith's address was one of practical advice to the young practitioner on how to succeed and what *not* to do. It was a homely, simple address.

Dr. Andrew H. Smith, twenty-fifth President, graduated from P. and S. in 1858. He had been Assistant Surgeon throughout the Civil War and had joined the Academy in 1877. He had served on the Committee on Ethics in 1880, was Vice President 1888–1890, and had twice been Anniversary Orator, in 1887 and 1902. He was sixty-six years old.

This year the scientific papers were excellent. The Sections were taking their full responsibility and produced some very good meetings. The Sections on Obstetrics and Gynecology discussed the subject of puerperal sepsis, in five papers. The Section on Pediatrics presented a symposium on typhoid fever with papers by Drs. Morse of Boston, Crozer-Griffith of Philadelphia, and Blackader of Montreal, who discussed the value of the Widal reaction; at another meeting, tuberculosis in infants was discussed by Drs. P. S. Sabine, H. M. Biggs, and Ravenel of Philadelphia. This was followed by a meeting arranged by the Section on Laryngology and Rhinology on "Tuberculosis of the Upper Air Passages."

The Section on Genito-Urinary Surgery offered a meeting on

"Surgery of the Prostate," at which Dr. P. Thorndike of Boston discussed the "when and how," and Dr. O. Horwitz of Philadelphia the results of 141 radical operations. The Sections on Otology, Surgery, and Ophthalmology also provided interesting meetings.

Among the "independent" papers may be mentioned Drs. Piffard's two on the value of ultra-violet rays, and on radium; E. Eliot, Jr., on the behavior of the costal arch in abdominal diseases; E. L. Opie (Baltimore), "Lesions of the Pancreas and Their Clinical Aspect"; J. A. Blake, "Treatment of Diffuse Peritonitis."

Dr. Ridlon (Chicago) discussed the "Ultimate Results of the Bloodless Replacement of Congenital Dislocated Hips." The Council had decided not to invite Dr. Lorenz to speak. His operation in a prominent Chicago family had received too much lay publicity.

Dr. H. W. Wiley, U.S. Department of Agriculture, discussed the "Influence of Preservatives and Adulterants in Food upon the Public Health."

The Carpenter Lectures were given in 1903 by Dr. J. S. Thacher, "The Diagnosis of Fevers," and the following year by Dr. Isaac Adler, "Primary Malignant Neoplasms of the Lungs and Pleura."

Dr. W. G. Thompson gave the Anniversary Address in 1903, "The Economic Value of Medical Science," and in 1904, Dr. W. H. Thomson, on "Internal Secretions." This was the third time he had delivered the Anniversary Address.

The Academy's activities in public health matters were not so numerous as in former years. The city's sanitarium for early cases of tuberculosis, Raybrook, had been authorized by the Legislature three years before, but completion was delayed because of insufficient funds. Resolutions were sent to the Governor, state officers, and the Legislature, deploring the delay and asking for suitable appropriations for immediate completion. A committee of seven appointed to attend hearings reported later that $115,000 had been granted for the purpose.

Dr. Knopf called attention to a bill that had been passed and was now before Governor Odell. The bill required the consent of the County Supervisors and Town Boards before a hospital for tuberculous cases could be established in any area. Resolutions were passed urging the Governor to veto it, because it would result in the loss of "thousands of lives, and increase the spread of tuberculosis in crowded districts in cities and towns."

An attempt having been made by real estate interests to annul the advances made in tenement house control (elimination of inside dark bedrooms, installation of fireproof stair wells, and so on), the Academy sent a protest to the Governor and to chairmen of committees of the Legislature.

Dr. Ernst J. Lederle had been Commissioner of Health under Mayor Low, and the incoming Mayor McClellan had threatened not to reappoint him. At a special meeting of the Council, long and strong resolutions decrying the removal of Dr. Lederle and praising his administration were offered, but the Council decided it was contrary to the Academy's policy to support, as a body, any individual candidate for public office.

Toward the end of 1903 the President and Dr. Jacobus, long in its service, presented their ideas on improving the Academy's position. Both recommendations were ordered printed and distributed to the members of the Council. The President felt the most urgent need at present was an increased membership, not only for more income but to improve the influence, power, and dignity of the Academy. Dues pressed heavily upon young men with restricted professional incomes, and the policy of the Academy practically offered a premium upon an unethical attitude of non-members. He suggested that new members' dues for the first three years be $10 instead of $20; for the next two years $15, and after that $20; and that it be optional to pay the whole initiation fee at once, or in five annual installments. The injustice to those who had always paid $20 was a matter of sentiment and not business. It was better for all concerned to accept reduced dues from new members for the first five years rather than to dispense with new members altogether.

Dr. Jacobus recommended an increase in membership of the Academy and proposed a committee of fifteen to twenty-five to select from physicians in New York and vicinity about 200 whom it would be desirable to approach, preferably by personal appeal and endeavor, with an invitation to join.

The By Laws should be amended so that the public could use the Library until 1 P.M. instead of 6 P.M., thus giving members more space and freedom. If dues were to be $20, Fellowship should be limited to 1,000; if $15, to 1,200. The object of limiting membership was to increase its value and desirability and to create, as in clubs, a waiting list from which to select desirable members. The restriction of the hours for the use of the Library by non-members and a limited membership filled to overflowing would result in fewer delinquents and fewer Fellows to be dropped, as well as a larger list of applicants.

An effort should be made to acquire the library and building of the Medical Society of the County of Kings, either through purchase or by close cooperation, and to interchange books and periodicals between the two libraries.

A small branch library, open only to Fellows, should be established in Harlem near 125th Street and Sixth Avenue, convenient to the underground station, and later another should be opened, perhaps in Staten Island. Dr. Jacobi recommended purchasing, if possible, No. 15 West 43d Street, which would provide increased space for books and reading rooms, a larger office for the Nurses' Bureau, a larger coat room, a place in the basement to store coal and to set up a new and larger dynamo. The top floor should be converted into a large and suitable apartment for the resident librarian.

The first and most pressing need was increased membership for there were probably less than 750 good paying members, and a thousand were needed to meet running expenses.

There is no record of any action on all these recommendations.

By the end of 1903 the Treasurer was in trouble again, in spite of the fact that the Trustees were paying for coal and the janitor's salary. The loan from Dr. Jacobi had been paid back, but another $1,000 was advanced by Dr. Smith, and with that the Academy paid all its bills and had $484 in the bank.

Resignations were continuing and new members did not offset them. Legal Counsel was consulted and rendered an opinion that if the Academy desired it could close the Library to the public after

2 P.M. It was decided to do so. This brought forth in the *Medical Record* an angry protest from a Dr. Tracy (he was not a Fellow), who went to the extent of writing to the Tax Commissioner asking why the Academy was permitted to maintain a "public library" that was not open all day. Dr. Jacobi replied that Dr. Tracy was neither a member of the Academy nor of the County Society or County Association: "Perhaps this was why he felt competent to criticize public medical affairs. Men of good standing and of ample means, when asked to join, would say not they! They would not think of paying for what the Academy gave them gratis. Books were taken out by non-Fellows, which were wanted by Fellows." Another Fellow wrote that if Dr. Tracy was too busy to come to the Academy in the mornings he must have a large practice, in which case he could afford to pay for the privilege of using the Library. In a later issue of the *Record* the letters from Counsel on the subject were published in full, on authority of the Council.

The Library Committee was asked to consider critically its list of periodicals, with a view to reducing the number; the Committee was able to convince the Council that this would be unwise.

It was voted that the privilege of removing books from the Library be restricted to Fellows in good standing. The Council later voted to extend the privilege of consulting the Reference Library after hours by issuing a card, good for one year, to accredited representatives of Fellows and publishers of medical books and periodicals, officials of public departments of the city, and members of the First District Dental Society. The Council also voted to establish "annual subscribers," who, on payment of $20 a year in advance and if approved by the Library Committee and Council, were entitled to all the privileges of the Library, including the circulating department.

Dr. Jacobi was appointed a committee of one to look into the question of the most economical method of lighting, whether to continue using the nine-year-old dynamo and gas, with street current when but little current was used, or to take all current from the Edison Company, or to install a larger dynamo. He reported use of the Edison Company would cost about $3,000.

The Superintendent of Buildings for Manhattan ordered the erection, forthwith, of fire escapes on the north and east walls of the Academy. This was referred to Dr. Jacobi, again with power to act; he reported that a reinspection of the building brought a second and more moderate order from the Department. He had an estimate of $149.50 for the work necessary.

Another blow to the Academy was an order from the Commissioner of Licenses directing it to procure a license for the Bureau of Nurses, as per law enacted in March, 1904. It was voted to discontinue the Bureau, as it was not deemed advisable to take out a license. Drs. Jacobi, Sayre, and Jacobus were appointed a committee, with power, to confer with the Commissioner of Licenses and make an equitable arrangement with nurses already registered, before the law became operative. One hundred and eighty-six nurses were still on the roll. The Committee was also authorized to rearrange salaries of those affected by the closing of the Bureau and to drop any employe not needed after the Bureau was closed. Dr. Jacobi later reported that the Commissioner of Licenses was willing to permit the Bureau to continue without a license until the expiration of the term of those who had registered prior to August, 1904; at that time the Bureau would be closed, and no new nurses would be registered.

In 1903 finally appeared the last volume of *Transactions* published by the Academy. The first 81 pages were given over to an account of the Semi-Centennial Celebration, with copies of all notices sent, the program, and the papers read, in full, and with a reproduction of President Cleveland's Address, in manuscript. This is followed by a list of all officers of the Academy from 1847 through 1896. The rest of the volume of 471 pages contains the Carpenter Lectures 1896–1901; Anniversary Addresses 1896–1901, except Dr. Welch's; Dr. Bryant's Valedictory and Dr. Janeway's and Dr. Weir's presidential addresses, and the memorial addresses for Drs. W. T. Lusk, J. L. Smith, Joseph O'Dwyer, and S. S. Purple. It also contains the list of officers of the Academy and Sections and the titles of all papers read at Stated Meetings 1896–1901.

The Council authorized the reprinting, separately, of the Semi-Centennial Celebration, "provided the expense was not in excess of appropriations made for the purpose." The reprint was, of course, in excess, by $772, which Dr. Jacobi paid.

As plans for future *Transactions* were given up, the stenographer employed to take down discussions was dispensed with.

A committee appointed to consider securing new Fellows was also instructed to suggest names for Honorary Fellowship. Dr. Jacobi was chairman of this committee. Thirty-three persons were recommended, five from America: Drs. Reginald H. Fitz of Boston; W. W. Keen of Philadelphia; William Osler of Baltimore; Victor Vaughan of Ann Arbor, Mich.; and W. H. Welch of Baltimore. All were unanimously elected.

Dr. Northrup, on behalf of numerous donors, presented a portrait of Dr. O'Dwyer, and Dr. Bryant one of ex-President Weir.

The only death reported which affected the Academy was that of Dr. T. Gaillard Thomas, Recording Secretary 1859–61, Orator, 1877, Vice President, 1878–81. He had read many really valuable papers at the meetings, and as one of the leading physicians of his day had contributed much to the Academy's success. He was seventy years old at his death; a memorial was presented by Dr. H. D. Nicoll.

As more room was still needed for the stacks the Council recommended the purchase of 15 West 43d Street. This was referred to a special committee of three to consider.

The only charges brought before the Academy were those of Dr. W. L. Carr against Dr. Fremont Swain, for publishing a public leaflet advertising certain treatments. Dr. Swain was given a chance to answer and his resignation was then accepted by the Council.

The Library was enriched by a gift of $3,000 from the Physicians of the German Dispensary, the amount received from the sale of its library. The gift was accepted and designated the German Hospital and Dispensary Fund, the interest to be spent for the Library.

The Academy closed the year 1904 with $940 in the bank, thanks to another loan from Dr. Jacobi of $1,500. Dr. Smith's loan had been paid back, and the collector had obtained $760 of back dues. Unpaid dues amounted to $1,358.

Dr. Smith was an interested and active President. He presided very regularly till mid-April 1903, and then was absent till October. He failed to preside at eight of the thirty-two meetings.

1905–1906

Charles L. Dana

DR. SMITH's Valedictory was a long and dreary account of the death and autopsy findings of the late President Garfield, assassinated in 1881.

Dr. Dana, in his Presidential Address, said medical literature was now so profuse, and the number of medical societies so great, that the profession in self-defense must take some measures to save time and, "unless it wished to be swamped by the exuberance of its own fertility," should master the art of presenting what it desired to record with accuracy, clearness, and dispatch. He suggested the appointment by the Council of a permanent Committee on Public Health and Medical Economics—which should be a large and varied one. It was a fine direct address and the *Medical Record* remarked editorially:

In his inaugural address the new President of the Academy of Medicine used the words "lucid brevity" as describing the characteristics he wished to see in the communications laid before that body. "Never," writes an ex-president of the Academy [Jacobi?] in a note to the *Medical Record*, "were two words more aptly put together. Would that they might be woven into the web of all medical discourses, and water-marked on every page of medical writing."

Dr. Charles Loomis Dana, twenty-sixth President, was a learned man of fifty-three, much interested in public health matters and in the history of medicine. He was a noted collector of engravings of medical men from the Father of Medicine down. He had joined the Academy in 1886, was chairman of the Section on Medicine in 1887, Orator in 1894, and Vice President 1901–3.

In spite of his interest in public health, there was less discussion and action on such matters in Dr. Dana's tenure than in several previous years. Dr. Wiley, Chief of the Bureau of Chemistry, U.S. Department of Agriculture, read before the American Association for the Advancement of Science a paper on "Diet in Tuberculosis," in which he advocated the use of alcohol. Resolutions were offered condemning his views as giving an impression that alcohol plays an important or even necessary part in the treatment of tuberculosis, that the promulgation of such ideas was likely to cause harm to the individual and to the anti-tuberculosis crusade, which relied on sanitation, good food, and pure air. The Council appointed Drs. A. A. Smith, Jacobi, and W. G. Thompson a committee to consider the matter; they recommended no action at the present time.

Dr. Peabody, Professor of Materia Medica at P. and S., offered a long preamble, emphasizing the evil caused by the widespread use of preparations of medicines of unknown and harmful composition, the result of widespread unscrupulous advertisement thereof, not only in the daily press, but often religious and otherwise respectable medical journals, and a resolution calling upon physicians in general and Fellows of the Academy in particular to cease ordering such preparations. He urged cooperation with the American Medical Association and its Council on Pharmacy and Chemistry in its efforts to inform the profession on all those fraudulent medicines. He called upon the state and city Boards of Health to do all in their power to protect the public from such secret remedies.

This was approved by the Academy and referred to the Council for action. Drs. Peabody, Fowler, and Jacobi were appointed a committee to promote legislation for the proper labeling of all medicines containing narcotics.

It must be confessed that this preamble and the consequent resolutions were not examples of "lucid brevity."

An ordinance had been issued by the Board of Health concerning unnecessary smoke, but its inspectors had been ordered not to issue summonses for non-compliance therewith. A protest against this action was presented and Drs. Bryant, W. B. James, and Robert Abbe were instructed to report on the subject. They recommended that the Department of Health give a public hearing to those who desired to appear to complain of nuisances in the city caused by the "discharge of smoke," and that the complaints lately received by the Council be referred to the Health Department, with the recommendation that the complainants submit in writing to the Health Department the "evidence relative to the discharge of smoke."

The Academy voted its approval, and the *Medical Record* commented:

> At the meeting of the New York Academy of Medicine—a body which under the present public-spirited and intelligent administration is well fulfilling its mission as the guardian of the people's health—held March 1, resolutions were passed reminding the Health Department of its duty in the enforcement of the law against pollution of the atmosphere by coal smoke. It is full time something was done to abate this evil unless we are content to sacrifice the beauty of our Italian sky to the greed of wealthy corporations. The records show that there has been a progressive decrease during the past few years in the number of complaints by Health Department inspectors, yet it is apparent to even the casual observer that the number of offenders against the smoke law is steadily increasing. Electric light is a great convenience, and even a necessity, but we need not barter our glorious sunlight to obtain it. There are some nuisances entailed by modern progress which must be endured, but for the smoke nuisance there is no excuse. Bituminous coal can be burned without this wilful waste of carbon, and it is strange that those in charge of power-houses and other large consumers of soft coal should not see that the prevention of smoke by suitable devices, or even by more careful stoking, would effect a very appreciable economy in fuel. They should be made to see it. One by one the great cities of the East are being devoured by the black smoke beast—even tidy Philadelphia is becoming grimy and soot-soiled—and if New York is to be saved, speedy and energetic action must be taken by the Health Commissioner. We have gone back to dirty streets, but let us at least keep the air clean.

A very important step was taken by the Council in 1905, when it appointed Drs. Bryant, W. G. Thompson, and Peabody a committee to consider public lectures on health matters to be given under the auspices of the Academy. The first lecture was given December 29, 1905, by Dr. Thomas Darlington, Health Commissioner, who spoke on "Pneumonia and Cerebro-spinal Meningitis," describing the findings of two commissions appointed by the Department the previous spring.

This was the first public lecture under the auspices of the Academy. It brought forth strong editorial commendation from the *Medical Record:*

Hitherto the newspapers have been forced to rely for their information regarding medical topics of public interest upon interviews with individual physicians, a system liable to great abuses, and one exposing the complacent "interviewees" to the often unjust accusation of "advertising." These public lectures under the auspices of the Academy of Medicine will do away in a measure with the newspaper need of individual interviews, but the principle might, we think, be extended with advantage.

The writer went on to say that, if properly arranged, such lectures would be to the laity what the Harvey Lectures were to the profession.

The Harvey Society was founded "to diffuse scientific information in selected chapters on anatomy, physiology, pathology, bacteriology, pharmacy and physiological and pathological chemistry through the medium of public lectures by men who were workers in the subjects presented." The Academy granted it the use of Hosack Hall for its meetings, which were announced in the Bulletin as "under the patronage of the Academy." The first meeting of the Society was held October 7, 1905, and after that all meetings were announced in the folder.

In 1906 the Nurses' Bureau wound up its affairs. Established in 1894, it had rendered definite service to the community. It was instigated by Dr. Jacobi and was constantly under his watchful and critical eye, as chairman of the Executive Committee. While there were occasional complaints of individual nurses, that could not be helped. Several hundred nurses had been provided each year, about one-third of them on night calls. Felix Wesstrom, the faithful janitor, was provided with a cot in the Bureau's office, so he could attend to the night calls. From the very start the Bureau was more than self-supporting, in spite of paying $360 each year as its assessment for expenses for rooms. While the license requirement was the immediate cause for discontinuance, the need had declined considerably as the various hospitals were establishing their own nurses' registries.

The subject of the training of nurses—what and how they were taught—interested the profession greatly. There was much criticism of the curricula in some cases, and the Council was requested to consider the problem and bring it before the Academy, in order that physicians' views might be heard. After some delay, the matter was referred to Dr. W. G. Thompson for report. We search the minutes in vain for this report.

Matters of ethics disturbed the Academy very little. A printed article relating to Dr. H. W. Mitchell's treatment of tuberculosis by a remedy (the formula of which was not given) was referred to Drs. A. A. Smith and W. G. Thompson. The formula was published later and the matter dropped.

Dr. I. L. Hill, a recent Fellow, was reported to be exhibiting "signs" at his office in 76th Street. He was communicated with and failing to answer, was requested to "show cause why he should not be dropped." He apparently "showed cause," for the charge was "dismissed."

In May 1906, Dr. I. S. Haynes presented a patient who had been shot through the abdomen, liver, and spinal cord, but recovered after laparotomy and laminectomy. Dr. Haynes read a paper on "Gunshot Wounds of the Spinal Cord, a Plea for early Myelorrhaphy." This case appeared in the lay press, mentioning also another surgeon. Both wrote saying neither had given any information to the newspapers. Dr. Haynes was informed his explanation was accepted and he was asked to try to find out how the typewritten copy of his address could have reached the newspapers.

The Council then took an action too long deferred, and ordered that folders of the Academy should not be sent to the newspapers except to announce a public meeting (such as the Anniversary Address or the Wesley M. Carpenter Lecture) or a program expressly intended for the public.

The Sections were producing creditable meetings each year, as required, but the Council did not seem satisfied with the work of the Sections themselves. A Committee appointed to consider their administration recommended, in general, that a list of all Sections be sent to each Fellow after he signed the Constitution, asking him to check the Section or Sections to which he would like to belong. The election of Section officers should take place in December, the nominations having been made at the preceding meeting. Only those assigned to a Section should be allowed to vote or be eligible for office. The Sections were to organize in January. In that month, and again in October of each year, the President should call a meeting of the Chairmen and Secretaries of all Sections for a general conference, to outline a harmonious program for the scientific work of the Academy and of the Sections, and to inform the officers of the Sections of the rules of the Academy. This was adopted.

As the Academy did not pay for the postal notices of Section meetings, the Sections augmented their income for this purpose by receiving "subscriptions" from non-Fellows. The Council instructed the Secretary to "express forcibly" to the chairmen of Sections the Council's disapproval of this custom, reminding them that non-members had no status in the Sections.

Two new Sections were authorized—on Dermatology and on Public Health. That was as near as Dr. Dana got to his suggestion of a standing committee on the latter subject.

In 1905 the Council again took up the subject of publishing the *Transactions*. Assigned to investigate, Drs. W. G. Thompson, Jacobi, and Huddleston reported that the *New York Medical Journal* would supply a stenographer and three copies of the minutes for $12 per meeting; but no recommendation was made and we hear nothing more of the matter. In 1906 an offer was made to provide stenographic reports of the Stated and Section meetings for $1,200 per annum. The whole matter was referred to Drs. Jacobi, Sayre (Treasurer), and Huddleston (Secretary). They apparently recommended that nothing be done.

The responsibilities of the Executive Committee were many and doubtless irritating. In the Trustees' minutes of 1905, we find this note: "It was voted that no regular employe of the Academy be permitted to act regularly as a collector of dues, or to receive any commission of any kind from the Academy, or from any firm or person, for any purpose whatsoever."

This Committee was also responsible for keeping track of the condition of the building and making recommendations for repairs and improvements. In 1906, a serious strike among the coal miners was attended by a rise in the cost of coal. The Treasurer was authorized to purchase a sufficient supply for immediate use pending a settlement of the strike.

Dr. Cheesman was appointed Executive Librarian in 1906. He reported to the Council that the Library was very well run, the card catalogue was full and in excellent shape. He was asked to look over the collection of instruments, pick out those desirable for exhibition, and dispose of the rest. Dr. Cheesman was later allowed $100 to purchase a cabinet for those he selected as worth keeping.

The Library was crowded with duplicate and triplicate volumes, and was seriously cramped for space. Cooper Medical College in San Francisco had made an offer of $6,000 for unnecessary duplicates. This was considered a fair offer and was accepted. But then came the San Francisco earthquake and fire. The matter was held over until it was ascertained if the offer was still good. Cooper College was more eager than ever to have the books, and they were sold, "ready for shipment." When the check came, some thousand dollars was deducted for transportation charges, but this was settled and the Academy added $6,000 to its Library Fund, which also received a bequest of $1,000 from Dr. A. W. Warden.

The Fellowship had now reached its constitutional limit; a number of applicants had been approved by the Committee on Admissions for whom there was no place. Those awaiting election were ordered notified by the Secretary they had all the privileges of the Library, pending election, except taking out books.

A minute of the Council is of amusing interest—the Faculties of Columbia University *other than the Medical Faculty* were allowed to use the Library at other than public hours. The "physicians and scientists" of the Rockefeller Institute were also granted the use of the Library.

Mr. Carnegie was very active in founding libraries. Dr. Jacobi communicated with him and reported the "negative answer he had received thereto."

In 1905 and 1906 the Library was granted its requested appropriation of $5,000. This was a unique experience for the Library Committee! And another almost unique experience was that it did not overspend its budget allowance. The $5,000 was for the upkeep of the Library—subscriptions to journals, binding, repairing, furniture, and so on. New books were bought from the income from the Library Fund, which could only be used for that purpose, and over $3,200 was so spent.

A special meeting of the Council was called to decide what to do in the San Francisco disaster. A committee was appointed to confer with the County Societies of Greater New York on raising a fund for medical sufferers. The Academy voted $300; together with the County Societies of New York and Richmond, $7,474.58 was raised and sent to San Francisco from 440 individuals and 14 medical societies.

After prolonged discussion in the Council, the Constitution and By Laws were amended. The objects were now declared to be *the Investigation* and Promotion of the Science and Art of Medicine and the maintenance of a Public Medical Library. Fellows residing in the city were limited to 1,000, and non-residents to 150. In 1904 *total* membership had been limited to 1,000, with not more than 250 non-residents of New York city.

A class of "Junior Subscribers," not yet three years in practice but otherwise eligible, had been suggested. They were to be elected for one year, pay $10, and have all the privileges of the Library and scientific meetings. The Council considered this "unwise."

The position of Treasurer of the Trustees was abolished, and to the Council was assigned definitely the duty of attending to the *executive* business of the Academy, and to the Trustees, the *financial.*

The official year was to begin the first day of January, and all officers assumed their duties on that day.

The Academy *might* be divided into twelve Sections—new Sections on Dermatology and Public Health being added.

All nominations were to be made at the *first* meeting of *November*, elections to take place the *first* meeting in *December*, and the annual reports presented the first meeting of January.

While amendments to the By Laws were under discussion, the question was raised whether the Executive Committee of the Council should be continued, and a special committee—Drs. Dana, Bryant, and Huddleston—was appointed to consider this matter. It recommended:

1. That the Committee be not abolished;
2. That to the profound wisdom, the great experience, and untiring energy of the chairman of the committee be added the attainments in this respect of the other members of the Executive Committee.

With this object in view, it is further recommended that the members of the Committee shall meet at their earliest convenience and so organize themselves that each member may bear an equal share of the responsibilities of their respective stations and shed accordingly the light of their combined wisdom on the proceedings of the Council of the Academy.

Dr. Jacobi, as President of the Board of Trustees, had been on this Committee for years, and the lion's share of work was done by him. How he ever had time to do anything else is a mystery. He may have had something to do with suggesting its discontinuance; after all, he was seventy-five. The Committee was given definite duties in regard to the administration of the Academy.

The clause permitting a candidate to be presented and voted on after the Committee on Admissions had refused to recommend him disappears from the By Laws. Dr. Calkins had lost after all (see pp. 14 and 25).

All other changes were chiefly in wording and clarifying existing rules, except one that made it possible for Fellows dropped for non-payment of dues to be reinstated by the Council within nine months, on written application of the delinquent *and* the payment of all indebtedness, including the current year's dues.

Financial affairs were better, although the Academy had to watch its step very carefully.

The Board of Fire Underwriters demanded improvement in the

electric wiring of the building. This cost $505. In Hosack Hall the lighting was changed to an overhead system of eighty-odd lights, and the large central chandelier and side lights were removed. New glass over the platform skylight replaced the painted glass. Altogether in these two years the Academy spent over $3,000 for repairs and replacements.

In spite of all this, in 1905, after repaying the loan of $1,500 to Dr. Jacobi, the Treasurer closed the year with a balance of $733, the first time he had been out of the red in a number of years.

In 1906, under the new Constitution, there was only one Treasurer and things were run in a more sensible manner. The Trust funds were the most complicated problem. Dr. Collyer had been a most efficient Treasurer for six years; but when his term of office terminated in 1905, Dr. R. H. Sayre, who had been Treasurer of the Trustees, also for six years, was elected Treasurer of the Academy and served for twelve years. The year ended with a balance in the Treasury of $3,133.

The Scientific Sessions were very full. During the two years, seventy-five papers were read, too many to list. They were on widely different subjects. Along public health lines Drs. W. H. Park read on "Colds and Grippe in 1904 and 1905," W. P. Northrup on "Roof Playgrounds," George A. Soper (by invitation) on the "Air in the Subways"; there was a symposium on the "Health of the New York School Child," and a group of papers on visual defects and their prevention. Baron Takaki of Tokyo spoke on "Medical Education in Japan." A reception was tendered Dr. Takaki by Dr. Jacobus.

Dr. John Rogers discussed the treatment of Graves' disease by a specific cyto-toxin; Dr. Flexner, dysentery toxin and mercurial colitis; "The Use of Adrenalin in Asthma"; the "Treatment of Cerebro-spinal Meningitis by Diphtheria Antitoxin"; the value of anti-gonococcus serum in gonorrheal arthritis; "Anaemia from Intestinal Parasites"; the function and disorders of the parathyroids, and the significance of persistent high blood pressure (Dr. T. C. Janeway) called forth much discussion.

The Nauheim system of treatment in diseases of the heart roused considerable interest. Gonorrheal infections in children, a big hospital problem in those days, was the subject of a symposium.

Many from out of town read or discussed papers—Drs. J. C. Munro, R. W. Lovett, R. C. Cabot, and C. J. Blake of Boston; de Schweinitz, J. B. Deaver, James Tyson, and C. K. Mills of Philadelphia; J. T. Johnson and J. Wesley Bovée of Washington; Lucien Howe of Buffalo; and Arthur Holding of Albany.

Dr. Simon Flexner delivered the Carpenter Lecture in 1905, "On the Etiology of Syphilis," and Dr. Harvey W. Cushing of Boston that of 1906, "A Discussion of Some Early and Some Late Cranial Injuries and Their Treatment, Based on the Histories of Three Illustrative Cases."

The Council appointed a special committee to assist in arranging programs: Drs. W. G. Thompson, Bryant, Peabody, and the Secretary, Dr. Huddleston.

The Academy made much of its Anniversary Addresses. In 1905 Dr. A. G. Gerster spoke on "The American System of Hospital Economy," which was followed by a reception. The expenses of this meeting were $235.90. The next year Dr. Roswell Park of Buffalo described "Medicine and Surgery in Classic Art and Satire," with illustrations. The Academy really splurged a little on this meeting. The Treasurer's account shows:

To collation for 350 persons	$225.00
Flowers for the President's table	2.50
2,600 sets of invitations, tickets, outside and inside envelopes, printing and postage on same	97.50
5 musicians	35.00
Awning on sidewalk	8.00
	$368.00

Dr. A. H. Smith's portrait was presented by some of his friends, and Dr. Peabody made an interesting presentation speech. He started off by referring to a book, *A Study of Life and Death*, which stated that fear of death was due to the dread of being forgotten. Dr. Smith thought nature's methods were as usual the best; death and oblivion were just a part of the cycle of life. But there were exceptions, and he quoted Jacobi as saying fame should occasionally fall to the lot of one who saved human lives and alleviated suffering as well as to him whose highest aim was to destroy life. He mentioned Dr. Smith in the last few words, as one who would survive through his writings.

A portrait of Dr. F. N. Otis was presented on behalf of his family, with a fine eulogy by Dr. Bangs, and Dr. Knopf presented one of Dr. Dettweiler, distinguished German scientist.

Dr. Jacobi presented the portrait of Dr. P. F. Mundé, elected a Fellow in 1875, Corresponding Secretary in 1885, and active in Academy affairs.

The Academy lost another old and faithful servant, Dr. John H. Hinton. He had become a Fellow in 1856, was Assistant Secretary in 1860, Recording Secretary 1861–64. His greatest activity was for the Library. Executive Librarian 1865–76, he was a member of the Library Committee from its inception in 1875 to 1883. He had also been a generous contributer to its funds. He died at the age of seventy-eight.

Dr. George R. Fowler, a Fellow since 1886, and elected Vice President in 1905, died in office. He had been Orator in 1896. He was only fifty-seven at his death. A memorial address was delivered by Dr. A. T. Bristow of Brooklyn. The eulogy was ordered printed, on motion of Dr. Jacobi.

The election of officers aroused more interest than in several years. No less than seven candidates, including Dr. Jacobi, were proposed for President; four were nominated for Vice President; four for Trustee, and three for the Committees on Admissions and Library. There was no contest for Secretary and Corresponding Secretary!

Dr. Wyeth was elected President, and Dr. Dana, Trustee.

Dr. Dana was an excellent President. The Academy made real advances and was on a sound financial basis. He presided at all but two meetings.

1907–1910

John A. Wyeth

In his farewell address, Dr. Dana said the custom of having a retiring address was not a common one, but not an unwise one if the President retired "without too much forensic effort," and told what his experience as an executive officer had suggested for guidance and inspiration. He ended his term of office convinced that the Academy was an organization wisely planned, unselfishly and effectively organized to bring out what was best in scientific and practical medicine. It was an Academy, or its equivalent, that humanized and elevated the profession.

He emphasized that meetings must be interesting to a busy doctor or he would not come. The appointment of a group which met at least twice a year to lay out plans for subjects of most interest was yielding good results. To a large extent clinical or descriptive medicine, and even gross pathology, was a finished story. (This in 1907!) The modern clinician had to work with a laboratory at his side. In the fields of prevention and therapeutics much remained to be done. Perhaps the only clinical field left was the interpretation of subjective symptoms. It was easy enough to recognize a crepitant râle or a cardiac dilatation, but not so easy to explain a persistent pain in the back. It was a great mistake to think that if "nothing could be seen, heard, felt or precipitated in a test tube," nothing was the matter.

He closed by emphasizing the Academy's need for $200,000 to enlarge its plant, and the same amount of endowment to allow the publication of its proceedings.

Dr. Wyeth gave an account of the value and gradual development of organization in medicine.

As announced in the "folder," the Academy inaugurated a new feature at this annual meeting: Dr. Stephen Smith, a Fellow for fifty-three years, spoke on surgical practice in the early days of the

Academy, and Dr. Jacobi, a Fellow of only two years less time, on medical practice in those years. Both the addresses, much enlarged for publication, appeared as special articles in the *Medical Record*.

Dr. John Allen Wyeth, twenty-seventh President of the Academy, was born in Alabama in 1845. He served during the Civil War, and was a prisoner for fifteen months. At its conclusion he became a farmer, but decided to study medicine, working for three years as a river pilot and captain to earn necessary funds. He studied at the University of Louisville and completed his course for M.D. at Bellevue Hospital Medical College in 1873. After two years as prosector and instructor at Mount Sinai, he went abroad for two years and returned to New York in 1880.

In 1881 he was one of the founders of the New York Polyclinic Medical School, the first postgraduate medical organization in this country. He also had been president of the New York Pathological, in 1885–86, New York State Medical Society 1901, and A.M.A. in 1902.

Apart from scientific matters, the problems of space and the needs of the Library occupied a great deal of the Academy's time and attention during Dr. Wyeth's administration.

If the Academy could have afforded to keep the building for its own uses, depriving the State and County Societies, as well as others, of the rooms for which they paid their share of the upkeep, it might have been possible to get along. But that was contrary to the accepted object—making the building the center of all medical activities in the city.

For several years the Library's need for more room had been increasingly evident. This was not only for the stacks, but for the actual readers. In 1907 the Council room was thrown open to Fellows, and shelf space there and also in a room directly above the stack room was provided. Two years later the Council room was also opened to Library subscribers.

In April, 1907, the Trustees authorized Drs. Wyeth and Jacobi to negotiate for the purchase of 15 West 43d Street, a small four-story brownstone building to the east of the Academy. But 1907 was a bad year in the money market, and in October, owing to the financial stringency, it was voted to postpone the matter temporarily.

Meanwhile the crowded conditions of all parts of the Academy were becoming unbearable. To relieve the congestion in Hosack Hall, the Trustees voted to narrow the platform from front to back and increase its width from side to side, thus increasing the seating capacity of the platform as well as of the auditorium, the cost to be $75. Also, it voted to place an additional front row of seats in Hosack Hall, and individual armchairs at sides and rear of the hall, to increase its capacity by 76 to 80 seats. The costs were estimated at $399. These changes were made during the summer.

Things lay dormant, in regard to increased space, till 1909, during which time $5,000 was spent on repairs and improvements.

In 1908 the Library Committee again sang its song of woe: pamphlets were now being stored in the Duplicates room. The Council directed Drs. Jacobus and C. M. Williams to consult with the architect as to possible relief. Nothing was accomplished.

In the fall of 1909 the Committee warned the Academy that disaster threatened the Library. At the present rate of increase there was barely room for two years' accessions. Stagnation was in sight, and resulting loss of efficiency. Books would have to be piled on the floor, or be in double rows on the shelves, where that was possible. New pamphlets were now being placed on the floor or window sills, as all cases were full. A large part of the duplicate collection was also now on the floors. The Committee criticized the Academy's policy of giving such a small allowance for journals, and so on, and while the Library had lived within its budget it only did so by failing to buy important new books, including the Paris Theses, which was a great loss.

In 1909 a committee on increased facilities made a very serious report, and it was voted to appoint a committee consisting of the Council, Library Committee, Chairmen of Sections, and living ex-Presidents, to report at the next meeting as to what to do. That was a cumbersome committee and it is not strange that it did not report.

In May, 1910, the President announced as a committee to consider ways and means of raising funds to increase the facilities of the Academy Drs. Bryant, chairman, A. Jacobi, Janeway, Holt, Gilman Thompson, Polk, and R. H. Sayre.

A committee on selection of a site had a hard time. At a special meeting called on July 6, 1910, to hear this committee's report, the Trustees voted to purchase the premises at 15 West 43d Street for not more than $100,000. Drs. Sayre, Wyeth, Dana, Polk, and others offered to advance the $5,000 necessary to bind the contract, which offer was accepted with thanks. The vote to buy was unanimous.

It was then voted to approve also the purchase of No. 10 West 44th Street, at a price not to exceed $120,000. The vote was unanimous, except for Dr. A. A. Smith who, on the ground of business policy, wished to be recorded as voting no.

A special meeting of the Academy was held on July 14 and immediately went into executive session, all non-Fellows being excluded.

The Committee on Site reported that it had considered:

1. Increasing the size of the present building by new construction from new foundations, practically doubling the present stack and meeting room facilities. On advice of two competent firms of architects, this was considered inadvisable.

2. Buying property elsewhere, upon which to erect a building. This was the popular idea for some months, and options were obtained upon several pieces of property. The total cost for any property which would in any way equal the conveniences of the present site, and the loss of facilities involved in moving and the prohibitive expense of a suitable new building, caused the abandonment of that plan.

3. Acquiring the building 15 West 43d Street at not more than $125,000 and 10 West 44th Street, immediately back of it, for not more than $125,000, were decided upon and the contract for the purchase of these properties at $100,000, and $120,000, respectively, was now in the hands of the lawyer. On all grounds it was considered this was the most advisable.

The Council had voted unanimously that the report be transmitted to the Academy, with its approval. It had also voted to recommend to the Academy that the Trustees be authorized to take a mortgage not to exceed $225,000 on the present property, at not more than 4½ percent interest, in order to finance the transactions.

The Academy adopted the plan recommended; the properties were bought and a mortgage of $220,000 was placed on the Academy's building. The Trustees appointed Drs. Sayre, Jacobi, and Jacobus to prepare a budget for 1911, and they reported probable income of $30,000 from all sources and estimated expenses of $31,246, including $6,500 for the Library. The Trustees promptly cut the Library appropriation to $4,500.

The Academy took immediate possession of the 44th Street property, ordered access to it by a cut through the yard of 17 West 43d Street, installed a new water meter, and granted permission to the Janitor and Assistant Janitor to live on the property.

The President announced the appointment of Dr. Haven Emerson as chairman of a committee on plan and scope for a new building, with power to select other members, and this committee was made responsible to the Board of Trustees.

By October 26, the Treasurer reported he had received pledges for $53,500 to pay off the mortgage; $6,620 was already paid in. Forty-seven pledges were for $1,000 each.

To go back to the Library. In 1907 Dr. Cheesman resigned as Executive Librarian. He submitted a report stating that in his estimation the office of Executive Librarian would be superfluous if each of the five members of the Library Committee did a reasonable amount of work each year. He thought it advisable to continue the policy of rotating the chairmanship each year; after four years of service the senior member should make an intelligent chairman. A new member of the committee should spend his first year as Secretary and should also solicit want lists from the Sections. A second-year member should preserve and arrange for exhibits of instruments and the like, and solicit and care for photographs of Fellows. The third and fourth-year members should examine and report on all books sent on approval by publishers and importers, and those suggested by Sections, as well as solicit donations from authors and publishers. As Chairman, in the fifth year, a Fellow would be ready to attend to the administration—heating, ventilation, cleaning, and so on—and make his reports to the Council.

Dr. Charles M. Williams was promptly appointed Executive Librarian and gave excellent service for eleven years.

It was voted that the Executive Librarian and the Librarian of the Academy be directed to visit, between May 1 and October 15, the medical and principal institutional libraries of Boston, the New York State Library at Albany, others in New York City, Philadelphia, and Baltimore, as well as the Congressional and Surgeon General's Library in Washington, to obtain information regarding proper conduct of an up-to-date scientific medical library. What they were to look for is given in detail. They were instructed to report at the regular meeting in October and to present three typewritten copies of the report, one of which was to be given to the Board of Trustees, another to the Committee on Library, and a third to be filed in the Library of the Academy for the use of the Executive Librarian and Librarian. Two hundred dollars, or as much of that as should be necessary, were appropriated for the actual expenses incurred in making the investigation.

The new Executive Librarian and Mr. Brownne acted in concert, and were determined not to overspend the sums appropriated, but in April, 1909, the Library Committee reported it had spent all but \$400–\$500 of its funds for the year, and asked for another \$1,000. The hard-hearted Treasurer showed that the condition of the funds would not permit the additional sum, but later he found that \$500 could be spared for the Library, and this was voted.

In the fall of 1909 the Committee presented another detailed statement of affairs, and in January, 1910, gave to the Trustees a report which was received while Dr. Jacobi was at the meeting of the State Medical Society. The report called attention to the difficulties experienced in living within the appropriation while meeting the increased demands on the Library. In the Committee's view, the salary list, paid out of the appropriations, was unduly large; the Resident Librarian received \$3,600 yearly "besides rent, heat, light, coal and elevator service," which was equivalent to another \$2,000. By contrast, at the College of Physicians in Philadelphia and the King's County Medical Society the salary was \$2,000, while at the Boston Medical Library it was only \$1,500. Even at the Surgeon General's Library in Washington the pay was only $3,500, and that was according to the Army rank of the Librarian. The Committee felt that even taking into consideration the higher cost of living in New York—due mostly to rent—the Academy was paying double or treble the market price, which was unnecessary. It recommended that the office of Resident Librarian be abolished, his functions to be divided among the present staff, and that an "assistant or cataloguer" be added at $500–$800 a year; this plan was entirely feasible, would result in greater efficiency, and save the Academy nearly $3,000 a year.

In view of the long and valuable services of the Resident Librarian the Committee suggested "that he might be allowed a pension for a short term of years, as a token of appreciation and esteem."

Action was postponed to an adjourned meeting five days later, by which time Dr. Jacobi would be back. After a long discussion, the matter was referred to the Chairman of the Board for a complete investigation as to the salary of the Superintendent Librarian and the salaries of other librarians of other institutions, the cost of coal and light for the Academy, and as to the advisability of discontinuing the Academy's dynamo and purchasing all light, the Chairman to report at the regular meeting February 23.

Dr. Jacobi made a very thorough investigation. It was finally voted that, in order to meet the increasing needs of the Academy, the salary of the Resident Librarian should be reduced by $1,000 per year from March 1, 1910, the Chairman to inform the Superintendent Librarian of the reduction in his salary.

The other matters were laid on the table until specially called up.

In 1910, at Dr. Dana's suggestion, the Library Committee was requested to compile a catalogue of all the busts in the Academy and to place the name on each. The same year it was voted that the Library should establish a "card catalogue of current committee and commission investigations along medical and medico-social topics, with a collection as far as possible of the actual reports," and $100 was requested from the Trustees to start the work. It is to be feared the work was never started.

Much of the Library staff's time was taken up by checking up on Fellows who kept books out too long, imposing fines, and so on.

The By Laws were amended to read: "Any Fellow, Associate Fellow, or other person violating the rules of the Library, shall, in the discretion of the Committee on Library, subject to approval of the Council, be suspended from the privileges of the Library for a period of time and shall be liable to a fine."

One Fellow withdrew some bound volumes of a journal, which he submitted as evidence in a civil law suit. The judgment was appealed and all exhibits impounded, including the Academy's bound volumes. After repeated letters, his lawyer explained the situation. The Fellow was deprived of his rights in the Library for a year, and the Academy sustained the action of the Library Committee. He was later asked to replace the volumes at his own expense.

Another Fellow was suspended from Library privileges for a full year for failure to pay any attention to letters asking the return of books long overdue. When he appealed to the Council it sustained the action of the Library Committee.

The Academy adopted a resolution passed by the Council that the Treasurer notify members who had not paid their dues on or before April 1 of any year that they would be deprived of the privilege to remove books from the Library or to consult the Library between 2 and 10.30 P.M. This resolution was to be sent out with the bills to members on January 1, 1911.

In 1910 the Alumni of Bellevue Hospital Medical College presented $1,200, through Dr. Sayre, to found the "Austin Flint, M.D., LL.D., Memorial Library Fund" for the purchase of medical books. Dr. Sayre took particular pains to emphasize "that the Dr. Flint referred to was born in 1812 and died in 1886" and suggested that "Natio 1812. Obiit 1886" be printed on the bookplate. (He was not to be confused with Dr. Austin Flint, Jr., who resigned in 1886 after the attack on Dr. Fordyce Barker.)

The Library Fund was also increased by a check for $120.26 from Dr. Ricketts, Professor of Pathology, University of Chicago, part of the $270.56 he had received that year for the Carpenter Lecture. He probably only kept enough to pay his expenses.

In July, 1910, Trustees of the Mott Memorial Library, previously installed as a separate library at 64 Madison Avenue, offered to the Academy the collection of books, instruments, and so on, with a check for $750 to pay for transportation; the gift was accepted.

In 1907, the Section on Public Health, reorganized after eleven years, offered resolutions in regard to milk regulations, which were passed by the Academy. Compulsory pasteurization of all milk was not considered necessary, but users of milk not "certified" or not proven "thoroughly inspected and wholesome" were advised to boil it for three minutes, especially if for children's use. The supervision of farms, dairies, creameries, milk during transit and delivery, and at distribution points ought to be continued. Official Bureaus and Departments should cooperate in prevention of communicable disease in cattle and their handlers. These resolutions were to be sent to the Committee on Public Health of the Board of Aldermen, to the Committee considering the Reese bill, and to the medical and lay press.

In 1898, because of differences of opinion on the subject, the Academy had taken no action in regard to regulating midwives. In 1907, however, it concurred in the Recommendations of the Association of Neighborhood Workers who in conference urged a state law regulating midwives and providing for examination, inspection and license. (That same year the Board of Health adopted fairly stringent rules and regulations for their control.)

Also, the Academy voted its cooperation with twenty organizations, mostly civic, in promoting cleaner streets. The resolution stated that public health required clean streets; that public indifference and ignorance was as much to blame as inefficiency of city officers; that the problem was a difficult one in engineering and administration, with financial and legal complications, which must be overcome. It recommended a careful study of the problem, and appointed Dr. Jacobi, and Dr. W. G. Thompson alternate, as a delegate to a joint committee, which memorialized Mayor McClellan.

In 1909 the Women's Municipal League asked the opinion of the

Academy on the competency of present statutes relating to cruelty to animals in, and publicity of results of, experimental laboratory work. Dr. Simon Flexner wrote the answer which the Council sent:

1. The present laws of New York are adequate to confine the practice of animal experimentation to proper persons and to punish all cases of cruelty, and

2. That the wide and full publication in scientific and medical journals of the results of animal experimentation, and the free access to the laboratories which custom prescribes for credited and properly interested persons, are sufficient to refute the charges of secrecy in laboratories in which experiments on animals are performed.

A statement concerning congestion in hospitals for tuberculosis, deploring the great lack of accommodations for advanced tuberculosis cases and earnestly requesting the Board of Estimate to take proper steps to relieve this immediate need, was sent to the Mayor, Comptroller, and President of the Board of Aldermen. A committee of five was authorized to present this resolution in person to the Mayor.

Dr. W. Gilman Thompson described the official city hospital situation in New York, and a committee of nine or more was authorized to report on the matter. This Committee recommended the charter of the City of New York be amended to provide centralization of the hospital system, and the Council authorized the Committee to continue its work in association with other committees of the city in the endeavor to incorporate the desired measures in the charter.

The Academy endorsed the resolutions of the Board of Trustees of the New York Public Library, protesting against a 25 percent tariff *ad valorem* on books, which did not exempt those for libraries but only those for use of the United States and for the Library of Congress.

A committee to study the question of filtration of the city water supply made a report which the Council approved and ordered read to the Academy and to be given to the Press. There is no copy of that report in the Academy.

On recommendation of the Public Health Section, and with the approval of the Council, the Academy passed these resolutions:

Resolved, That the Academy of Medicine requests the Department of Health to prepare for the examination of specimens of smears for gonococci, and request the Department send to all physicians in Greater New York a letter stating that they are prepared to examine smears of pus for gonococci for the purposes of diagnosis, and that the Department, after examining specimens of pus, send to the physician by whom the specimen is sent, a circular of information as to the care of gonorrhoea, syphilis and chancroid. And, further, that the Department of Health furnish to the physicians, cards for voluntary reporting of cases of gonorrhoea, syphilis and chancroid, to be mailed by the physician in a sealed envelope and kept by the Department for statistical purposes, the card to be so arranged as to furnish the Department with the age, sex, and civil condition of the patient, but not to disclose the identity of the patient.

The Section also presented to the Council:

WHEREAS, It has been convincingly demonstrated by recent investigations that an appreciable amount of infectious material is transmitted in thickly populated communities by the fly, and

WHEREAS, The greater number of these flies of which over 98 percent occurring in houses belong to the species musca domestica, breed in stable manure, therefore be it

Resolved, That the New York Academy of Medicine, recognize in the fly both a nuisance and a menace to public health, and therefore recommend to the Department of Health of New York City, that measures be taken for the prevention of the breeding of flies in this way by suitable measures directed toward the handling and disposal of stable manure in thickly settled parts of the city, and further recommends that measures be taken to prevent the ingress and egress of flies to and from the infectious cases of illness in the city hospitals, and also recommends that that portion of the Sanitary Code (Section 46) dealing with exposure of food to dust and flies in public places be made still more comprehensive to prevent the transmission of infectious material in this way.

The Council voted that the Secretary present the resolution informally to the Health Department and report its attitude at the next meeting. There is no record that this was done.

The Academy also endorsed the Owen Bill to establish a Federal Department of Health.

In 1910 the possibility of publishing in one place a list of all medical meetings to be held in New York was taken up, and a committee was appointed to confer with societies holding meetings in the Academy. Nine organizations discussed the matter but did not come to any conclusion.

The Council voted that a committee of ten be appointed to represent the Academy at the hearing on the budget estimates of the city for 1911, to secure proper recognition of the health needs of New York and provisions to meet them. The President appointed the "available ten members" of the Council on this committee.

The Section on Public Health had requested the Librarian to obtain copies of bills dealing with health which came before the Legislature. He arranged with the County Medical Society to send copies to the Library.

The scientific sessions were carefully planned and well carried out. Each Section presented a program, and symposia were the rule in all meetings. The discussions included typhoid fever, the possible sources of infection, three small epidemics in Pennsylvania, and nutrition in typhoid fever; the recent epidemic of poliomyelitis, and a paper on experimental poliomyelitis by Drs. Flexner and Lewis; the problem of pellagra; "Serum Treatment of Cerebrospinal Meningitis," by Drs. Flexner and Jobling; "Recent Advances in Syphilis, and Demonstration of the Spirocheta Pallida," by Dr. James Ewing.

Many papers were read by guests from other cities. Tuberculosis of children was discussed by Drs. McCrae of Montreal, Hamill of Philadelphia, and Morse of Boston; exophthalmic goitre by Drs. L. B. Wilson of Rochester, Minnesota, W. S. Halsted of Baltimore, and Alfred Stengel, of Philadelphia.

New methods in the study of the diseased heart were discussed by Dr. W. B. James, the first physician to import an electrocardiograph. Other subjects were malignant endocarditis, its bacteriology, and possible surgical treatment; vasoconstriction and vasodilatation in arterial disease; anaesthetics, including rectal anaesthesia; thoracic surgery and intratracheal insufflation.

Matters of public health were also discussed—street cleaning and its problems, and open-air treatment in homes and hospitals. The whole long list is an interesting collection.

From the folders of the Academy we learn that public lectures were given on a number of topics, chiefly by laymen.

The Anniversary Meeting in 1907 was again made much of. The Council voted $400 to pay expenses, and spent $406.25. Colonel Gorgas spoke on sanitation of the Canal Zone, and invitations were sent to President Theodore Roosevelt, ex-President Cleveland, and Governor Hughes, none of whom attended.

The next year the Academy was forced to be economical; special invitations "with outer and inner envelopes" were given up, for the total expenses were only $21.75. Major Charles Lynch spoke on the "Medical Service in a Modern Army in War," as exemplified by the Japanese Army in the Russo-Japanese War.

In 1909 Dr. Louis Livingston Seaman described his personal observations of the sleeping sickness in Uganda, with an illustrated talk on a short safari to the sources of the Nile; and in 1910 Dr. William H. Welch of Johns Hopkins presented proposals for furthering legislation to regulate animal experimentation.

The Carpenter Lectures were given regularly. It had been the custom to reprint them in various sizes, from the journals which published them; the Trustees decided hereafter they should appear in a uniform size, the same as the *Transactions*.

In 1907 the Lecture was on "The Mosquito as a Sanitary Problem," by Dr. Edward A. Ayers. The next year Dr. G. S. Woodhead of Cambridge University spoke on "Some Phases of the Evolution of Modern Preventive Medicine, Illustrated by the Present Campaign against Tuberculosis."

The 1909 Lecture was on "Some Aspects of Rocky Mountain Spotted Fever, as Shown by Recent Investigations," by Dr. H. T. Ricketts, University of Chicago, and in 1910 Major F. F. Russell,

M.C., U.S.A., reported on "The Control of Typhoid Fever in the Army by Means of Vaccination."

The Committee on the Gibbs Prize Essay reported that nine essays had been submitted, and some were of much merit. The most praiseworthy one was incomplete—so announced by the author—"for lack of times." The Committee was inclined to award a portion of the prize to this essay, but as $2,000 had been offered, they recommended the prize be not awarded. It was suggested that in the future, discretion be given the Committee to award a part of the prize to one or more meritorious essays, according to the degree of merit. The Trustees decided to vote a part of the whole sum, if the donors agreed, and it was also voted to try to persuade them to change the terms of gift, substituting "to promote *research* in the cause, pathology and treatment of diseases of the kidney."

The donors agreed to the $500 payment, and this was awarded to Dr. Norman E. Ditman, in collaboration with William H. Welker, "in partial recompense for the expenses undertaken in the study" connected with "Deficient Oxidation and Nephritis."

Dr. Sayre later criticized the announcement of a part award, as made, and it was then voted to send a formal letter to the donors of the fund, stating that the conditions had proved impracticable after numerous endeavors, and that the fruit of the recommendations of successive Prize Committees and the mature deliberation of the Council was that a committee of five should be appointed by the Council from eminent physicians and laboratory workers, and that this Committee should chose one, two, or three workers in various laboratories, giving the grant for their work, and publish the work as a Gibbs thesis.

After some conferences, the donors agreed to the changes and the following then appeared:

The Council of the New York Academy of Medicine desires to announce that the income of the Edward N. Gibbs Fund, amounting to $500 a year, will be granted for a period of years to any qualified worker to be selected by the Council from those who may apply, for its use in research in the clinical, pathological or chemical problems of diseases of the kidney. Applications stating the qualifications of the applicants and the topic which he proposes to pursue, should be sent to the Secretary of the Council of the New York Academy of Medicine, 17 West 43rd Street, New York City.

James Ewing
George E. Brewer
W. Gilman Thompson, CHAIRMAN

The award has been made on this basis ever since.

During this period, matters of ethics were of very minor importance. Dr. L. A. Conner called attention to an advertisement of Glycothymolin with a letter written by Dr. Justin Herold, a Fellow of the Academy. To the request for an explanation, he replied, and the Council took no action.

Charges were presented against Dr. John Sedgwick Billings. Dr. Dana was appointed a committee to see the Fellow bringing the charges, and they were withdrawn.

Newspaper clippings of a public lecture at the Skin and Cancer Hospital were submitted, in which Drs. L. D. Bulkley and W. S. Bainbridge were quoted. Both Fellows were asked for an explanation. They submitted letters, and were informed the Council urged every possible precaution be taken to avoid such publicity in the future.

Some Fellows were becoming sensitive about their names appearing in the papers. Dr. Frederic Griffith did not wait for charges to be brought. He wrote regretting some publicity of which he had no previous knowledge. The Council replied that his position had not been injured by actions performed by others.

The following brief minutes of the Council are interesting.

"Voted that nothing be hung on the walls of the Council Room without the authority of the Council."

"Voted that the three comic pictures on the walls of the Council Room be removed." We wonder what the pictures were.

In 1907, Dr. Bryant, after serving ten years on the Board of Trustees, declined reelection. The Trustees adopted the following:

WHEREAS, Dr. Joseph D. Bryant has declined renomination as Trustee of the Academy and thus disappears from our councils after twelve years of uninterrupted service in this body, and

Whereas, In his wide range of contacts with the community, both in his official and in his personal relations to it, he has been of very special value to the Academy in furthering its best and highest aims, and has always striven for its advancement, not only in its scientific activities, but also in its more direct duty to the public at large, and

Whereas, Its present temporal welfare is in no small degree due to his example and his efforts, therefore be it

Resolved, That the Trustees make this record upon their minutes, of their appreciation of Dr. Bryant's services to the Academy and their sense of their personal loss in his withdrawal from their councils.

A. Jacobi
George L. Peabody

Dr. Gorgas was elected an Honorary Fellow in 1908.

In the same year ex-President D. B. St. John Roosa died at the age of sixty-nine and Dr. Dana delivered a eulogy. And in 1910, Dr. A. H. Smith died. The President, Dr. Wyeth, delivered an address in his memory.

During the Hudson-Fulton celebration in 1909, the Academy extended the privileges of the Library to the Surgeons of the visiting fleets, during their stay.

The engineer of the Academy wrote, calling attention to his eleven years of service with but one raise of wages of $5 per month in all that time. He asked for a raise also on the ground of extra service in the way of repairs, and so on, outside of his regular duties. It was voted to raise his salary from $80 to $90 per month.

A number of small, interesting gifts were presented. A mortar and pestle belonging to Dr. Daniel W. Kissam, born 1763; from Dr. Osler, a facsimile of the diploma granted William Harvey by the University of Padua in 1602; a record of vaccinations and inoculations of smallpox at Milton, Mass., in 1809; a replica of the bronze medal presented to Dr. Jacobi by the Alumni Association of Mt. Sinai Hospital on completion of fifty years of service. The American Gynecological Society also presented a medallion, struck to commemorate the first ovariotomy by Ephraim McDowell in 1809.

In March, 1910, the President was authorized to reserve all meeting rooms and halls in the Academy on May 6 for a reception given by the State Medical Society in honor of Dr. Jacobi on his eightieth birthday.

"At least 800 persons were present at the meeting," the *New York Medical Journal* tells us, including Surgeon-General Wyman, Drs. James Tyson and Willard of Philadelphia, Isaac Abt of Chicago, Woods Hutchinson of Asheville, N.C., H. D. Arnold of Boston, and a number of others from various cities in New York State.

Dr. Bryant presided and made a few brief remarks, saying that the State Society had forestalled Dr. Jacobi, who had hoped to give a little "get together" himself; but that this gathering was in line with his own ideas. He concluded, As their friend was older in time than all but a few of them, younger in activity than most of them, virtuous and public spirited as the best of them, larger in experience than any of them, it was fitting on his eightieth birthday that they should transmit to enduring substance the likeness of Abraham Jacobi.

Dr. Jewett, President of the State Society, then took over, and after a few words of appreciation of Dr. Jacobi, said "wishing to show the respect and affection they bear you in the name of the Medical Society of the State of New York, I present you with the likeness of one of the world's most eminent citizens and most venerable men." A bas-relief portrait of Dr. Jacobi was then unveiled by his granddaughter; it is today one of the treasures of the Academy.

The report goes on to say that

Dr. Jacobi was very much affected by the expressions of regard from the speakers, and it was with some difficulty that he controlled his feelings in accepting the gift. He said that this conspiracy of friends had begun in the House of Delegates of the Medical Society of the State of New York. No objections had prevailed and the responsibility was theirs. . . . He was the beneficiary of their goodwill and old and young friendships, with nothing left him except an old heart full of gratitude and no words sufficient to express it.

He said he intended to collect a number of the eulogies lately pronounced, so as to learn what he should have to live up to in order not to disappoint or disgruntle his friends in coming days or months, or, preferably, years. He made a fine, brief address full of pride of what had been accomplished by the profession and full of hope for the future.

The Council proposed to make Dr. Jacobi an Honorary Member, after all these years of service, but feared he might not be eligible for office as a Trustee, so the Counsel of the Academy was asked for an opinion. His opinion was election of a *Fellow* as an Honorary Fellow did not disqualify him for the office of Trustee. Dr. Jacobi was promptly elected Honorary Fellow and continued as President of the Board of Trustees.

Dr. Wyeth served two terms as President. He was not opposed for reelection. He presided very regularly, only missing six meetings, two of them being special meetings during the summer of 1910. He was not a very forceful President and was not elected a Trustee on retiring.

Dr. W. M. Polk was elected President for the next two years.

1911–1914

William M. Polk

DR. WYETH in his Valedictory gave a detailed report of the activities of the Academy, scientific and administrative, during his term of office, emphasizing the growth of Section activities.

Dr. Polk spoke of the revolutionizing era of medicine in which the Academy had developed, deplored the mercenary motive, regrettably increasing in the profession at large, and urged hospitals to develop their usefulness by adopting social service activities as was being done at Massachusetts General Hospital. Both addresses were later published in full in the *Medical Record.*

They were immediately followed by a paper by Dr. John B. Murphy of Chicago, President of the American Medical Association, on "Surgery of the Joints."

Dr. William M. Polk, twenty-eighth president, was a man of sixty-seven. A Southerner, like Dr. Wyeth, he had fought through the Civil War in which his father, General (formerly Bishop) Polk, had been killed. After the war, he gave up his work as superintendent of an iron foundry to study medicine at the University of Alabama, later completing his course at the College of Physicians and Surgeons in 1868. He had been connected with both Bellevue Hospital Medical College and New York University, and from 1898 was Dean and Professor of Gynecology at Cornell University Medical College. He was a Fellow of the Academy from 1873, Orator in 1889, and Vice-President, 1895–97.

In many ways the next four years were the most active the Academy had experienced. An imposing array of papers was presented, among them, the value of X-ray in the early diagnosis of carcinoma of the stomach, and gall bladder infections with pyloric adhesions, illustrated by a "cinematographic demonstration of gastric peristalsis," in which Dr. Lewis Gregory Cole took a leading part; congenital pyloric stenosis and the results of surgical treatment by gastro-enterostomy; and bone grafts in ununited fractures.

Three papers were read on alcohol and alcoholism. The psychological problems of medicine brought forth four papers, one by Professor Heilbronner of Utrecht, delivered in German. The psychopathies of children and psychoanalysis with special attention to Freud and his theories were interesting subjects.

A meeting was given over to the criminal (including the defective child), from social, legal, and medical viewpoints, and at the next meeting Dr. Stephen Smith reviewed recent court decisions on malpractice. Judge Clearwater and Dr. Dana entertained the Academy with papers on "Expert Medical Testimony."

Salvarsan, its value and methods of use; the study of the functional capacity of the heart and the use of the "Micrograph" were also discussed; phenolsulphonephthalein and renal function was talked about, and reviewed again three years later. Occupational diseases was a very important subject and a special notice for that meeting emphasized that "The public are invited." Five important papers were presented.

Public health and allied subjects were very prominent during Dr. Polk's term of office. Surgeon-General Wyman, U.S. Public Health and Marine Hospital Service, gave an address on present-day public health activities. One thousand extra invitations were ordered sent out by the Trustees.

Another meeting for which special cards of invitation were issued to the public, and for which the Fellows were asked to give the widest possible notice, was given over to "National Quarantine," discussed by Dr. Leland E. Cofer, U.S. Public Health and Marine Hospital Service.

At a meeting to discuss nursing education, five papers were read, three by heads of nursing organizations. Resolutions were passed and referred to the Council, urging a study of the whole subject. The Council referred it to the Committee on Public Health, Hospitals and the Budget.

Hospital and dispensary facilities for the treatment of venereal diseases brought forth papers by Drs. Biggs, Homer Swift, E. L. Keyes, Jr., S. S. Goldwater, and W. T. Longcope. Resolutions were adopted and published opposing a new Health Department clinic for treatment until it was proven existing clinics were inadequate, but approving the diagnostic service through its Department of Laboratories for those unable to pay, and the establishment of a Department of Health hospital for treatment in certain stages of venereal diseases. It was also recommended that private hospitals admit acute cases of syphilis and establish a special department for treating them. An association of clinics for venereal diseases was suggested, perhaps in connection with the Associated Out-Patient Clinics. A reduction in the cost of salvarsan was recommended, by lifting the customs duties, and newspapers were urged to discontinue the use of obscure terms and to speak frankly of gonorrhea and syphilis.

At a meeting in 1913 Professor Adami of McGill University discussed the "Cancer Research Institute," and Professor W. F. Wilcox of Ithaca gave cancer statistics. Dr. Willy Meyer emphasized the importance of public education on the subject, and Dr. Howard C. Taylor, Sr., introduced resolutions approving such education, which were approved by the Council and published.

Other meetings were given over to the purification of the waters of New York harbor, the value of different types of food and changes caused by canning. The education of the crippled brought forth several papers from heads of institutions for that purpose.

Programs were arranged by the Rockefeller Institute for Medical Research twice, by the Department of Laboratories of the Health Department, one by the College of Physicians and Surgeons on general studies and another by its Department of Surgery on experimental work, and by the Memorial Hospital on studies on cancer.

The Academy assigned one stated meeting to a joint session of its Section on Pediatrics and the New England and Philadelphia Pediatric Societies, at which one paper was read by a member of each.

In March the Trustees announced a special meeting for April 6, 1914, and authorized the Treasurer to rent a moving picture machine, and pay for a supper from the Loomis Entertainment Fund.

There is no mention of this meeting in the Academy minutes, but a special notice announced:

A SPECIAL MEETING WILL BE HELD IN

HOSACK HALL

MONDAY EVE., APRIL 6, AT 8.30 O'CLOCK

Order:

I. A Study of the Movements of the Intestines. Under Artificial Circulation. Demonstrated by Motion Pictures.

II. Athletes in Action as Demonstrated by Motion Pictures.
Film from the Marey Institute of Paris.

Dr. Gustave T. Monod, M.D. (Paris)
M.R.C.P. (London)
of Vichy, France (by invitation)

Discussion by Drs. Jacob Kaufmann, Max Einhorn, George R. Lockwood, Edward Quintard, J. W. Draper, E. W. Caldwell and L. G. Cole.

A Collation (Loomis Entertainment Fund) will be served after adjournment, to which the Fellows and guests are invited.

Many outstanding workers from New York and other cities contributed or discussed papers.

The Anniversary Addresses were made a good deal of. In 1912 and 1914, at any rate, we know that engraved invitations were sent (there are copies on file) inviting to the "Anniversary Meeting and Reception." The addresses were as follows:

1911: Dr. James Ewing, "The Public and the Medical Profession."

1912: Dr. C. L. Dana, "The Doctor's Future in Its Relation to National Medical Insurance."

1913: Dr. Graham Lusk, "The Fundamental Basis of Nutrition."

1914: Hon. George McAneny, President of the Board of Aldermen, "Some of the Relations of the Medical Profession to the Municipal Government." (This was the first time the Anniversary Address was given by other than a medical man.)

The Carpenter Lectures were:

1911: Jacques Loeb, Rockefeller Institute, "The Role of Salts in the Preservation of Life."

1912: Max Rubner, University of Berlin, "Concerning the Life of a

Cell." (A special card was sent out for this meeting, stating the paper was "not as yet published.")

1913: Dr. W. H. Park, "Antitoxin Dosage, Anaphylaxis, Active Immunization against Diphtheria."

1914: Dr. W. B. Cannon, Harvard University, "The Physiological Equivalent of War."

The Gibbs Memorial Prize was awarded to Dr. Herman O. Mosenthal for research in diseases of the kidney.

In addition to the papers on public health measures, activities along these lines were many. The Academy sent resolutions to Governor Dix, recommending an appropriation so that Dr. Porter, Commissioner of Health, could investigate and study poliomyelitis "epidemic since 1907, and reportable since 1910."

On recommendation of the Council the Academy endorsed the proposed amendment to the Public Health Law abolishing the common drinking cup.

Also it adopted a resolution submitted by the Section on Obstetrics and Gynecology, urging State legislation requiring training, registration, licensure, supervision, regulation and control of women practicing midwifery. Fifty thousand births were reported annually in New York City by midwives, practicing without any required education or supervision. The recommendations of 1907 had not produced results.

The Section on Pediatrics recommended amending the Building Law to allow tenements with outside stairs to do away with the ventilating shaft, and allow toilets to open on this stairway. The Academy approved the plan.

The Section on Ophthalmology requested the Council's permission to cooperate with other medical societies in combating "evils arising from the advertisements of optometrists." The Council decided this was "inadvisable."

A committee, of which Dr. Dana was chairman, had been appointed to consider the hospital situation in New York. It was still active. Another committee to attend the hearings on the City Budget for 1911 was still in existence. Dr. Dana recommended this latter committee be discharged and its interested members assigned to the

Committee on Hospitals (which had received through the Bureau of Municipal Research a grant of money from Mrs. E. H. Harriman), in order that this Committee could keep in touch with the Board of Estimate and the various city departments associated with health matters. This was done.

Soon after, the Section on Public Health submitted a report to the Council, which a special committee considered, recommending that the Section be disbanded and that the Council appoint each year a Committee on Public Health to consider all matters in this field and report as occasion demanded.

Dr. Dana promptly reported for the enlarged Hospital Committee, and presented the resignation of all its members. The Council then appointed an interim "Committee on Public Health, Hospitals and the Budget," the functions of the resigned committee being assigned to it. This original Committee, to serve until the January, 1912, meeting of the Council, consisted of:

C. L. Dana, Chairman
A. T. Bristow
R. J. Carlisle
A. G. Gerster
S. S. Goldwater
L. E. Holt
J. H. Huddleston
A. Jacobi
T. C. Janeway
S. Lloyd
J. A. Miller
W. G. Thompson
L. R. Williams

And so was appointed what is now known as the Committee on Public Health Relations of the New York Academy of Medicine. The functions and duties of this committee were announced as follows:

I. PUBLIC HEALTH

a. To maintain a bureau for the collection of facts in regard to public health, sanitation, and hygiene.
b. To endeavor to establish an active cooperation with all public health activities in the city.
c. To keep the medical profession advised of current public health conditions.
d. To render to the health, school and other public authorities and to

the community at large an authoritative medical opinion on public health matters. This is to include frequent conferences with officials of various City Departments, the holding of public meetings, the giving of lectures, the distribution of literature, and other methods of publicity.

e. To undertake and suggest special researches looking to the solution of vital public health problems, such as an investigation of industrial diseases, etc.

f. To make a comparative study of methods and results of public health activities in other cities, both in this country and abroad.

g. To cooperate with the Library Committee in maintaining the literature in the Academy Library upon the subjects of public health, sanitation, and hygiene, in a high degree of efficiency.

II. MUNICIPAL BUDGET

a. To utilize facts obtained by the study of public health and hospital conditions for practical application in the preparation of the annual municipal budget.

b. To assist actively the various departments of the city government which relate to public health and hospitals in the preparation of their tentative budgets.

c. To take an active part in the budget hearings before the Board of Estimate and Apportionment.

III. HOSPITALS

a. A study of hospital and dispensary conditions in New York City, including public and private institutions in all the boroughs. This study to be made from a standpoint of: (1) Construction; (2) Equipment; (3) Administration; (4) Medical Efficiency.

b. To plan for the future development of hospitals and dispensaries according to the distribution of population and to further the efforts already being made to raise the standards of dispensary work.

c. To undertake a comparative study of hospitals and dispensary conditions in other cities, both in this country and abroad.

d. To cooperate with the Library Committee in establishing and maintaining a section in the library of the Academy for the collection of all forms of literature relating to hospitals and dispensaries.

IV. REPORTS

a. From time to time reports of this Committee shall be presented to the Academy.

This was a big program, but the Committee not only lived up to it, but in its many years of service has enlarged its field. Dr. E. H. Lewinski-Corwin was its active, efficient Secretary from the first.

For several years the Academy had urged raising the standards of expert testimony in the courts. A committee had been appointed to further such efforts. Dr. Dana was its chairman, and he naturally referred its findings to the Committee on Public Health. This Committee presented a long and favorable report and urged again, in brief, that medical experts be paid by or through the court, and that they have certain minimum standards of qualification. The Public Health Committee recommended that the report be adopted, and the Academy did so unanimously. It was very favorably commented on by the *Medical Record.*

The records of the Academy are full of the reports of this Committee and its activities for the next three years. There were approved a bill to promote the efficiency of the Public Health and Marine Hospital Service; a report on health conditions in public schools; and a resolution against a special city hospital for children, a separate service in general hospitals being considered much preferable.

In February, 1913, the Committee recommended, in a long report, the formation of a State Board of Control to have general supervision of the mentally defective from birth throughout life; this was approved by the Academy. It was a very comprehensive and rather complicated program, outlining what should be done for those who are non-self-supporting and those who could be made self-supporting.

The Assembly bill requiring coroners to file reports of autopsies with the State Department of Health was discussed and approved. After discussion, Dr. Soresi proposed the following: "As we physicians realize the immense importance or better, absolute necessity of performing autopsies, all physicians should pledge themselves to leave their body for autopsy; such conditions should be made essential for everyone who wants to enter a medical school in future." Strangely enough, there was no seconder, so no action was taken.

The Public Health Committee prepared an argument in favor

of the establishment of a hospital for communicable diseases in the Bronx, which was adopted. The hospital was never built because of opposition from real estate owners.

The Council presented, from this Committee, and the Academy adopted the following:

Resolved, That the plan of investigation of the Food Inspection Division of the Health Department, outlined by the Public Health, Hospitals and Budget Committee, at the invitation of the Health Department, be approved by the Council, on the following conditions:

1. That the form, method, extent and means of investigation be accepted in writing by the Health Department.
2. That the form, method, extent and means of investigation be accepted by the Bureau of Municipal Research.
3. That no expense in the investigation be incurred by the Committee.
4. That no publication of the report or its conclusions be made without the approval of the Council.

In December, 1913, during an outbreak of typhoid fever, the Academy voted to issue a statement of the efficacy of immunization against the disease, and endorsed the efforts being made to protect all exposed to it, either by their own physician or by the Department of Health.

In 1914 the Academy voted to endorse an Assembly bill to substitute a Chief Medical Examiner for the inefficient system of coroners. It had taken this step several times before. The next year the Committee on Public Health took active part in drafting and securing the passage of a bill which established in 1918 the office of Chief Medical Examiner.

It also opposed a Senate bill amending the Public Health Law in regard to habit-forming drugs and another amending the State Charities Law in relation to dispensaries.

The Committee, after a special study of tonsillectomies as performed in dispensaries and hospitals, recommended certain rules, which were adopted. Also the Academy approved of a conference with the Mayor, heads of various city departments, and other civic bodies interested in street cleaning.

A case of tuberculosis occurred among the employees of the

Academy. The Committee was promptly requested to make a physical examination of all employees.

The following announcement appeared in the folder during this time:

TO THE FELLOWS OF THE NEW YORK ACADEMY OF MEDICINE:

Inasmuch as one of the objects of the Academy is the promotion of the public health, it seems advisable to call attention to the activities of the Academy along these lines.

The President appoints a Committee on Public Health, Hospitals and Budget each year. This Committee investigates matters on its own initiative and serves as a source of information to organizations of citizens and departments of City government which are concerned with the public health. The range of matters which come before the Committee for consideration and action is very wide. The Committee calls upon the special Sections of the Academy from time to time for authoritative statements upon special matters concerning which their opinion is asked.

It is well known that there are many Fellows in the Academy who are always ready and willing to bear their share in any work for which they are specially equipped when the public welfare is at stake. The amount of work asked of the appointed committee is often so large as to become a serious burden. It is suggested, therefore, that those Fellows who are willing to be called upon by the Committee to take up matters on request as the need arises, should send their names to the Secretary of the Committee, Dr. James Alexander Miller, with an indication of the kind of public health activity with which they would wish to be associated.

All these things, some of which required prompt action, were often done under great difficulties. Everything the Committee undertook—every report and investigation—had to be approved by the Council and then voted by the Academy. This consumed valuable time. In December, 1914, it was proposed:

that the President be authorized to appoint each year a Committee to be known as the Public Health Committee, and to fill such vacancies as may occur in it or make such additions as may seem best. This Committee shall be authorized to cooperate with public health activities and to make studies of and issue statements upon matters pertaining to public health and hospitals, but such statements shall not be issued until approved by three-fourths of the Committee and by the President of the Academy. Subject to these provisions, and in pursuance of these objects, the Committee is authorized to appear before any committee, board, legislature, or other body, in order to make statements and express opinions on matters relating to public health and hospitals.

This proposal was announced in the folder for the next meeting, and in January, 1915, authority was officially granted to the Committee, which also abolished its cumbersome name.

And so began the activities of the Committee on Public Health as an integral part of the Academy, independent as to its activities, but always responsible, in the end, to the Academy. For more than three decades it has so served the Academy. Its complete story is an epic by itself. It has acted in an advisory way when advice of a medical or public health nature was wanted. The Mayor, the Commissioners of City Departments, the Board of Education, the Board of Health, the Governor, and members of the State Legislature and the Congress of the United States have all had occasion officially to seek its advice.

It has undertaken endless surveys and inquiries into existing conditions. It has acted as an educational body, by conferences, lectures, published articles and books, focusing the attention of the profession and the laity on health problems and the methods of meeting them. (See *Thirty Years in Community Service*, 1911–1941.)

And so carefully has it confined itself to authorized activities and course of procedure that in all the years of its existence there has never been more than an occasional trivial objection to its action.

For some time the subject of an Academy bulletin of clinics and meetings had been discussed and studied. A committee appointed to formulate a plan felt that the difficulties of getting information and the cost of publishing were too great. Meanwhile an independent group had formed as the Society for the Advancement of Clinical Study in New York, and it now applied for quarters in the Academy for an Information Bureau. After mature deliberation, arrangements were made to grant the Society quarters free of charge, to allow it to put up a bulletin board, to allow Mr. Brownne to appoint a clerk, all from funds provided by the Society. This arrangement was to last one year, on trial. With true economy, the Academy stipulated that the clerk while on duty should operate the general switchboard of the Academy!

This was the forerunner of the Academy's Committee on Medical Education, established twelve years later.

In October, 1911, the Academy voted the following:

Resolved, That the secret division of a fee with any person who may be instrumental in influencing a patient to apply for operative care or professional advice, is unworthy of any member of the medical profession.

Resolved, That any member of the Academy who promises, offers, or gives, or causes to be promised, offered or given, any money or other valuable thing to any person for inducing or influencing a patient to apply to such member for operative care or professional advice, shall be reported to the Academy by the Council, with a recommendation for his expulsion from membership.

Strange as it may seem, this was not approved by either Drs. Jacobi or A. A. Smith, than whom there were no more absolutely upright practitioners. President Polk was not sure the Academy had gone far enough. In his second Inaugural he stated the Academy ought to use its great influence to give the Board of Regents of the State a similar authority to that of the Appellate Division of the Supreme Court of the State, which could for sufficient cause expel an offender against legal ethics from the courts.

A committee had been appointed to consider improvements in the organization and programs of the Sections. In December, 1912, this Committee reported to the Council, recommending three things: 1) that a vice president be assigned to assist the officers of the Sections in efforts of cooperation and increased efficiency (Dr. W. B. James was appointed the following month); 2) that a member of a Section should not be entitled to vote or hold office therein or to receive postcard notices unless he "voluntarily" made the agreed-upon contribution to the Section for its support; 3) that each year Section members should receive notices asking whether they wished to enjoy the privileges mentioned in (2); and that if so, they would be called on to contribute.

These propositions were all approved and were subsequently added to the By Laws. This was a great triumph for the Sections, which had been trying for years to attain financial security.

This Committee was continued and, together with the Recording Secretary, was instructed to consider amendments to the Constitution.

In April, 1913, the By Laws were amended to read:

Article XXI, Section 3. Resolutions or reports concerning public questions not pertaining to the special objects of the Academy on which action is desired, shall be referred to the Council for its consideration, and reported at the first stated or special meeting following the next meeting of the Council. Such resolutions or reports shall be printed in full or in such abstract as shall indicate their purport, and shall be sent to each Fellow of the Academy with the notice of the meeting.

The Folders of Academy meetings show this was regularly observed.

The Committee reported, and in December, 1913, the Academy adopted a revised Constitution. The important changes were the addition of "The promotion of Public Health" as a third object; the removal of certain details on library management, responsibility for which was delegated to the Library Committee, who were to make and announce the rules; and the rules, noted above, pertaining to Section affairs.

In November, 1911, it was announced by Dr. Jacobi that about the middle of the next September several hundred German physicians and teachers would arrive in New York to study medical practice, hospitals and institutions in America, while en route to the International Congress on Hygiene and Demography. Their presence bid fair to be "epoch making" and was an illustration of the fact "that America is taking its rank among teaching nations." Dr. Jacobi thought the Academy should do something, and was promptly made its representative in the matter. A circular letter was voted sent to the various institutions and officials concerned, to be signed by the President and Recording Secretary.

An interesting note is that of December 28, 1910. The privilege of using Hosack Hall and two other rooms on February 20, 1911, from 9 A.M. to 6 P.M. was granted a committee to examine candidates for positions on the House Staffs of New York, Presbyterian, Roosevelt, and St. Luke's hospitals.

The Library, of course, was having a harder and harder time. The Trustees had insufficient funds to fulfill its needs. The cost of periodicals was considerable, and the Trustees were not sure whether the interest from the trust funds "to be spent for new books" could be spent on periodicals. They asked Counsel for an opinion, and he ruled that current journals came under the head of new books, and that the income from each and every fund, mentioned by name, could be spent legally for subscriptions. This helped out considerably. But binding and temporary shelf room cost money, and the appropriation from income of the Academy never exceeded $5,000 in any year. (This did not include salaries.) Mr. Brownne, Executive Librarian, asked for $60 a month for one or two assistants to work on a "shelf list" of books and periodicals. This was left by the Trustees to their Chairman and the Treasurer, with power, "if the finances of the Academy would justify the expense."

For 3,000 duplicate books and periodicals, chiefly the latter, sold to the State of New York for its library, the Academy received $3,500. The Council approved the Library's plan to exchange its books on natural history for medical books from the Public Library.

The libraries of the late Dr. E. B. Coburn and Dr. Charles S. Bull were received. Dr. Everett Herrick, a great friend of the Academy all his life, left $25,000 to the Library Fund in 1914. A small residue of a fund to give a dinner to Dr. Biggs, recently appointed Commissioner of the reorganized State Department of Health, was also turned over to it.

The Council approved the purchase of 605 volumes of Theses of the University of Paris, at $1.00 per thesis.

The Library Committee was permitted to open the Library to Fellows on Sundays and legal holidays from 10 to 5, when it seemed desirable, with of course the approval of the Council. This was done at the end of the year.

The Academy ran into serious difficulties in regard to the enlargement of plant and facilities. In January, 1911, the Council received this recommendation from its Committee on Finance:

WHEREAS, A Committee on Finance of the Academy is endeavoring to raise money from the Fellows to pay for the property recently purchased to enlarge the Academy site, and

WHEREAS, It is desirable to have a new structure erected as soon as possible after plans are matured and adopted, and

WHEREAS, There is no money in hand or in sight for such a huge undertaking;

Resolved, That the President of the Academy be, and he is hereby authorized and requested to appoint a Committee on Ways and Means to solicit money from the beneficently inclined lay men and women for the purpose of erecting at an early date a new building for the New York Academy of Medicine and its valuable Library on its old and recently acquired premises, 15, 17, 19 and 21 West 43rd Street, and 10 West 44th Street, New York City.

The Committee to have power to add to its members, such other well disposed physicians, or lay men, or women, as it may think necessary and advisable, to help obtain the large amount of money needed for the new structure.

A report read by the Committee on Plan and Scope recommended that it was in the interest of the Academy to so plan to use the entire area in its possession that it should ultimately have a building new from the foundations up, first erecting a structure upon the lot at 10 West 44th Street eight or ten stories high, to house the power, heating, lighting, and ventilating plant in the cellar, offices for administration and for reception of books and supplies on the main floor, and stack room for as many stories overhead as seemed necessary; two or more of the upper stories to be reserved temporarily for reading and meeting rooms during the period of destruction of the present building and the one at 15 West 43d Street and the reconstruction upon this large area of the main new building. The Committee referred to the fact that six months had already elapsed since the new lots were acquired and that it would take at least six months constant application by some building committee and an architect to develop plans which could be accepted, before the building upon the 44th Street plot could be considered, and a year to bring the first wing of the contemplated building to completion. To the end that progress be made, the Committee urged upon the consideration of the Board the early selection of an architect.

The Trustees, having heard the report of this Committee, adjourned to attend the meeting of the Council and then reconvened at 10. 50 P.M., the Council having approved of the report.

A circular of information, giving the facts to date and the plan, was ordered sent out to the fellowship.

The appointment of a Committee on Ways and Means was considered unwise by the Council, "at the present time."

But now began real trouble. York and Sawyer were selected as architects and submitted three sets of plans with a long explanatory letter, which stated in part:

May we call your attention to the following general considerations.

(1) A cube is the most economical figure to build and to administer; it is contained in the least superficial area.

(2) Such a solid as that bounded by the lot lines of your northern property is so far from a cube that it is disproportionately expensive to build, inconvenient to administer, requires additional stairways, an excessive number of stack stories and cannot be adequately lighted.

(3) Other things being equal, the stories of the cube, the main building, are a better proportion, much better lighted, more flexible in their possible subdivision, more generally available than the floors of the extension and,

(4) Since you will in any case have half a dozen stories on 43rd Street and since the elimination of an extension on 44th Street will mean the addition of upper stories to the main building, and since under such conditions as obtain in your location, with the proper elevator service which you must have in any case, these upper stories will be better lighted and ventilated, quieter, cleaner and more desirable than the lower floors (even those of the main building) we conclude

(5) That, in general, without regard to specific conditions or plans, it is better to carry up a compact main building, concentrate areas, have short runs from the stairs and elevators to the rooms and offices, short horizontal delivery from the farthest stack to the book lift; that it is preferable to get up in the light, air and quiet rather than to extend

a plan of irregular form into a space uneconomically prolonged and narrow.

The cost at 40 cents a cubic foot, for the same area provided in all three plans, amounted to $540,000.

Toward the end of May the Committee on Plan and Scope handed in its report, signed by Dr. Haven Emerson, Chairman.

The Committee studied the three tentative plans and agreed that one of the three, while not by any means perfect, embodied so much that was desirable and so far improved upon the others that the architects were to be advised to continue working upon this plan.

This conclusion of the Committee led to their passing a motion to the effect, that it is not desirable to use the property at 10 West 44th Street for the purposes of building for the Academy.

Our Committee was appointed to study and plan for provision for increased facilities for the Academy.

After considerable discussion and with the benefit of the expert opinion of the architects we agree unanimously that to retain the 44th Street property is inadvisable from the point of view of economy of construction, convenience of administration and permanent cost of maintenance.

Your committee on site being ignorant of many of the problems, factors and causes concerned in the construction of a complicated building upon lots of various shapes, and fearing that we might find ourselves at the mercy of adjoining owners of property decided that the 44th Street property ought to be bought at the same time that the lot at 15 West 43rd Street was acquired.

The meeting of the Academy called to authorize the purchase unanimously approved of the decision of the Committee on Site.

As I was a member of the Committee on Site I feel that some explanation is needed for a reversal of the decision of that Committee by the Committee on Plan and Scope.

The letter of the Architects, the motion passed by the Committee on Plan and Scope after looking at all sides of our needs and possibilities of accommodation will, I think, convince you that we are right in urging the sale of the lot at 10 West 44th Street.

The Trustees agreed, the Council agreed and the Academy later agreed. It was rather a blow and slowed things up, for the time being, till other factors came into the picture later.

Pledges for Academy Extension Fund amounted to $105,658 by

the end of 1914, and the fund had $76,095 on deposit. The mortgage had been reduced from $220,000 to $200,000, and was renewed for three years, but at 5 percent instead of 4½ percent.

The Academy held a mortgage for $7,500, which it had been obliged to foreclose. "The unsettled state of the real estate market" made it impossible to sell, so the Trustees had spent $4,500 on improvements, and the property was now leased "to advantage."

The Trustees had spent as little as possible for renovations and repairs "because of the probability of having a new building in the near future"; but boilers had to be renewed and many other smaller repairs made.

Several Fellows requested the Trustees to install electric fans. They replied it should be done as soon as finances permitted.

It was voted to publish in 1911 a list of all officers and Fellows past and present, which was to be the first of a series of "Quinquennial Catalogues." It appeared, and was the first—and last. There is no printed record of membership, except of active Fellows, after 1911.

November 7, 1912, Dr. Abraham Jacobi presented his resignation as Trustee to become effective December 31, 1912, with a request for immediate acceptance so that nominations for the place would be possible. The minutes tell us:

> On motion of Dr. Jacobus, it was voted:
> That the resignation of Dr. Abraham Jacobi, as Trustee of The New York Academy of Medicine, an office which he has filled as President of the Academy ex-Officio and as Trustee by election, together, since January 1885, nearly twenty-eight years, with great ability and fidelity and with invaluable benefit to the Academy, be accepted with sincere regret and the heartiest wishes for his good health and happiness in the future.

This event is more graphically described in an article in the *New York World* of November 8, under these headlines.

DR. JACOBI TOO OLD FOR ACADEMY WORK

Great Objection to Loved Leader Resigning Trusteeship, but His Wish Prevails

The official connection of Dr. Abraham Jacobi with the Academy of Medicine, the development of which he has fostered for half a century, was ended last night when his resignation as trustee was accepted unwillingly. Advancing years and his duties as President of the American Medical Association were given and taken as the reason for the step.

The meeting was thrilled when the Secretary, Dr. John H. Huddleston, read Dr. Jacobi's resignation. Dr. Arthur M. Jacobus promptly objected. He said that Dr. Jacobi's foresight and tact had largely resulted in procuring the site of the Academy's building at No. 17 West Forty-third street, and bringing about its construction. Dr. L. Emmett Holt, Vice-President, who was presiding, denied Dr. Jacobi the floor until Dr. Tobias had said of him "age cannot wither nor custom stale his infinite variety," and Dr. Joseph D. Bryant had averred that of all men he knew Dr. Jacobi had the keenest sense of obligation.

With tears in his eyes, Dr. Jacobi then rose to ask that his resignation be accepted. He told how he had vainly sought several times to resign, so that a younger man might succeed him.

"Every one of us must die," he said, "Probably I shall soon pass away. But the Academy must live. I have worked to the best of my ability. I hope you will find a better man in my place. But somebody must do the work. You and you and you—" and he pointed to several other members. He pleaded that he be permitted to withdraw, and there was a dramatic unanimity in the vote, "Aye." He bowed his thanks.

Dr. Jacobi had been elected President of the American Medical Association in June, at the age of eighty-two.

He attended his last meeting of the Trustees December 23, faithful to the last in his duties.

In 1911, Dr. E. G. Janeway, President in 1897–98, died at the age of seventy. He had had a very distinguished career and had been a strong supporter of the Academy. A memorial meeting was held in April and Dr. Francis Delafield spoke of him as a physician, Dr. William H. Welch as a pathologist, Dr. A. Jacobi as a consultant, and Dr. Joseph D. Bryant as a friend. It was a very impressive meeting.

In 1914 three Fellows who had been of great value to the Academy passed on. Dr. Everett Herrick, a Fellow since 1867, Trustee, 1882–97, and Vice President, 1897–99, had worked hard for its advancement. He was eighty years old and had been inactive for several years. He left the Academy $50,000, half for the Library and half for the Endowment Fund.

Another great loss was Dr. Joseph D. Bryant, LL.D., a Fellow since 1875, President 1895–96, and Trustee for ten years thereafter. The Council recorded at a special meeting: "During all these years his sound judgment, convincing personality, and rare executive ability made him a leader in its councils. Always foremost in the advocacy of scientific progress, a teacher of exceptional attainments, his loss will be greatly felt by the Academy and the profession."

Dr. Bryant left one-seventh of his residuary estate to the Academy, to be paid "upon the death or re-marriage of his widow."

The third loss was Dr. Egbert LeFevre, Corresponding Secretary since 1911. He was only fifty-five years of age when he died of scarlet fever. He had been a Fellow since 1889. The Council recorded: "He was learned and helpful as a councilor, inspiring as a teacher imbued with scientific zeal, active in philanthropic work, and in measures for civic betterment." He received his M.D. from New York University in 1883, and degrees of Doctor of Science were conferred on him by Rutgers in 1910 and Doctor of Laws by New York University in 1911.

Dr. Simon Baruch, in February, 1912, presented in behalf of many friends, a portrait of Dr. Wyeth by J. Campbell Phillips. He read several letters from the contributors, including those of Drs. Jacobi, Isaac Adler, and W. J. Mayo.

Dr. Polk was an excellent President. He gave much time to Academy affairs and, in spite of an enormous practice and teaching demands, he presided at all but thirteen of the sixty-three meetings during his terms of office.

1915–1918

Walter Belknap James

THE NEW ADMINISTRATION was ushered in by an unusual inaugural celebration. Dr. Polk's Valedictory was brief and Dr. James, accepting gracefully his new duties, reminded the Academy it was well occasionally to get away from strictly practical medical and surgical problems. This year was the four hundredth anniversary of the birth of Vesalius and it was fitting and proper that the Academy should recognize that event. He introduced Dr. William H. Welch, who spoke on "Vesalius and the Spirit of His Time." It was an interesting if, as stated, unprepared address. Dr. Welch was followed by Dr. Fielding H. Garrison, Librarian of the Surgeon General's office, Editor of the *Index Medicus*, and one of the most learned authorities on medical history; his talk was illustrated with lantern slides.

Dr. Harvey Cushing spoke of the influence of the Renaissance on anatomical illustrations, showing pertinent examples by Leonardo da Vinci, Michelangelo, and Raphael, and then showing portraits of Vesalius.

In connection with this meeting there was an exhibit of original and early editions of the works of Vesalius, of his contemporaries and teachers, his followers and imitators, and also those of his critics and opponents. There were forty-nine volumes on exhibition from the Academy's own library and from those of the King's County Medical Society, Drs. Cushing, Garrison, Streeter, Coley, and Pilcher. A two-page "catalogue" of the exhibit was printed with a reproduction of an engraving of Vesalius. It was the first of many exhibits the Academy has produced, and was a very creditable one. It lasted four days.

Dr. James, the twenty-ninth President of the Academy, was a highly educated man, of great versatility and endless energy. He had been a Fellow since 1889, but had not been very prominent in its affairs, and had never held office except that of Vice President, 1912–14. He had succeeded Dr. Francis Delafield as Professor of Medicine at the College of Physicians and Surgeons, and had been connected with Bellevue, Presbyterian and Roosevelt Hospitals. A man of great personal charm, of established professional and social position, he presided over the Academy during one of its most difficult periods of development.

World War I was in full swing and Germany was in the ascendant. One of the first things the Academy did was to appoint a committee to cooperate with others to receive donations for the relief of physicians and their families in overrun Belgium. There were so many other committees for the relief of Belgium that the committee did not have striking success.

During the first two years the scientific programs continued very much as usual. They were well arranged. Two were from the Rockefeller Institute, the first, describing some of their studies on pneumonia, and the role of serum, digitalis, and optochin, in its treatment; and the second, on meningitis, with Dr. Flexner's paper on the "Varieties of Meningococci," the effects of intraspinal injections of serum by Dr. Ayer, and other interesting reports.

The City Department of Health provided a program; Dr. Matthias Nicoll, Jr., spoke on the "Diagnosis and Treatment of Tetanus," Dr. Park on recent developments in prevention and treatment of diphtheria, Dr. Emerson on the new Sanitary Code of the City, and other papers were read.

The State Department of Health presented a long program with papers by Drs. Hermann M. Biggs, Commissioner, L. R. Williams, Deputy Commissioner, C. E. A. Winslow, Division of Publicity and Education, A. B. Wadsworth, Division of Laboratories, Cressy L. Wilbur, Division of Vital Statistics, H. L. K. Shaw, Division of Child Hygiene, and F. M. Meader, Division of Communicable Diseases.

Two consecutive meetings were given over to the latest views on syphilis, including serum diagnosis and the colloidal gold test. At other meetings the discussions included:

"Vitamines, a New Factor in Nutrition"; "Typhus, Endemic in

New York" presented by Dr. N. E. Brill and described by him as "unwisely called Brill's Disease"; "Treatment of the Failing Heart," with papers by Drs. Theodore B. Barringer, Cary Eggleston, N. B. Potter and J. S. Thacher; the "Management of Chronic Renal Disease" by Dr. Theodore Janeway, Johns Hopkins; and, after the widespread epidemic of poliomyelitis in 1916, one by Dr. Lovett of Boston, who had been called upon by Dr. L. R. Williams to organize the state campaign "to minimize the ultimate disability" therefrom.

The importance of Saratoga Springs as a health resort occupied another meeting. Alcohol, its psychological effects and its effects on personal efficiency, were discussed at another.

Many papers were read by authorities from other cities; Drs. C. B. Walker and W. B. Cannon of Boston; J. G. Clark, Edward Martin, Thomas McCrae, and W. L. Clark of Philadelphia; John Howland, L. F. Barker, L. V. Hamman, and Hugh Young of Johns Hopkins; E. C. Rosenow of Chicago; and E. R. Baldwin of Saranac.

A special meeting was held April 20, 1915, to urge the transfer of the Quarantine Service at the Port of New York from state to national control. The Academy had been interested in quarantine since 1887, when it made a study which was instrumental in having the disgraceful existing conditions corrected. In 1892 it made another study and in 1893 sent a committee to Washington to urge the nationalizing of quarantine. In March, 1915, the matter was acute again. The World War made it seem probable that a great deal of infection would be carried by refugees to our shores. The Public Health Committee asked permission to circularize the Fellows to use their influence in securing support of the transfer. The Council decided it was "inadvisable" to do so, but asked the Public Health Committee to take such further action as would secure the transfer.

The result was a special meeting, at which Hosack Hall "was ompletely filled, with an audience which remained throughout e meeting, and manifested considerable enthusiasm." Dr. James ade a very clever introductory speech, and read a few of the 38 letters of approval he had received, including one from Surgeon-eneral Gorgas. The "Present Health Conditions in Europe and

Their Relations to This Country in the Coming Months" were described by Mr. Henry James, based on observations in Servia. Dr. William C. Woodward, former President of the American Public Health Association and Health Officer of the District of Columbia, and Ex-President Taft made interesting addresses.

The Academy also passed resolutions requesting the State Legislature to have a Census taken in 1915, and decided to take part with the city and state Departments of Health and the American Museum of Natural History in the exhibit of hygiene, in celebration of the fiftieth anniversary of the foundation of the Department of Health of the City.

In April, 1916, it was voted:

> that the New York Academy of Medicine views with regret the inadequate provision made for the medical service in the bills now before Congress for increasing the Army of the United States, which gives less than five medical officers to 1,000 combatants, whereas experience in the present war in Europe indicates that ten medical officers to 1,000 combatants are necessary under conditions of actual warfare. The ratio in the Army of the United States in peace time should not be less than seven medical officers to 1,000 combatants, to be increased to ten per thousand in wartime.

In this period the Library was not heard from quite so often. The Council approved of granting quarters to a stenographer for those desiring to dictate. This was to be tried out for six months, the Fellows using the service to pay the expense. It was not a success.

The Council also recommended to the Trustees that the Library should collect and file press reports of the Academy's activities, together with programs of meetings which might be valuable to preserve. The Trustees appropriated $25 for the purpose. This was ordered at an unfortunate time. The Library had all it could do to run its own affairs. It is to be regretted, however, that no such file of clippings was collected and filed.

Library space was overcrowded, but one result of the war temporarily helped that. There was a cessation of German and French periodicals. The Library Committee asked for no appropriation for 1916, as there was a considerable unexpended balance on this account.

But there was the continued cry for more shelf space; books were already being stored on the floors. Accommodations for readers were inadequate. Their number had steadily increased during ten years from 14,124 to 27,203. In the three years the Library had been open on Sundays and holidays, to Fellows only, the number using it had increased from 763 to 887.

The Committee reported later it had found no solution to the lack of accommodations for readers, except that the Librarian, finding anyone standing, instructed such person to go upstairs to some other less convenient room.

In 1915 through the efforts of Dr. Bernhard W. Weinberger, the First District Dental Society began an association with the Academy which has resulted in total donations of over $13,000 for books and binding, and in the Academy's acquisition of an outstanding collection on dentistry.

The Trustees were having their troubles—plenty of them. Unsatisfactory conditions were not confined to the Library. The Society of Medical Jurisprudence complained of the uncomfortable hardness of the seats in Dubois Hall and its very bad ventilation. The Council replied in view of the radical changes contemplated it seemed unwise to make any changes in that room.

The ventilation of Hosack Hall continued to be complained of and the Trustees finally authorized its House Committee to spend "not more than $50" to improve it!

The next year the County Society's Comitia Minora complained of the ventilation, lighting, and heating of Room 48, assigned to them, and asked the Trustees to do something about it.

The Fellows were complaining of inability to park their cars in front of the Academy, as the space was occupied by those visiting Stern's and Aeolian Hall, on the opposite side of the street.

And, finally, the Treasurer reported a communication from the Borough President, stating that 43d Street was to be widened, and all vaults, bay windows and other obstructions would have to be removed within a few months. The necessary changes eventually cost the Academy $2,500.

The plans for enlarging and rebuilding the Academy had been constantly discussed by the Council and Trustees. These years of European War were not ideal for raising money. The President discussed the situation with the Trustees and it was voted his report be printed and sent to the Fellows, which was done. It was his official report for 1916, before he started his second term of office, and is the first printed report on record.

He gave a very clear and concise account of matters since 1911. When the project was started, subscriptions were to be paid in five annual installments. By 1916 they would all be paid and the lease on 15 West 43d Street would expire at that time. He then outlined the plan to build first on 15 West 43d Street and later to remodel the old building, removing some of its defects. Such a building would meet the Academy's needs for another twenty years. More money would be needed and the Trustees and Council were considering how it could be raised.

And so 1917 started. It was obvious that the United States would inevitably be drawn into the European War, and that at no distant date. The Army Medical Corps had already organized an Officers' Reserve Corps, and a number of Fellows had joined it. In March, 1917, the Council considered a suggestion to amend the Constitution to continue the first stated meeting each month, to make the second meeting of each month subject to the call of the President or Council. This was voted referred to the Academy, but there is no record of its ever having been voted on.

In November, 1917, however, it was voted: "In view of the large number of active Fellows of the Academy who are away in military service, it would meet with the approval of the Council if the scientific paper should be omitted from such stated meetings of the Academy during the coming year as in the judgment of the President seems wise." It is to be noted papers were read at every meeting in 1918.

Also the Council decided that, owing to the extraordinary conditions created by the war, the Chairmen of the various section be permitted, with the assent of the President, to omit a meeting.

The Academy increased the limit of Fellows resident in New York City from 1,200 to 1,300, and made five years in practice necessary instead of three.

Although in April the United States declared a state of war to exist, in May the Academy considered at a special meeting, a resolution

for the purpose of meeting the growing needs of its Library and readers, the New York Academy of Medicine hereby approves the project of erecting an addition to its building on the lot No. 15 West 43rd Street, already in its possession, and that the Board of Trustees is hereby authorized to proceed with the erection of this building according to plans to be approved by them and at such time as they shall deem it wise to so build, considering the current cost of building and other existing conditions, and that the Board of Trustees is hereby authorized to sell, for a price that shall seem to them wise, the lot No. 10 West 44th Street.

The Council also reported: "Although the present time is not considered by the Council a favorable one for building, yet it believes that action upon the matter should be taken now, in order that, if the Academy approves, detailed plans and specifications may be prepared in advance, so that advantage may be promptly taken of a favorable building market whenever it occurs."

Dr. Jacobi opened the discussion. Proposed changes in the old building and floor plans of the proposed addition were shown by lantern slides. The Academy adopted the resolution and approved the report of the Council.

The County Medical Society proposed to cooperate with the Academy in looking after the interests and the families of physicians who had been called to the war; the Council thereupon appointed a committee of five authorized to extend its benefits beyond the membership of both the County Society and Academy. By April, 1918, this joint committee had received $35,289.96 for this purpose. Requests for funds appeared in the Academy and County Society folders, from April 18 through December 5.

Dr. Gilman Thompson was appointed to represent the Academy on the Advisory Committee of the Council of National Defense.

He was appointed, at his own request, to represent the Academy on the American Committee for the rehabilitation of destroyed French and Belgian cities and towns, and was requested also to act as a committee of one to present to the Council a plan for the proper recording of the interesting collateral activities of the Academy during "this year" of war.

Throughout the war the Library was open to all men in uniform. Hosack Hall was offered free for all meetings for purposes connected with the war, and rooms were provided for examination of candidates for the Medical Reserve Corps.

The war hit the organization of the Academy pretty hard. By May, 1917, Drs. C. M. Williams, Executive Librarian; R. H. Halsey, Assistant Secretary; and F. T. van Beuren, Recording Secretary, had all been granted "indefinite leaves of absence." As several of the officers of the Sections had also left to enter the Service, the President was authorized to appoint temporary officers to fill their places. Drs. Haven Emerson and R. S. Haynes were appointed Acting Recording and Assistant Secretaries, but it was not long before they, too, left to go abroad. By the end of 1917 two hundred Fellows were in Service. The question of hanging out a Service Banner was left to the Trustees.

The Academy, at the suggestion of the Council, amended the By Laws, Article X, Section 12, by adding: "It [the Council] shall be empowered during the continuance of the war to remit wholly or in part, or permit the postponement of the payment of the dues of any Fellow now in active service, or to transfer Fellows in such service from Resident to non-Resident membership." As no printed Constitution and By Laws were issued between 1914 and 1920, by which time this was inappropriate, the amendment does not appear in any printed copy.

In May, 1918, Dr. Dana, Chairman of the Public Health Committee, appealed to the older Fellows, who were not available for military service, to help relieve the shortage of dispensary physicians, which was causing serious curtailment of their activities, as their contribution to the war effort.

In October an appeal was received from the Commissioner of

Health, and endorsed by the Public Health Committee, to attempt to secure volunteer physicians for service among the sick poor during the current influenza epidemic. Assurances were sent to the Commissioner that the Academy would at once do all in its power to help him. It was voted that the Executive Secretary of the Public Health Committee interview the Commissioner of Health and suggest to him that the Academy would send out a notice to all its members, calling for volunteers; a list of their addresses and the hours at which they would be available would be deposited with the Health Department, and the physicians would be summoned directly from that body. The details of the matter were entrusted to the Executive Committee of the Public Health Committee. The records show that thirty-nine Fellows offered to answer calls from the Commissioner.

Similarly, an appeal was received from the Red Cross for physicians to work among "the stricken people of Perth Amboy," with what results we do not know.

The scientific sessions were kept up very well, but the Sections were not able to arrange programs as they had been doing. It was therefore up to the President to see the meetings went through.

In January, 1917, reports were read on typhus fever, the results of expeditions into Mexico, the Balkans, and Russia. The isolation of the bacillus of typhus from the body louse and the methods of protection and immunization were described.

In March the Section on Medicine arranged a session on influenza, and, in December, Laryngology and Rhinology arranged a paper by Dr. H. L. Lynah on "Treatment of Stenosis of the Larynx and Trachea after Diphtheria." In April, 1918, Genito-Urinary Surgery arranged a meeting with four papers on "Prostatectomy and Surgery of the Urethra." Those were the only Section-arranged meetings in two years, except that of Pediatrics mentioned below.

Groups of papers were read on influenza; modern aspects of tuberculosis; the treatment of inoperable cancer, with the then status of radium and X-ray; and the study of crime and the criminal from the point of view of modern psychiatry.

Dr. S. S. Goldwater discussed "the care of the sick in a modern community"; Dr. J. E. Goldthwait of Boston, "The Challenge of the Chronic Patient"; and Dr. M. S. Gregory, "The Modern Conception of the Nature of Inebriety."

In May, Dr. A. E. Taylor (Department of Agriculture) discussed "Food Supply in War Times," and in November Dr. Alexis Carrel, "The Principles of the Treatment of Wounds."

During 1918, most of the meetings centered about the war and war problems. The Medical Staff of Camp Upton gave a series of papers on their experiences: Majors Magnuson and Murray discussed physical reconstruction, and Dr. Pearce Bailey, Lt. Col., M.C., "Neuro-Psychiatry and the Mobilization."

Dr. C. L. Gibson, recently returned from France, spoke on "Surgery and Actual Surgical Conditions at the Front." Professor Pierre Duval spoke, in French, on "Modern Aspects of Lung Surgery"; his address "was kindly translated by Lt. Col. Raffaele Bastianelli," who then read a paper on the same subject. Dr. Bastianelli had had much experience in portable surgical hospitals in the Italian Alps, where patients were transported to the hospital through space by overhead cables. Sir Thomas Myles spoke on some of the later phases of lung surgery with special reference to the work at Base Hospitals.

Another group of papers was on "Medical Problems in Aviation."

The Public Health Committee arranged an important meeting on the "Prevention of Disease in War Industries," and resolutions were passed, urging greater attention on the part of medical schools and hospitals to the study, prevention, and care of occupational diseases.

The Section on Pediatrics presented the problem of child welfare work in France, with papers by George Vincent of the Rockefeller Foundation and Ralph Pemberton of the Red Cross. The Section also, with the approval of the Council, established a "Committee on War Time Problems of Childhood of the New York Academy of Medicine" and arranged with Secretary Lane, Department of the Interior, to publish a series of articles which this committee would provide.

It was a thoroughly war year.

The Sections did extremely well and only Medicine, Obstetrics and Gynecology, and Laryngology and Rhinology cut out more than one meeting, except Historical Medicine, which had no meetings.

The Carpenter Lectures were given as usual:

1915: Dr. G. W. Crile, "The Kinetic Drive, Its Phenomena and Its Control."

1916: Dr. Philip Kreuscher, "A Clinical and Experimental Study of Metastatic Arthritides."

1917: Dr. W. J. Mayo, "The Relation of the Spleen to Some Obscure Clinical Phenomena."

1918: Professor Graham Lusk, "The Scientific Aspects of the Inter-Allied Food Situation."

The Anniversary Addresses were rather unusual. In 1915, the subject of "Disease and Crime, an Anthology," was presented by Messrs. George W. Wickersham, President of the Bar Association, T. M. Osborne of Sing Sing, and Judge Harry Olson, Chief Justice of the Chicago Municipal Court.

In 1916, Hon. Chauncey M. Depew spoke on the "Art of Growing Older" and the value of an interest in public life.

Henry Fairfield Osborn delivered the 1917 address, on the "Origin and Nature of Life" and in 1918 Edwin G. Conklin spoke on the "Biology of Democracy with Especial Reference to the Present World Crisis."

As the President was always authorized to select these speakers, Dr. James may be given credit for originality.

Naturally the program for the addition to the Academy was in abeyance all through the war. But general plans had been drawn, and were exhibited for many weeks in the smoking room. Dr. James reported on retiring as President that these plans were being completed and specifications were expected to be ready before the next spring, so that "as soon as building costs and conditions make it possible" work could be begun.

The use of 10 West 44th Street having been given up for building purposes, an offer was received from Louis Sherry to rent the property for $5,000 a year for ten years, he to pay all taxes, assessments, insurance and repairs, with option to purchase within five years for $100,000. The Academy had paid $120,000 for it, and the Trustees were at first not inclined to accept the offer, but on the advice of a special advisory Finance Committee, composed of two bank presidents, it was finally accepted. The upkeep was costing the Academy at least $5,000 a year.

This action caused more complications. The tenant desired immediate possession, so the duplicate books stored in the building were removed to 15 West 43d Street, without proper arrangement. This was a great inconvenience and a thorn in the side of the Librarian for years. It was not worse, however, than conditions today when the duplicates are stored in cases in the tenements to the east of the Academy.

Felix Wesstrom, the "janitor" of the Academy, lived at No. 10 West 44th Street, and lost his quarters. He was granted $30 a month increase in salary in lieu thereof.

A Section on Historical Medicine had been established in 1917, and seventy-five members were present at its first meeting. It was promptly requested by the Council to examine all pictures, portraits, statues, and collections in the Academy and, as far as possible, to classify, rearrange, catalogue, and label all needing that attention.

A statistical Secretary was appointed in 1863. His duties had been gradually increased and now were to keep a record of every former and present Fellow, Associate and Honorary Fellow, with date of birth and graduation; educational attainments; offices held in the Academy; date, place and cause of death, with "such other circumstances as shall fully illustrate the vital statistics of the Academy." He was to report each death with obtainable biographical data, and make an annual report to the Council each year. He had done his work very well.

The Academy now amended the By Laws to change his title to "Historical Secretary," and add to his duties the following:

> He shall record all gifts to the Academy (other than moneys and books, as elsewhere provided for in the Academy records) such as collections of instruments, portraits and other pictures, apparatus, medals

or any similar donations, together with the name of the donor and circumstances of presentation.

He shall record the public organizations which have held meetings during the current year in the Academy building, together with a memorandum of the general purpose of such meetings.

He shall record any other general purposes for which the rooms of the Academy have been used during the current year apart from the regular meetings of the Academy, its Sections, or committees.

He shall summarize, particularly, any general public activities of the Academy not comprised within its routine functions. He shall present to the Academy in writing, at its annual meeting, a comprehensive report of all topics recorded as above specified, designed to afford a complete historical record of its collateral functions, its gifts, and any other matters pertaining to its historical interest.

He was, of course, a practicing physician!

Ethical problems were few. The Committee on Admissions reported that several Italian physicians had been refused nomination because of publishing professional cards in the lay press. The Council voted this was a proper cause for exclusion.

Portraits were received of Dr. Francis, second President of the Academy (by bequest); ex-President Dana, by Cecilia Beaux, from the Charaka Club; ex-President Polk through Dr. Stewart; Dr. L. E. Holt from a group of pediatricians; and Dr. C. H. Knight, Librarian from 1887 to 1891.

Dr. W. J. Morton, a Fellow, presented a bust of his father Dr. W. T. Morton, of anaesthesia fame, together with an autograph letter of his, and descendants of Dr. Vacher, a surgeon in the Revolution, gave instruments used by him in that war. Other gifts were an army medical chest found on the Battlefield of Bull Run, an antique clinical thermometer, and the scalpel used by Surgeon General Bliss in operating upon President Garfield in 1881.

Dr. Ramon Guiteras, a Fellow since 1890, left $5,000 to the Academy "for any purpose that may be desired."

The Academy lost a number of very active and useful Fellows during these years. Dr. J. H. Huddleston died of pneumonia in 1915, at the age of fifty-one. Elected in 1897, he had delivered the Carpenter Lecture in 1902. He had been Assistant Secretary,

1898–1900, and Recording Secretary for ten years thereafter. He was elected a Trustee in 1913. Resolutions were passed stating:

Dr. Huddleston served the Academy of Medicine in the whole-hearted, faithful way in which he did everything which came to his hand, performing not only the regular duties of his office, but giving much time, thought, and energy to the many committees on which he was appointed. His lovable personality and genial manner endeared him to those Fellows with whom he was brought into intimate contact, while his scholarly attainments and broad grasp of the principles of medical science commanded the respect of the whole Academy. To the trustees and to the council his sound judgment and firmness of character were of inestimable value, while their deliberations were enlivened by his genial companionship.

Dr. A. A. Smith also died in 1915. A Fellow since 1876, he had been a member of the Council more than fifteen years and had succeeded Dr. Jacobi as Chairman of the Board of Trustees. Resolutions were passed by the Council recording his "constant service to the best interests of the medical profession. His energy was untiring, his judgment was of rare value, and his influence most beneficial, while his genial personality and strong Christian character made a deep and lasting impression upon all who enjoyed the privilege of his friendship." The Academy also passed strong resolutions.

In the summer of 1915 Dr. Francis Delafield died at the age of seventy-three. He had contributed much to the Academy's scientific meetings. He had delivered an address at the memorial meeting for Dr. E. G. Janeway in 1911. A memorial meeting was held for him and the address was made by Dr. T. C. Janeway, son of Dr. E. G., his pupil at the College of Physicians and Surgeons. It was a fine tribute to Dr. Delafield, and concluded as follows:

Gentlemen, when Francis Delafield passed away last summer, in his seventy-fourth year, New York City lost one of the really great figures which it has contributed to American medicine. The profession of New York should cherish his memory by following his example: to care not for fame, but for fact; to spare no labor in the ascertainment of fact; to use to the full each new method which will put us in possession of new facts; to impart these facts in language which shall be unequivocal; to face facts with uncompromising honesty to the reality outside ourselves and to our own mental integrity, and to face situations with unswerving fidelity to others. In one thing only would I have you diverge from his precepts—I would have you not cease to remember, nor forget to honor the name of Francis Delafield.

In 1916, Dr. A. B. Judson died. He had been a very important and constructive Fellow of the Academy. Elected in 1872, he had served on the Committee on Ethics in 1880 and had been Statistical Secretary from 1886. The resolutions adopted by the Academy state:

Dr. Judson was a man of lovable personality, prone to see that which was good in every man, and overlooking his failings. He was glad to extend a helping hand to the younger men in his specialty, and if he differed from his confreres on any topic did so in a way that did not give offense. Whatever Dr. Judson started to do he did it with his whole heart and he did it thoroughly. In nothing was this more clearly shown than in his connection with the New York Academy of Medicine. From 1886 until the time of his death Dr. Judson was our statistical secretary, and to his diligence and painstaking accuracy we owe the exact record which we possess of the part which every fellow of the Academy has taken in its activities. While Chairman of the Section of Orthopedic Surgery, he had full records made of the transactions of the Section, and saw to it that these were published in full in many journals both in this country and abroad, as well as being filed on the shelves of our own library, and in this and many other ways he made this section one of the most widely known throughout the medical world.

In his death the New York Academy of Medicine has lost one of its most faithful and conscientious officers, and in acknowledgment of his services the Council of the Academy desire this record of their appreciation to be spread upon the minutes and a copy sent to his family and to the medical press.

Dr. Judson, a graduate of Brown University, was attending lectures at Jefferson Medical College when the Civil War broke out. He promptly joined the Navy as Assistant Surgeon. Promoted to Passed Assistant Surgeon in 1864, he received his degree from Jefferson in 1865, and was made Surgeon in the Navy the next year, serving till 1868, when he received a degree of M.D. *ad eundem* from Bellevue Hospital Medical College. He worked for the Health Department for several years and in 1887 assisted in forming the American Orthopedic Association, of which he was Vice President in 1889 and President in 1890. He was sixty-nine years old.

In March, 1916, Dr. Wisner R. Townsend died at the age of sixty. A Fellow since 1889, he had been a member of the Committee on Admissions, 1904–8, and a Trustee since 1913. The following resolutions were passed by the Academy:

. . . the Academy of Medicine has lost one who for ten or twelve years had devoted a large part of his time and strength to its service and whose usefulness it is impossible to overestimate. As a member of the Board of Trustes and Council and as secretary of the former body, he took upon his shoulders a large part of the burden of the practical administration of the institution. Scarcely a day passed when he failed to report here to attend to any business that might arise, he being a member of the house committee. His wise judgment, his cheerfulness and unfailing tact made him always beloved by his fellows upon the board.

Few men have devoted more time and labor to the welfare of the profession, while his sympathy with its younger members and his kindnesses to them gained for him their warm affection.

The New York Academy of Medicine, mindful of his great services to it and mindful of his high character as a man and Physician, hereby records the sense of loss and conveys to Dr. Townsend's family its sincere sympathy in their sorrow. . . .

Another prominent figure retired from the Academy's activities. At the annual elections, Dr. Reginald H. Sayre declined to serve again as Treasurer. The Council adopted these resolutions:

It would be difficult for the Academy to express its obligations to Dr. Reginald H. Sayre.

For eighteen years he has been its Treasurer and for the same period has occupied a seat on the Board of Trustees and the Council.

During this time the Academy has suffered no loss in its investments. Under his management its financial position has steadily grown more stable.

His watchfulness and his integrity has given a feeling of security to all of those concerned in and responsible for its management.

In short, he has been for all these years an ideal treasurer, his interest suffering no relaxation during this long period of service.

As a Trustee and Councillor his wisdom, good sense and kindliness and his devotion to the Academy have made him almost indispensable in the deliberations of the two Boards.

Only the memory of his long term of faithful and successful service meets the keen unwillingness of his fellow-members to lose his presence and his aid, and makes us realize that he has earned the right to honorable retirement.

He will carry with him always the affection and respect of all the officers and employees and the gratitude and good wish of every Fellow of the New York Academy of Medicine. Therefore be it

Resolved, That as a token of its affection and appreciation the Council of the New York Academy of Medicine orders that the above minutes be spread upon the record of this meeting, and that they be transmitted to the Academy at its next meeting and read there as the action of the Board of Trustees and Council.

In 1915, Dr. Rudolph A. Witthaus died. Although not a Fellow of the Academy, he left his whole estate to its Library Fund, in trust, however, until the death of a beneficiary to whom during life he left $300 a month. To this beneficiary he also left his portrait. Dr. James was requested to communicate with her and say that the Council would appreciate any efforts on her part to see that the portrait of Dr. Witthaus eventually came to the Academy. The Academy received regularly the income of the estate, minus the $300 a month until 1934, when the principal of the fund, amounting to over $200,000, was turned over. The portrait was never received.

From the income of this Trust however, the Trustees agreed to pay to the divorced widow of Dr. Witthaus, "in indigent circumstances," the $50 he had given her each month. This amount was gradually increased and ultimately—at the time of her death about 1932—the Trustees were paying her $150 each month.

In January, 1918, the Trustees held a special meeting to discuss the coal shortage. Their supply would only last till March. It was voted to place on the doors of the elevator, "Those who wish to use the Library are requested to walk upstairs. In coming downstairs, everybody is requested to walk. The elevator is to be used only for reaching floors above the Library. By carrying out the above, the Academy will save about half a ton of coal per day."

The Treasurer reported that there was a deficit for the year of $7,900, and a deficit of $5,000 from 1917, making the total $12,900.

The Public Health Committee reported that Mrs. Harriman had decreased her contribution for the coming year and the Public Health Committee was facing a deficit of several thousand dollars. Another letter announced that, pending Mrs. Harriman's pledged subscription for the current year, the committee was without funds and unable to pay the salaries of the staff as well as meet other expenses. The Committee requested the Trustees to loan to the Committee the funds necessary to meet such obligations, the loan to be paid as soon as Mrs. Harriman's check was received.

Library affairs were fairly quiet, except for the acute shortage of stack room. Dr. Gerster suggested that a dictaphone be provided, to obviate the necessity of carrying books away from the Library. There is no record of the purchase. He also criticized the accumulation of dust in the journal room, and had noticed it was removed with a dry duster. The House Committee reported at the next meeting dusting was now being done with a damp cloth and not with a feather duster.

There were other little troubles. The Public Health Committee wanted more room provided for it in the plans for the new building and complained of the ventilation in its cramped quarters. Dr. Corwin called the Trustees' attention to the habit of male inhabitants in the rooming house in the rear exposing themselves either naked or in scant attire at the windows, much to the annoyance of the female employees of the Academy.

The Public Health Committee also was not getting satisfactory cooperation. Its request to the Section on Otology for an opinion on the effects of the dictaphone on the hearing of operators had met with a distinct rebuff. The Council decided the Public Health Committee was perfectly within its rights in asking opinions of any Section, and that Sections were expected to cooperate as far as possible in the solution of any problems that came before the Public Health Committee.

Dr. Walter James was a very attentive and capable President. He rarely missed a meeting of the Trustees or Council, except in the winter of 1918, when he was ill for three months. He may be given credit for introducing several new ideas into the proceedings. He was elected a Trustee and rendered valuable service for several years.

1919–1924

George David Stewart

Dr. George David Stewart, thirtieth President of the Academy, was born in Nova Scotia of Scotch parentage. His father died when he was six, and he was brought up by his grandfather, from whose library most of his education was obtained. At fourteen, he ran away to go to sea. Six weeks before the mast were sufficient to cure that longing, and he returned to study under a rare teacher who showed him how to teach himself. He taught at several small schools, and attracted the attention of the Rector at Saint Francis Xavier's, Antigonish, who did much for him. Intending to enter the ministry, his friendship with the local doctor led him to study medicine, and he graduated from Bellevue Hospital Medical School in 1889.

After service at Bellevue for two years, he returned to Picton, Nova Scotia, to allow a friend there to take a postgraduate course in Edinburgh for one year, as he had promised. He then returned to New York.

He was fifty-seven when elected President and was Professor of Surgery at University and Bellevue Medical College, Visiting Surgeon, Third Division, Bellevue, and President of the Medical Board, as well as Visiting Surgeon at St. Vincent's.

Dr. Stewart was a man of great personal charm. With a Scotch burr he never lost, and a wonderful sense of humor, he was a most popular speaker and had a host of friends. One of them, George F. Baker, endowed the Chair of Surgery at the University and Bellevue Medical College with one million dollars, in his honor.

A great lover of the poetry of Robert Burns, Dr. Stewart could recite his Scotch verses by the hour and was president of the Robert Burns Society in New York. He was the third, and last, President to serve three consecutive terms.

No record can be found of Dr. James's Valedictory or Dr. Stewart's Inaugural, which were followed by "The Experiences of a Surgeon in the War Zone," by Dr. G. E. Brewer, Colonel U.S. Army Medical Corps.

The first February meeting was arranged by the Public Health Committee, on the "Control and Prevention of Venereal Diseases." Five papers were read and resolutions of the Public Health Committee were presented: 1) urging the Department of Health to exercise its full powers for their better control and eventual eradication; 2) approving facilities offered by it since 1912 for laboratory diagnosis; 3) favoring compulsory reporting of all cases to the Department of Health; 4) urging admission of cases of syphilis in the communicable stages to general hospitals; and 5) the same for active cases of gonorrhea. These resolutions were voted on at the next meeting and were all adopted except (3).

In July, 1919, during the summer "vacation" of the Academy, Dr. Abraham Jacobi died, in his ninetieth year, at his summer home on Lake George. The official records of the Academy are silent about his funeral, but the papers tell us that, after private services at his town home, for the family only, "the auditorium of the Academy of Medicine . . . was crowded to the doors" for the public services. The body was met by Dr. R. H. Sayre, Vice President of the Academy, and by Major Putnam, both lifelong friends, who led the procession, followed by Mr. and Mrs. George L. McAneny, his son-in-law and daughter, and other close friends and relatives. While a quartette from St. Thomas' Church sang "Abide With Me," the body was carried to the platform from which he had spoken so many times, and placed in the center.

Dr. Sayre spoke feelingly of Dr. Jacobi, who, driven from his own country as a young man, came to the United States where he started at the bottom of the ladder and won every honor the profession could bestow. Invited to return later to occupy the chair of Professor of Pediatrics at Berlin, the highest honor Germany could offer him, he declined, because he would lose his American citizenship. Dr. Sayre said it was proper the funeral should be held in the Academy, which was a monument to Dr. Jacobi's wisdom, foresight and sagacity. He had served it for four years as President and twenty-three years as President of its Board of Trustees, and thereafter was a constant attendant at its meetings. His heart was wrapped up in it and he was ever watchful against anything which might injure it. For years he attended the meetings of all the Sections and what he said was worth listening to.

His voice was heard whenever he felt the city or country was menaced by any danger. Wherever he decided he owed a duty to the people of this nation, either as a man or physician, to raise a voice of protest against evils whether they had to do with the realm of medicine or not, he never hesitated to speak. He never talked at random, and so his words were ever listened to with respect, and his suggestions had a weight of authority seldom accorded to any. . . . Few people could say as much in a few words or say it to such good effect.

The choir sang "Lead Kindly Light" and Major Putnam spoke of him briefly, as a citizen, and the part he had played in developing civic life of the city. The choir then sang Tennyson's "Crossing the Bar," after which the audience rose and filed past the coffin.

It was an impressive occasion.

On May 6, 1920, a memorial service was held, that day being his ninetieth birthday. Dr. Stewart presided. Twenty years before, on his seventieth birthday, a bas-relief of himself was presented to Dr. Jacobi by the Medical Society of the State of New York. Mr. George McAneny presented it now, on behalf of the family, to the Academy, fulfilling Dr. Jacobi's wish. He stated Dr. Jacobi's love for the Academy surpassed anything of that sort he had ever seen. As years crept on, and signs of advancing age began to appear, "no matter what the state of the weather or his own state of body or mind Dr. Jacobi never permitted any of these things to keep him away from the Academy. . . . Here he served, here he was brought when he was dead. It is most fitting that he should express through this bronze reminder his continued presence with you, for his spirit must go with you in your work."

In accepting the gift Dr. Stewart called attention to Dr. Jacobi's having been a Fellow for over sixty years, "a member for more years than Pitt or Fox, Nelson, or Hamilton were permitted to live, and for almost twice the span given to Byron or Burns." He spoke feelingly of Dr. Jacobi's services to the Academy and closed by saying "though made of enduring bronze, [the bas-relief] is not nearly so imperishable as the spiritual legacies which he has left us and which will go on and on, for they are the very essence of immortality."

Dr. George E. Vincent, President of the Rockefeller Foundation, then spoke of the influence of Dr. Jacobi on his times. It was a fine scholarly address and concluded with these words: "Dr. Jacobi incarnated the scientific spirit, love of his fellows, unflagging devotion to his work, a firm conviction of its value, a clear vision of its larger possibilities, a deep sense of social comradeship and obligation."

Dr. Jacobi left the Academy his medical books and memorabilia, and $5,000, to be added to the Philippine Meyer-Ernst Jacobi Library Fund.

He was the greatest friend the Academy ever had.

During these two years after the close of the war, a considerable part of the papers dealt with war conditions. Influenza and its prevention; the functional reeducation of the French, British, and American soldier; the Genito-Urinary and Venereal Service in the A.E.F.; chronic arthritis in the Army, and efficiency and sanitation in the feeding of the Army. Prof. Stewart Paton of Princeton spoke before 150 Fellows on the "Present Emotional Unrest, Its Causes and Treatment."

There was a long program on the significance of blood examinations; "Moving Pictures in the Diagnosis of Tuberculosis"; a meeting on thrombo-angiitis obliterans, and another on encephalitis lethargica. There was a very fine session on the deaf—adult and child—their training and what could be done for them. Several meetings were given in cooperation with outside organizations, one with the Association for the Prevention and Relief of Heart Disease. The Peter Bent Brigham Hospital put on a fine program, and Dr. W. H. Wilmer came from Washington to speak on the "Injurious Effects on the Eye of Various Toxaemias." Another program of four interesting papers was arranged by Dr. W. H. Park, Bureau of Laboratories of the Department of Health.

The Committee on Library presented a program, with Dr. Stewart speaking on "Feeds and Needs of the Library of the Academy"; the story of "A Great Consultation in the 16th Century," by Dr. Dana; and "Medical History, a Safeguard against Medical Fads," by Dr. J. J. Walsh.

A special meeting was held in memory of Sir William Osler. Addresses were made by Dr. Stewart and by Drs. F. J. Shepherd of Montreal, Thomas McCrae of Philadelphia, E. C. Streeter of Boston, and W. H. Welch of Baltimore.

The Public Health Committee was very active. Its report on the dispensary situation in the city resulted in an offer by the United Hospital Fund to continue the study of the problem. The Committee also reported on the medical aspects of the Workmen's Compensation Act in the State (at the request of the State Industrial Commission); on birth control; the bill introduced to establish health centers; and the use in New York State of Federal grants to stimulate venereal disease control; and assisted in preparing a scientific program for a Milk and Child Health Exposition, which was a great success.

The Carpenter Lecture as given in 1919 by Sir Arthur Newsholme on "The Increasing Socialization of Medicine," and in 1920 by Sir Berkeley Moynihan, on "Gastric Ulcer and Its Treatment." The minutes tell us that, at the latter, "the audience filled the hall to capacity."

The Anniversary Addresses were well attended. In 1919, Rev. Dr. Charles A. Eaton's discourse on "New Men for a New Age" called forth "a rising vote of appreciation amid hearty applause." The following year Hon. James M. Beck discussed "One Cause of War Neuroses."

The Library, after staying well within its budget allowance for 1919, had to expend considerable to pay for the journals and books that had accumulated during the war. The Trustees authorized the Librarian to purchase fourteen incunabula which were on the market, but they were bought and presented by Mr. James B. Ford.

Dr. Alfred Meyer proposed, again, that the Academy establish a branch medical library in the Bronx or Harlem. The Council appreciated his interest but were unable financially to do so. Triplicate copies of books would be gladly lent to such a library, if Dr. Meyer started it.

The Library readers registered in 1920 were 24,475, an increase of nearly 4,000 in one year. The shelves formerly in the Council Room were removed and placed in the hallway above the Library. The Public Health Committee had moved to No. 15, and its former quarters were now full of shelves and books.

A committee studied the Constitution and By Laws for amendment and reprinting. Their recommendations, adopted by the Academy, were unimportant.

In 1919, the elevator, which for two years had only been used for service to floors above the Library, was restored to its former usefulness.

Dr. Stewart was reelected for a second term, without opposition. His inaugural was the report of the President for the previous year. He stressed again the overcrowded and distressing condition of the Library and the fact that it was only by the most rigid economy that the Academy was approximately living within its income.

In January, 1921, the Academy increased the Resident Fellowship to 1,350; and, in March, the roll of non-residents with offices in the city was increased to 300. Thus the Academy gained an additional $2,000 income. The Council decided to budget each of its departments, and each was required to live within its allotment. Commercial organizations were required to pay $100 for the use of the Library and other subscribers were to pay $20, the same amount as Fellowship dues. (In 1922 Resident Fellowship was increased to 1,400.)

In April, 1921, the Treasurer reported that for the first six months of the fiscal year expenses had exceeded budget allowances in many items, and the Academy was in a precarious financial condition. He repeated his warning in May. In October he anticipated a deficit of about $13,000 and was authorized to make such temporary loans as might be necessary.

The Library reported that because of lack of funds it had been unable to buy from 75 to 100 books needed and seventeen journals; it had been ordered to stop binding journals and books for the remainder of the year.

A special meeting of the Trustees called to consider Library affairs voted that, while they did not wish to diminish the value of the services of the Library by curtailing the purchase of books, the Library Committee should so arrange its budget in the future as to "conform to the income of the Academy." The chairman of the Committee stated that the Library could be made more efficient if the Fellowship were assessed $5 a year for the next two years. This was considered "not advisable."

The Council voted to publish a ten-year report of the Public Health Committee. That Committee recommended increasing the annual dues $5, in order to obtain additional financial support. This was not received favorably either.

By the end of 1921 the apparent deficit had been reduced to some $4,000. The lot of the Treasurer could not have been a happy one.

Scientific meetings were well arranged and attended. Cooperation with other organizations was a striking feature. In January a meeting was held with the Society for Experimental Biology and Medicine and the Harvey Society in memory of Dr. Samuel J. Meltzer, with Dr. Gary N. Calkins of Columbia University presiding. Dr. Welch was one of the speakers.

The Rockefeller Institute provided the program on four occasions: experimental measles, typhoid carriers, and S. pallidum infection in rabbits and its relation to problems in human syphilis, in 1921; and bile flow and bile Stasis in 1922.

When the Mayo Clinic presented a program on thyroid pathology, and surgical treatment, "an appreciative audience filled the hall to capacity." A meeting was held with the First District Dental Society at which the interrelationship between physician and dentist was discussed. Dr. Barker of Johns Hopkins, Professor Johnson of the Chicago Dental College and Professor Miner of Harvard read papers.

Another meeting was held with the Association for Prevention and Relief of Heart Disease, at which five papers were read, mostly by Fellows of the Academy.

The Sections on Obstetrics and Gynecology, Dermatology and Syphilis, Genito-Urinary Surgery, Neurology and Psychiatry, Laryngology and Rhinology, and Otology provided good programs during the two years. The Public Health Committee presented its Survey of New York Hospitals, with other papers by Drs. George B. Wallace and S. S. Goldwater.

Endocrines in otology was discussed, with Dr. Sajous of Philadelphia reading a paper. Other meetings were given over to X-ray in diagnosis and therapeutics; digitalis and the value of cardiograms in diagnosis; The Port of New York, its health and sanitary problems. Drs. Joslin of Harvard and L. H. Newburgh, University of Michigan, discussed the present treatment of diabetes, and in December, 1922, Dr. F. G. Banting spoke on "Pancreatic Extracts in Diabetes Mellitus."

Many other interesting papers were presented.

The Carpenter Lectures were given by Sir Harold J. Stiles, "Surgical Tuberculosis in Children and Its Relation to the Milk Problem," in 1921, and by Dr. Raffaele Bastianelli, on "Diagnostic and Therapeutic Importance of Some Typical Tender Bone Points," in 1922.

Dr. H. S. Pritchett of the Carnegie Corporation gave the Anniversary Address in 1921, on "A Layman's View of Medical Progress," and Prof. E. G. Conklin of Princeton on "Problems of Organic Adaptation" in 1922.

Dr. Stephen Smith, after having been an active member for sixty-eight years, resigned in his ninety-ninth year of age, and was promptly elected an Honorary Member. It was he who led the fight in Albany to establish the first Metropolitan Board of Health, and formed the American Public Health Association. He was acknowledged the "Father of Public Health." He died that same year, missing his hundredth birthday by a few weeks.

The matter of proper newspaper publicity of the work of the Academy was discussed at length by the Council, but no conclusions were reached.

At the end of 1922 the Trustees reported that for the first time in a number of years the Treasurer's report showed no deficit.

The Library was $2,000 overdrawn, but was within its budget.

The Rockefeller Foundation asked the Academy to donate its triplicate volumes for distribution in European countries for libraries stripped by the war. The Academy wisely consented to do so, and a notice was published in the bulletin for several months asking unwanted journals for that purpose.

The Historical Secretary recorded that six societies had offices in the building, fifty-two held their meetings there in 1921, and in 1922 ten societies were housed there.

In 1921 the Academy cooperated with the Public Health Education Committee of the County Society in giving an excellent series of five free public lectures on health education.

Dr. Stewart was elected President for the third time. His report for 1922 was a most important and impressive one. To appreciate what it meant we must briefly review the subject during the previous thirteen years.

In November, 1909, the Library Committee reported that, at the existing rate of growth, by Janauary, 1912, the stacks could contain no more books, and urged a new building to meet the needs of the Academy. At the meeting December 2, 1909, it was decided to provide a larger building. A number of sites were considered, and in two years the Academy had collected $130,000, a sum utterly insufficient for the purpose. When in 1910, Mr. J. S. Kennedy, President of the Public Library, left that institution two and a half million dollars, Dr. Delavan suggested to President Polk that, as the Library of the Academy was practically the medical part of the library system of the city, it might perhaps receive a portion of the income from the Kennedy legacy. This was, of course, found legally impossible.

In 1911, No. 15 West 43d Street and the building directly behind it, 10 West 44th Street, were bought without architectural or builders' advice. Plans were developed to construct an addition on both lots, with ultimate rebuilding of the original structure at 17–21 West 43d Street, but the architects were very much opposed to such an irregular structure and the plan was abandoned. Three sets of plans were drawn, however, by York and Sawyer.

In 1915 plans were made to build a stack room, with temporary quarters for the Academy, on lot No. 15 West 43d Street while the rest of the plant was to be torn down and rebuilt. But war was on in Europe, prospects for financial aid were bad, and with our entrance into the conflict in 1917, the whole matter had to be postponed. In 1919 it was revived. Plans were again drawn, but architects and builders advised against immediate action on account of the great increase in construction costs. This continued through 1920, although another building committee was appointed in 1919.

Meanwhile the condition of the Library had become deplorable. Its duplicates and rarely used books were stored at 15 West 43d Street, to which a passage had to be cut for access to them. Books were accumulating in piles on the floors, all window sills having been full for a long time. In his Presidential Address in 1921, Dr. Stewart had spoken at length on the subject. The Council discussed the matter and the President was authorized to appoint another committee to secure funds for the extension covering No. 15.

Dr. D. Bryson Delavan, a member of the Council, was not satisfied with this viewpoint and wrote a long letter to Dr. Stewart, emphasizing that the Academy was an educational institution, and as such, an endowment was essential to its success; that the proposal was a makeshift which would be quickly outgrown; it was not worthy of the Academy or what it stood for.

This letter and a similar one from Dr. James were read to the Council. The President was requested to call a meeting of a group of members, including the Council and Trustees. He accordingly gave a dinner at the Lotos Club, March 21, 1921, to about thirty influential and interested Fellows, at which Dr. Delavan's plan was read. It was not enthusiastically received. Several felt the plan was "impractical" and "a dream." In April, Dr. Stewart gave another dinner to a largely different group of Fellows. A letter was read from Dr. W. B. James, stating that three or four years earlier the Academy had failed to secure aid from one of the Foundations, but he believed their attitude had now changed. A brief vigorous campaign should be carried out for a larger development; if unsuccessful, then a more modest one should be undertaken. He believed, however, that several pertinent arguments had not been presented to the Foundations.

As a result, the Trustees appointed committees on "Plan and Scope" and "Building and Finance." Dr. Delavan was made chairman of the former. The action of the second committee was naturally dependent on the decisions of the first. Dr. A. B. Duel was a member of "Plan and Scope" and Dr. W. B. James of both committees.

The first committee, appointed in March, held several meetings during the early spring but came to no conclusions, and in June Dr. Delavan prepared a detailed prospectus to be considered by its members in the fall. No definite plans resulted from all this, and in 1922 things were about as indefinite as before, except that a group of the officers and Trustees were quietly acting to interest the Carnegie Corporation and the Rockefeller Foundation in the plans for a greater Academy.

In January, 1923, Dr. Stewart announced that the Carnegie Corporation had promised a new building to cost approximately one million dollars, provided the Academy furnished the site, and the Rockefeller Foundation promised an endowment of approximately one and a quarter million dollars. The site had been secured and the Trustees would announce it when they asked the authority of the Academy to make the business transaction. Dr. Stewart added that, to secure the new property, approximately $250,000 more would be needed, and urged the interest of the Fellows of the Academy.

How this was started has never been told. Dr. Arthur B. Duel, in a personal letter to the Director, Dr. L. R. Williams, written in 1931, evidently in reply to some question of his, stated:

> Dr. Pritchett spent a week-end with me during the Fall of 1921 and, when we were shooting pheasants, he asked me if anything interesting or exciting had happened to me. I told him that the Academy of Medicine had just honoured me by asking me to become one of its Vice-Presidents. He was immediately interested and wanted to know something of what the Academy was.
>
> I told him then of its work and pointed out the possibilities of its improvement. I also spoke of our fine library that was then bulging and

housed in a non-fireproof building. We became much interested in the shooting again and nothing more was said about it.

A few days later he called me up and said he had been thinking seriously about the Academy of Medicine, and that he thought it offered a great possibility for one of the activities of the Carnegie Corporation. Angell of Yale had just resigned from the Presidency of the Corporation to take the Presidency of Yale and Dr. Pritchett was Acting-President of the Corporation as well as President of the Foundation. He asked me to talk with the members of the Council and arrange a dinner inviting him (Carnegie Corporation), Vincent (Rockefeller Foundation) and Butterfield (Sage Foundation) to meet and talk over the situation. Walter James gave the dinner at his house.

It resulted in Pritchett giving $1,250,000 for building—subsequently increased by a further addition as you know after Keppel had come in (probably due to Pritchett's pressure on him to finish the job), and a like contribution by Vincent for endowment. Vincent at the time said that he had no doubt that they would be open to additional grants as the needs of the Academy were shown to require them. Butterfield would do nothing: he said it was out of his line of endeavour. . . .

Now the Academy had something definite to work for. The Council authorized the President and Secretary to prepare and publish in the lay press the announcement of the gifts, together with a statement of the Academy's plans for the future. At a special meeting on January 15, Dr. Stewart outlined the situation in regard to site. A lot on the southeast corner of Park Avenue and 60th Street, 100 ft. 5 in. by 120 ft., costing $754,500, was recommended. Resolutions were presented and passed, January 18, authorizing the Trustees to sell all its property on 43d Street and all other property it could sell to purchase the lots at 60th Street. Dr. N. E. Brill, Secretary of the Trustees, put himself on record as being greatly disappointed that the site chosen was no larger than the one at 43d Street. To build on such a plot meant a tall building, expensive to run, and there was no parking space at 60th Street.

The first payment on the new property, $63,000, was due February 1, and the Treasurer was authorized to sell Liberty Bonds as needed. It was paid, but the Council felt it might be necessary to place a new mortgage of $100,000 on 43d Street, and the Academy so ordered. It was not necessary to do it however. In the meantime Mrs. Helen Hartley Jenkins offered $50,000 to purchase the site at 60th Street, if a tablet mentioning the fact be placed somewhere in the building. This was accepted.

In January the Council appointed a committee of five to approach Fellows of the Academy "and others" for subscriptions for the new building. The Committee was empowered to add to its number. Under the chairmanship of Dr. R. S. Haynes, and now enlarged to sixty, the Committee presented plans for a whirlwind campaign. Authorization was given to consult Mr. Ivy Lee, well-known fund raiser, and $5,000 were granted for expenses.

The campaign opened with an objective of $250,000 by May 1. The first public performance of Sacha Guitry's *Pasteur*, played by Henry Miller, was given at the Empire Theatre for the benefit of the Academy, before a full house. Every trick in money-raising was used. Form letters were sent—a new one every few days—announcing progress and appealing to every Fellow for 100 percent response, no matter how small the amount. Catchy broadsides with an imaginary diminutive figure holding out one hand to receive and the other pointing to the appeal, named GOGI ("Give or get it"), came out at short intervals. Most of the Sections sent out special appeals to their members. The Westchester County Society sent out a special notice to its members. A special letter was sent to the non-resident and associate members. A subcommittee on Hospitals wrote to all known Alumni Associations asking them to contribute *something*. Another letter was sent to all Fellows emphasizing the GI of GOGI, *Get it*.

As the campaign progressed a series of cartoons appeared, with two figures on opposite sides of a fence, one smiling and with his pockets turned inside out, the other frowning and with pockets intact, giving the percentage of Fellows who belonged to each category. A poster to be placed in doctors' offices was also provided.

A bulletin board in the entrance hall of the Academy listed the name of every Fellow contributing. A large dial with figures from 0 to 250,000 was also there, with the hand pointing to results so far obtained. Toward the end, a special letter was written to all who had not contributed, not asking for money, as the goal had been reached, but asking *why* they had not contributed. Dr. Stewart wrote two personal letters to the Fellows.

In May the Academy voted: "Resolved that the Fellows of the New York Academy of Medicine place on record their hearty appreciation of the work of the Committee of Sixty, and especially of its Chairman, Dr. Royal Storrs Haynes, for the energy and efficiency with which the campaign for funds for the building site has been conducted, and for its gratifying results."

The Committee of Sixty reported to the Council May 22, 1923, that subscriptions from Fellows amounted to $261,679.64 and from friends of the Academy $269,704.41, a total of $531,384.05, of which $456,266.70 had been paid in. A committee of thirteen had underwritten the expenses of the campaign to the extent of $6,500. The Academy only had to pay $297.44.

A building committee of twenty-one, with the President ex officio, was appointed with the energetic Dr. Duel as chairman.

The Counsel of the Academy, Mr. Van Sinderen, resigned and Mr. Frank L. Polk, son of the former president, was elected to the office. He served for the rest of his life, and his partner, Mr. J. W. Davis, is still the devoted Counsel of the Academy.

Plans were drawn for the new building and the Trustees discussed beginning operations in the fall, but both Foundations and the contractors and architects all advised postponement on account of the still high cost of building materials. Dr. Stewart was authorized to make a public statement to the Fellows by letter. These original plans would cost much more than the million given by the Carnegie Corporation. The Corporation was asked for an increased amount, but the Academy was told to go ahead with plans, cutting as much as possible.

By October the property was in the hands of the Trustees; $613,500 was paid in cash and a mortgage was taken for $141,000.

In November, 1923, the Council and Trustees took a most important step. The position of Director of the Academy was established, and a committee recommended Dr. Linsly R. Williams for the office. He had been suggested by Dr. A. B. Duel and the value of the suggestion was immediately apparent to Council and Trustees. Dr. Williams was promptly elected and from the first had the complete confidence and trust of both bodies—*and* the Foundations.

Dr. Williams had been a member of the Academy since 1904, had been chairman of its Section on Medicine, and had made suggestions for better organization of Sections, which the Council adopted. Appointed Deputy Commissioner of the State Department of Health in 1914, he lived in Albany. On the entrance of the United States into the World War, he resigned and was immediately sent by the National Research Council with a committee to study sanitary conditions in England and France; he presented a monumental report of these investigations. He then entered the Army and went with the 80th Division to France, ending up as Assistant to the Officer in Charge of Civil Affairs in occupied Germany.

In 1919 he was selected to succeed Dr. Livingston Farrand as Director of the Rockefeller Commission for the Prevention of Tuberculosis in France, remaining in charge of that work until 1922. When elected Director of the Academy he was Managing Director of the National Tuberculosis Association. He retained that position until December, 1928, combining it, by permission, with his new office. The Rockefeller Foundation agreed to pay his salary until the new building was functioning.

Dr. Williams was at once invited to attend all meetings of the Trustees and Council, and immediately plunged into studies and investigations which were of immense advantage to the Academy. The first thing he tackled was the plan for the new building, in an attempt to lower the cost without impairing the proper functioning of the Academy. Within a few months he had persuaded the Council and Trustees that the whole plan was extravagant and unwise. The Trustees held several special meetings to consider nine different parcels of land, offered for from $300,000 to $600,000. The replies to a letter asking all Fellows their choice of location were not very helpful.

Finally a site on Fifth Avenue at 103d Street was found available for $250,000. At a special meeting April 9, 1924, the Treasurer

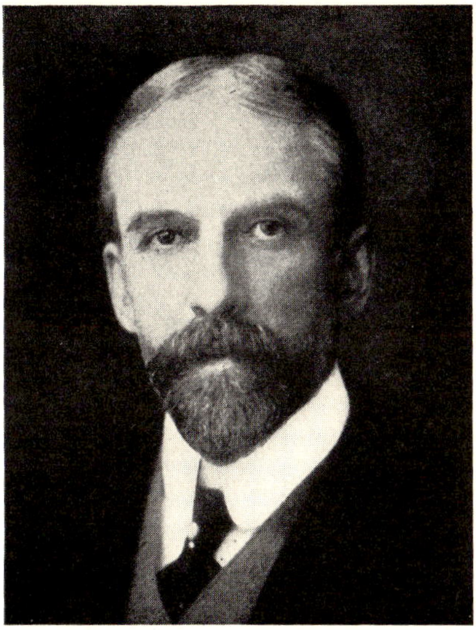

CHARLES L. DANA, 1857–1934
Twenty-sixth President, 1905–1906

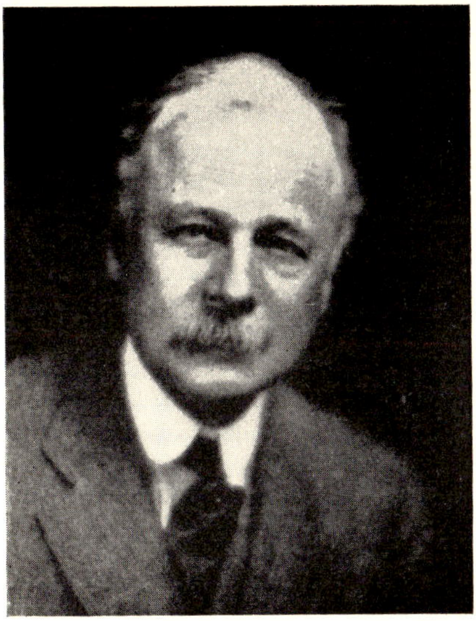

WALTER B. JAMES, 1858–1927
Twenty-ninth President, 1915–1918

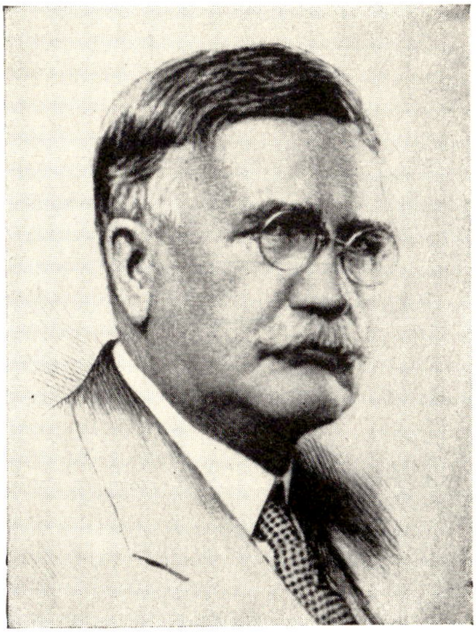

GEORGE D. STEWART, 1862–1933
Thirtieth President, 1919–1924

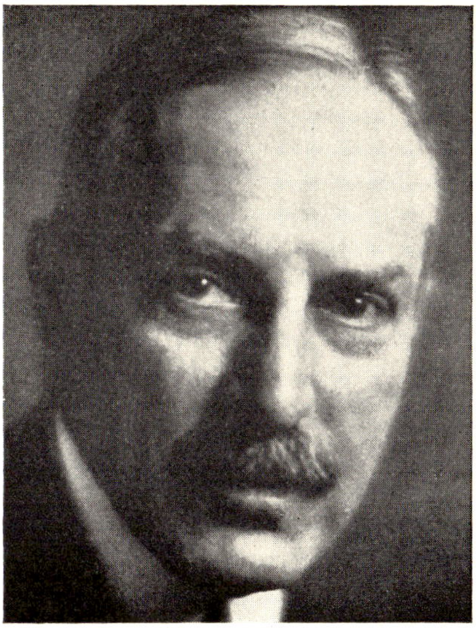

LINSLY R. WILLIAMS
1875–1934
Director, 1924–1933

was authorized, if the President approved, to secure an option on the property. The Carnegie Corporation was asked if there was any objection to selling 60th Street and buying elsewhere. There was none. The Board of Education had its eyes on this corner for a new high school. Dr. O'Shea of the Department of Education, "because of his great affection for Dr. Stewart, and his friendship for Dr. Linsly Williams" withdrew condemnation proceedings on the property, so the coast was clear.

At the Trustees' special meeting on April 14, 1924, the Director reported that Mr. Wheelock, the Academy's agent, had informed him the property at 103d Street and Fifth Avenue had been bought for $225,000. It was promptly resolved that "The Trustees do not desire to purchase the property at 103d Street and Fifth Avenue, as they have not disposed of the Park Avenue property." At another special meeting two days later to consider whether the Academy had actually purchased the 103d Street site, Dr. Williams reported he had arranged to have the property held for the Academy. What he did not tell the Trustees was that, so convinced was he of the wisdom of the purchase, and so sure the Academy would eventually be also, he had taken the responsibility of buying and holding the site until the Fellows accepted it. This was known to a few, but was never revealed during Dr. Williams's lifetime, at his behest. The purchase of the present site was approved by the Academy on May 1, 1924.

The life of a Trustee was not an easy one in the first nine months of 1924. Instead of the five meetings usually held, there were twenty-six, mostly in connection with the sale of the properties at 43d and 60th streets. After the approval of the Carnegie Corporation of buying on 103d Street and the Rockefeller Foundation's statement that the site had no relation to its endowment, an offer to sell the 60th Street lot for $1,030,000 was finally accepted, but the bidder failed to sign and it was eventually sold for $1,000,000, plus $2,500 from the buyer and $4,000 from the Academy to pay the bonus for canceling the mortgage on part of the property. The Academy therefore gained the price of the new site in this transaction. The 43d Street property was sold in 1925 for $745,000.

The Charter of the Academy was amended, April 25, 1924, to authorize an increase in the number of Trustees to not less than five or more than fifteen, one fifth retiring every three years. The income of the General Permanent Fund was now to be used only "for the purpose of advancing Medical Science."

Dr. Williams, entering upon his duties as Director, January 1, 1924, lost no time in making progress, and the Council and Trustees lost none in referring to him every question which would ordinarily have been referred to a slowly moving special committee. When one thinks of the number of problems, many of them very important—finances, policies, organization, and the details of administration—presented for settlement to the governing bodies of the Academy, which were composed of men actively and busily engaged in practice, one wonders that so few mistakes were made. The time lost in selecting a site and the amount of money spent on unused architects' plans, would have been largely avoided if a man like Linsly Williams had been giving *all* his time to the problems involved.

The Building Committee was instructed to have final plans drawn as quickly as possible. The new building was estimated to cost $1,550,000. At the end of the year the President, President-elect, Chairman of the Building Committee and the Director were appointed to present the plans to the Carnegie Corporation, and ask for another $550,000. It was eventually granted.

Drs. Dana, W. B. James, and Holden were appointed a committee on art to submit plans for the exterior and interior decorations of the building. An "acoustical engineer" and a consulting engineer were authorized to try to prevent such errors as existed in Hosack Hall.

It was seriously considered whether to buy the southern half of the block to acquire land for possible enlargement, but this was decided by the Trustees as unnecessary.

The Library Committee had been in sad difficulties during these two years. It had a large and steadily growing deficit, and was frightfully cramped. Shelves were put up in windows, and the floors were littered. Lack of funds prevented necessary binding; unbound journals suffered as a result. The Director advised accepting the deficit and borrowing, if necessary to keep the Library efficient. The Trustees in 1923 voted to transfer the salaries of the Library Staff to the Academy Account, thus reducing the deficit by some $9,000.

In addition to his other duties, the Director was requested to make a list of all Fellows who had served in the war, and who were killed during that period. He was also to report all deaths of Fellows immediately, so that the President could automatically appoint a committee on resolutions. He was instructed to cooperate with the County Society for a meeting on Health Examinations and to help arrange a series of lectures on pre-clinical signs of disease to be given by that society.

The list of casualties was prepared and is now cut in the wall of the Hall by the entrance to Hosack Hall, opposite the list of Benefactors.

IN MEMORY OF
RAE H. WIDDEN
THEODORE JANEWAY RICHARD WEIL CLARENCE FAHNESTOCK
MEMBERS OF THE NEW YORK ACADEMY OF MEDICINE WHO GAVE
THEIR LIVES TO THEIR COUNTRY DURING THE GREAT WAR
AND IN COMMEMORATION OF
THREE HUNDRED AND FORTY SIX FELLOWS OF THE ACADEMY
WHO RENDERED LOYAL SERVICE TO THE UNITED STATES
MCMXVII–MCMXIX

For a number of years the Society for Clinical Information and the New York Association for Medical Education had offices in the Academy. They had been issuing bulletins and were both active. In October, 1923, they held a joint meeting and voted to combine their efforts under a Committee on Medical Education to be appointed by the Academy. This Committee was made up of the members of the governing bodies of these organizations who were Fellows of the Academy, with an Executive Committee of which Dr. C. N. Dowd was chairman. The Rockefeller Foundation had pledged the Academy $12,000 a year for three years to maintain a Bureau of Clinical Information. This Committee on Medical Education published a daily bulletin of surgical clinics and operations and a weekly bulletin of medical clinics in twenty-four hospitals. It gave information to 436 visitors in 1924, from every state in the Union and from "every State in Western Europe except Portugal, and from Russia, Czecho-Slovakia, Armenia, China, Japan, India, Ceylon, Formosa, Australia, South Africa, Argentine, Brazil, Colombia, Chile, Panama, Hawaii, The Philippines and Canada." Dr. Frederick P. Reynolds was appointed Medical Secretary for the Committee in April, 1924.

The Council voted in 1924 to resume publishing a *Bulletin*, after a lapse of twenty-three years, and the Director was requested to formulate a definite plan. The Rockefeller Foundation was asked for, and gave, $3,500 to publish it. The *Bulletin* appeared in January, 1925.

In February, 1924, the Rockefeller Foundation granted $5,000 a year for the educational work of the Academy for three years, to begin January first, for general surveys, educational and informational work, which was to terminate when the Academy occupied its new building and received its endowment fund from the Foundation.

Much time was spent in simplifying methods of bookkeeping and procedure. A simplified classification of the various funds made things very much easier.

The Director informed the Trustees that the American Library Association asked for the cooperation of the Academy in the preparation of a list of all periodicals, the National Union Check List. It was recommended that the Council authorize the Director to make investigations in regard to securing money for this National Check List, and the Rockefeller Foundation was requested to give $2,500 for the purpose, which was granted.

Dr. Williams also brought up the question of taking over the publication of the *Index Medicus*, if funds could be secured from the Rockefeller or Carnegie Foundation. He was authorized to make further inquiries. The Carnegie Institute had published the *Index Medicus* for many years and continued to do so through 1926, when it was superseded by the American Medical Association's *Cumulative Index*.

The fiscal year for the Academy was changed in 1924 to correspond with the calendar year. The Treasurer's report for fourteen months showed a deficit of $6,091.71.

The Director presented the next year's budget of $131,796, with an estimated income of $159,630. He was authorized to expend the sums appropriated for the specific purposes mentioned and to make such transfers within each segregated item of salary or expense as he might deem necessary. This budget was to be assumed as a guide, but it was not to be exceeded in any one of the segregated items without the approval of the Trustees, and no change in salary was to be made in positions paying $2,000 or over, without definite authority from the Trustees.

In January, 1923, the Academy held a Pasteur meeting, at the end of an exhibition commemorative of the centenary of Pasteur's birth, which began December 27, his birthday. There were a number of celebrations in New York. The largest meeting was at the Museum of Natural History, sponsored also by a number of national and local organizations, including the Academy. Dr. Stewart spoke at that meeting. Columbia University also held a meeting, and the city designated January 10 "Pasteur Day," to be celebrated at all public schools.

The Academy's exhibit was a very creditable one; it contained many items of great interest loaned from all over the country and by the Pasteur Institute of Paris. The meeting which closed the exhibit was addressed by Professor Chittenden of Yale, Drs. Welch of Johns Hopkins, E. F. Smith of the Department of Agriculture, Simon Flexner, H. M. Biggs, W. W. Keen of Philadelphia, and Etienne Burnet, head of the Pasteur Institute at Tunis. A catalogue of the exhibit and the papers read were published by the Academy. A bust of Pasteur by Aaronson, which was exhibited for the first time, was offered to the Academy for $5,000, and declined, but was later presented by a daughter of the late Ward McAllister.

A Committee on Programs had been appointed, consisting of

Drs. George B. Wallace, chairman, Hartwell, and Van Beuren.

Many interesting papers were read, a large number, as usual, by outstanding men from other cities. Professor Yandell Henderson (Yale) discussed automobile exhaust gas as a health hazard. Dr. Archibald (McGill) spoke on the surgical treatment of pulmonary tuberculosis; Dr. D. F. Jones (Boston), "A Study of Carcinoma of the Rectum"; Dr. J. L. Gamble (Boston), "Alterations in the Acid-base Structure of the Blood Plasma Producing Acidosis." Dr. Hugh Young (Baltimore) spoke on urogenital tuberculosis, and Dr. E. B. Krumbhaar (Philadelphia) on the "Haemolyto-Poietic System in the Primary Anaemias."

Dr. Joslin, of Boston, spoke on diabetes treated with and without insulin. The talk took the form of a clinic, as his patients had volunteered to come to New York to illustrate his "methods."

The Sections did not arrange quite as many meetings as in previous years. Medicine gave two, one on "Certain Aspects of Leukaemia" by members of the Collis P. Huntington Memorial Hospital of Boston and the other on the "Therapy of Pneumonia," with papers by Drs. Huntoon, C. A. L. Binger, and R. L. Cecil.

Surgery, Otology and Genito-Urinary Surgery arranged interesting programs. Neurology and Psychiatry presented three papers by Drs. Frederick Tilney, J. Ramsay Hunt, and T. H. Weisenburg, of Philadelphia, on the influence of the cerebellum on motion, postural function and in disease.

Historical Medicine offered a paper on the rise and development of orthopedic surgery by Dr. E. G. Brackett of Boston, which was followed by an illustrated talk by Dr. L. P. Clark on the "Psychology of the Characters in Alice in Wonderland."

The Section on Laryngology, formerly the New York Laryngological Society, "the oldest society in that line," staged a Fiftieth Anniversary Meeting. Dr. A. B. Duel made the opening address and Dr. Delavan spoke on "New York the Birthplace of Laryngological Science." Mrs. Lefferts presented a portrait of Ludwig Türck of Vienna.

The Public Health Committee arranged a group of papers on various phases of child health work.

The Carpenter Lectures were given by Prof. W. B. Cannon, Harvard, on "A Consideration of the Nature of Traumatic Shock," with lantern slides, and by Dr. Thorvald Madsen, Director of the State Serological Institute of Copenhagen, and Chairman of the Health Committee of the League of Nations.

The Anniversary Address in 1923 was by Dr. W. S. Thayer of Baltimore on "Studies in Acute Bacterial Endocarditis," and the next year Dr. John H. Finley of the New York *Times* spoke on "Three Fields of Human Activity."

The Gibbs Prize of $1,500 was awarded in 1923 to Dr. J. Harold Austin of the University of Pennsylvania.

In February, 1923, the Academy passed, unanimously, this resolution:

Whereas, Numerous instances have been brought to the attention of the Council and the Public Health Committee of the New York Academy of Medicine of rebates being offered to, and accepted by physicians, from commercial laboratories, opticians, druggists and others to whom patients are referred, therefore be it

Resolved, That the New York Academy of Medicine condemns such practices on the part of those offering the rebates, as well as on the part of physicians accepting them, as being unethical and detrimental to the profession, and that violation of this rule will expose the member to expulsion from the Academy.

That was practically the only question of ethics brought before the Academy, although two or three minor issues were referred to the County Society, where they belonged.

Dr. Charles A. Powers, a former Fellow, who had moved to Denver to live, left one-half of his residuary estate to the Academy on the death of a beneficiary. That legacy has not as yet been paid in.

A portrait of Dr. W. B. James and a portrait bust of Dr. A. G. Gerster were received.

In March, 1923, Felix Wesstrom completed thirty years of service with the Academy, and the Trustees voted that funds which might be collected from the Trustees and Council should be spent on a watch, suitably engraved, to be presented to him. "Felix," as everybody called him, was well known to every Fellow at 43d Street. He had served the Academy in practically every position possible from elevator boy to assistant superintendent.

In December, 1924, it was voted that a suitable letter of appreciation be sent to the New York Bottling Company which had furnished bottled water to the Academy for over ten years, gratis.

In October, 1923, the chairman of the Public Health Committee asked the Trustees please to clean up their quarters, which had not been done in three years. Mr. Brownne was instructed to clean up the rooms.

At the annual elections Dr. Samuel A. Brown was elected President.

Dr. George David Stewart had been a fine President and had handled difficult situations with the greatest tact. His influence in the fund-raising campaign was great; Mr. George F. Baker's gift of $100,000 was given solely on his account. Dr. Stewart was an extremely busy man, but he presided over three-quarters of the stated meetings, and was very regular in his Council and Trustees' meetings.

At the end of the next year, an enthusiastic Fellow suggested, and an equally enthusiastic and appreciative Academy, voted:

> WHEREAS, Dr. George David Stewart, former President of the New York Academy of Medicine, has been very active in the affairs of the Academy of Medicine for many years, and
>
> WHEREAS, He has rendered brilliant and untiring service to the Academy in the acquisition of its new site, and
>
> WHEREAS, The present location was obtained only through his devoted and well directed efforts, therefore be it
>
> *Resolved*, That the Fellows of the New York Academy of Medicine tender a testimonial dinner to Dr. George David Stewart at some early date and that they present a token of their appreciation and esteem to Dr. Stewart on that occasion, the cost of said token not to exceed $1,000.

Nothing more is heard of this.

1925–1926

Samuel Albertus Brown

Dr. Stewart, in his Valedictory Address, emphasized the prominence of the Public Health Committee in the activity of the Academy, his hopes for the Committee on Medical Education, the needs for greater support of the Library and his ideas concerning the scientific programs of the Academy.

Dr. Brown recited briefly the history of the founding of the Academy and its various homes, its former financial difficulties, its present financial situation and his hopes for better things in the future.

Dr. S. A. Brown was fifty-one when he became thirty-first President. Graduating from University and Bellevue Medical College in 1894, he served at Bellevue for two years and started practice in 1896. He was later Dean of the University and Bellevue Hospital Medical College and was Attending Surgeon to Bellevue.

He joined the Academy in 1901, served on the Committee on Admissions 1917–21, and was appointed on the Committee on Public Health 1921–24, and on Medical Education in 1924, and had been Vice President since 1923.

Resolutions were passed authorizing the President to appoint each year a Committee on Medical Education, and permitting it to make studies of existing undergraduate and postgraduate courses offered in the City of New York and in such other places as it might deem wise; to study and issue statements thereon, but that such statements should not be issued until approved by three-quarters of the Committee, and by the President of the Academy of Medicine. This put the Committee on the same footing in regard to freedom of action as had been granted the Public Health Committee in 1914.

Even at the very beginning of 1925 the Trustees, and particularly the Director, realized that the financial situation was not very satisfactory—even with the splendid endowment made by the Rockefeller Foundation.

While the actual deficit for 1924 was only $6,091.71, the cumulative deficit amounted to $23,642.59. As the budget for 1925 was only $132,000 and the estimated income $159,000, it was thought that things would be taken care of. By May it was realized that more endowment must be secured—$40,000 more of income was needed. In May the President gave an informal dinner at the New York Yacht Club at which the situation was discussed. It was later voted by the Council that a committee be appointed to try to secure another million for endowment, but not by an open campaign for funds. The President was requested to ask certain Fellows to approach Messrs. George F. Baker, Jr., Edward S. Harkness, James B. Ford, George Eastman, and J. P. Morgan. The first three had already given $200,000 for the purpose, and there is no record of any further contributions at this time.

A long statement of the purposes and needs of the Academy was prepared by Dr. Williams and was printed and circulated. But the records show no more additions to the endowment during 1925 or 1926.

In April, 1925, the sale of 222 East 83d Street, secured on a foreclosure of a mortgage of $7,500 some twelve years before, was authorized: $4,500 had been paid at that time for legal fees in this matter, and repairs. In May the Trustees were informed that the original foreclosure had been declared invalid, so all commissions were ordered paid for the arranged sale, and a new foreclosure had to be started. The property was eventually sold for "a profit of $4,500."

Of course the planning for the new building and its actual construction were very important duties of the Director. He attended to the minutest details. Estimates for excavation were obtained and out of the nine received, that of the Crimmins Construction Company was accepted. The work was started in May, and was expeditiously and satisfactorily done.

But 43d Street was still troublesome. Dr. Williams was authorized to advise with a competent engineer, preferably the one appointed for the new building, in regard to heating the place.

A member of the Library Committee was wisely added to the Building Committee, which held frequent meetings—eighteen during the year. A special Art Committee was appointed to cooperate with it, consisting of Drs. Dana, W. B. James, and Holden, to recommend inscriptions to be placed on the exterior of the building, and also the details of decoration for the interior.

Dr. Dana took a great personal interest in the Latin inscriptions over the windows, and in the beautification of the building. In 1925 he presented to the Academy 121 lithographs, etchings, mezzotints, and engravings of medical men, and later added thirty-four more. Many of them hang in the Academy today. He also presented a collection of first editions of the works of Oliver Wendell Holmes.

As early as the fall of 1924, the future and development of the Library was given much attention. Dr. Fielding H. Garrison, Librarian of the Surgeon General's Library, was, by permission of the Surgeon General, appointed Consulting Librarian of the Academy. In the folder of February 2, 1925, appeared this notice: "Dr. F. H. Garrison, Consulting Librarian, will be at the Academy of Medicine on Saturday, February 21st, and will meet by appointment any member desiring assistance in bibliography, preparation of papers requiring research work, criticism, revision or reduction of manuscript for the press etc. At 4 P.M. Saturday February 21st, Dr. Garrison will hold an informal historical conference on Diabetes and Insulin."

As has been already mentioned the Academy voted to publish a monthly bulletin, which appeared March, 1925. It contained important papers and addresses, and much Academy news which the Fellows should know about. The Director was made Editor! Two dollars of annual dues were allotted to it.

Dr. Garrison contributed an article to most of the numbers during 1925 and in 1926. He was receiving an honorarium of $1,200 a year for his services. In 1927 finances would not permit of the Consulting Librarian—he was really no longer needed—and Dr.

Garrison was retained as an editorial writer at $500 a year. He continued his contributions for several years.

Mr. J. S. Brownne was now seventy-one. He had been appointed Librarian in 1880 and had served the Academy faithfully for forty-five years. He was retired on August 1, 1925, with the title of Consulting Librarian.

Up till 1880 the Library at 31st Street had been managed by a Fellow, without salary. Its possessions were not extensive. When the addition to the building was made and Dr. Purple contributed some 2,000 volumes, it was felt a full-time professional librarian must be secured. Mr. Brownne, who had been Assistant Librarian to the Astor Library, was appointed. Having a good education and practical experience, he was well qualified for the position. With indefatigable energy, he immediately began cataloguing the library. With little assistance he accomplished this in short order, and it was kept up to the minute to the very end of his services.

He lived in the building, and to his duties as Librarian were added, at various times, those of clerk, bookkeeper, and Superintendent. He attended to repairs, engaged the constant succession of janitors, and did practically everything. When the Academy moved to 43d Street, the library was moved and installed in an incredibly short time, all through his skill and management. He continued to live on the top floor of the Academy, as he had at 31st Street, brought up his family there, and built a sort of roof garden for his children to play in. The Academy was his home.

When the Academy acquired the Library of the New York Hospital in 1898, the 23,000 volumes were sorted, catalogued, and placed on the shelves in a few months, instead of the year it was expected to take.

For a number of years Mr. Brownne was in his office, accessible to Fellows wanting advice on where to look for things. He became quite an able bibliographic authority. Never having enough funds for the Library's needs, but undismayed, Mr. Brownne always made the best use of what funds he had, and in all his years of service the Library was well run and cared for.

He had always been assured by the Trustees, especially Drs.

Jacobi and Loomis, that the Academy would always be his home. A Committee composed of all the former chairmen of the Library Committee, some twenty-four in number, were appointed to obtain subscriptions for a fund to buy him a home just outside New York. It raised $5,318.00, which provided the home, and he was retired with a pension of $4,000 a year. The following resolutions were passed.

John S. Browne, Librarian of the New York Academy of Medicine for forty-five years, during which time the Library has grown from a small to a great collection of medical literature, is about to retire from active service with the title of Consultant Librarian.

By his untiring efforts he has obtained gifts and support for the Library. By his amiability and constant readiness to help, he has won the admiration and friendship of the Fellows and of the general reading public. The Committee on Library has benefited greatly by his wise counsel and his rare discrimination and judgment in the selection of books, and the entire Academy has profited by his devotion to the interests of the Library which he has done so much to foster and develop.

On behalf of the Fellows of the New York Academy of Medicine, and in recognition of his great service as Librarian for so many years, we desire to express to him our sense of deep obligation, to wish him long health and happiness, and to present to him a token of our appreciation and esteem.

Resolved, That by and with the consent of the Council and the Trustees, these resolutions be spread upon the minutes of the meeting of the Committee on Library and of the Council of the New York Academy of Medicine.

Mr. Browne, in all his years as librarian, accumulated material in a scrapbook, hoping to write a history of the Library, but he never did. This scrapbook was presented to the Library by his daughters in 1945, and has been of the greatest value in writing this history of the Academy.

In the interval Mrs. Laura E. Smith, who had been his capable assistant for 34 years, was made Acting Librarian. In October, 1925, Dr. Archibald Malloch was appointed Librarian—to begin his work January 1, 1926. He was abroad at the time in connection with the Osler Memorial Library.

Dr. Malloch was a graduate of Queens University, receiving his medical degree from McGill, where he had served as resident pathologist and bacteriologist and medical interne. During the war he had served with the Red Cross and in the Canadian Army Medical Corps. He had also been Beit Fellow in London. When appointed, he resigned as Demonstrator of Medicine at McGill, Assistant Physician at the Royal Victorial Hospital, and Assistant Editor of the *Canadian Medical Association Journal.*

Dr. Malloch's interest in library work was roused when he and Dr. W. W. Francis were selected by Sir William Osler to prepare a catalogue raisonné of the 8,000 volumes in the Osler Collection.

The formal laying of the cornerstone of the new building took place on Friday, October 30, 1925. It had been announced in the folder and all Fellows were invited to attend.

Dr. Brown spoke very briefly on what the Academy had stood for for nearly seventy-five years: the betterment of professional standards and professional ethics, the development of medical education, the furthering of public health functions of the city and country, and the Library. He thanked the Foundations and the generous donors who had made this building possible and promised to do everything possible to be worthy of the trust implied in their gifts.

After laying the cornerstone Dr. Stewart spoke, also very briefly, mentioning the former homes of the Academy, and how, when 43d Street was occupied, the speakers of the evening were confident that adequate quarters had been provided for the Library and all Academy activities for a long time. Yet, "in the span of one average professional life," the Library was so overcrowded that "many wonderful books have long been waiting on the floors for the time when increased room would permit their promotion to the aristocracy of the shelves."

He explained, for the benefit of the laity, who were "only vaguely aware of its existence, and almost entirely unfamiliar with the scope of its work or the direction of its aims," that the Academy was not a social club for relaxation and recreation, but a forum for the discussions in the realms of medicine, public health, social welfare, and biological sciences.

He concluded with a tribute to Dr. Pritchett of the Carnegie Corporation, "who saw in the Academy an opportunity to promote medical education by assisting and enlarging an institution created by the doctors themselves."

The builders, Mark Eidlitz and Son, had been well chosen. By December, 1925, the building was reported "30 percent finished, work continuing satisfactorily and financially within the original contract."

Mr. George T. Eddy was commissioned to find a Latin motto for the new building. He produced one, and an honorarium was voted to him. What it was is not stated, but presumably it is that over the front entrance:

POST MILLE SECULA PRAESCINDETUR OCCASIO ALIQUID ADJUCIENDI
(After thousands of ages the opportunity continues
of adding to our knowledge)

As early as October, 1925, a committee was appointed to have charge of the ceremonies to take place at the opening of the new building, and that same month the First District Dental Society was allotted space therein, the first outside group to be planned for.

It was decided to name the Auditorium "Hosack Hall" and the large Section Room on the second floor "Dubois Hall." Dr. Duel was to interview Mrs. Jenkins to ask if she desired to suggest a name for any room in the new building.

In September, 1926, the Trustees purchased the lot to the east, for future development.

During these two years of preparation and reorganization, the rules of the Trustees, and the Constitution and By Laws were amended several times. Hitherto anybody could start a special library fund with any amount. The bookkeeping on these funds of a few hundred dollars was complicated and time consuming. It was now ruled that a contribution of $5,000 for the Library could be a "named" fund for special purposes, stipulating the character of books bought, and so on, and a special bookplate would be provided.

Contributions from $1,000 to under $5,000 could be a "named" fund also, could be restricted for specific purposes, but no bookplate would be provided. Anything under $1,000 would go to the general Library Endowment Fund.

The question of who were resident and who were non-resident Fellows was troublesome. The By Laws were amended so that those who lived or *had an office* within twenty-five miles of City Hall, whether residing in New York or New Jersey, should be Residents and pay the regular dues of $20 per annum. Under this ruling 122 non-resident and 30 associate members were transferred to the resident list. Also twenty-eight associates were made non-resident members. The Treasurer wrote a special letter of explanation to each group and requested the balance of their dues. The Fellowship was increased to 1,625, probably to cover this change. The Director was requested to speak before each Section, explaining the change, and emphasizing the financial needs of the Academy.

The question of increasing dues was discussed for a long time, the Director insisting that it was absolutely necessary, but action was postponed.

Amendments were also passed simplifying the accounting for restricted funds, the limitations on investing of funds, and bonding of the Treasurer was eliminated.

The Committee on Admissions was having a hard time. It reported there were 127 applications for Fellowship, and no vacancies. In June, 1925, it sent a letter to all Fellows, which stated in part:

> . . . The constantly increasing number of applications for membership in the Academy which has been made during the last two years and the long waiting list at present, has thrown a heavy responsibility upon the Committee on Admissions. It is no longer a mere question of keeping out unworthy applicants. It has become a question of selecting from a large number of eligible applicants those most desirable to fill the few available vacancies. Membership in the Academy has always been a privilege. If, in the future, a careful selection of applicants be made, election to membership will soon be recognized as something of an honor. Such selection cannot be made unless the Committee on Admissions is furnished with full information about each applicant. It is there-

fore urgently requested that Fellows of the Academy interest themselves in aiding the Committee by the confidential expression of opinion of candidates, either by letters to the Committee or by communication with one of its members. . . .

Having these considerations in mind, the question that any endorser of a candidate ought to ask himself is, "Will this man be a worthy addition to the Academy?" The question is not, "Is there any reason why this man should not be elected?," but, "Is there a reason why he should be elected?"

. . . It is believed that the interests of the Academy will be best served if the following qualifications be considered: That in addition to qualifications as to character and behavior the candidate has made some contribution of recognized value to medical literature; or, that he be actively engaged in medical teaching; or, that he hold some hospital position or medical post of importance; or, that he has shown outstanding professional ability as a practitioner.

This brought such satisfactory results, it was sent out again the next year.

The Committee on Admissions was authorized when a candidate had insufficient endorsements after six months, to notify his endorsers, and also if, after six months a candidate had definite opposition, to give his endorsers the opportunity to withdraw his name.

Dr. Nellis B. Foster was Chairman of the Committee. The Council passed the following resolution:

Resolved, That the services of Dr. Nellis B. Foster to the Committee on Admissions and to the Academy have been of such an exceptional character that the Committee feel that Dr. Foster is in a very large measure responsible for the present policies and practices of the Committee, especially in respect to raising the standards for membership.

The Council voted that the Program Committee should consist of the three Vice-Presidents and the Director; and the selection of a Carpenter Lecturer and the person to give the Anniversary Address were left to it.

The name of the Committee on Public Health was changed to "Committee on Public Health Relations." There had been so many changes that a committee was appointed to suggest other changes and rewrite the whole Constitution and By Laws. The new edition was adopted in February, 1926.

The Standing Committees were increased from two to four: Education, and Public Health Relations, which had hitherto been committees appointed by the Council, were made Standing Committees of the Academy. Each was to consist of thirty members appointed annually by the President, subject to the approval of the Council, and their powers and duties were defined in some detail.

There is no longer mention of an "Anniversary Meeting"; for it, there was substituted "at least one meeting shall be held annually to which the public shall be invited." The "Anniversary Discourse" was mentioned for several years, however.

A Nominating Committee for officers was authorized, to consist of three Fellows, no one of whom should be a member of the Council.

The number of Fellows residing within twenty-five miles of the City Hall was now limited to 1,625, and those outside those limits 400. Members of the Army, Navy, and Public Health Service were not counted in the total. Associate Fellows were limited to 400. (In October, 1926, the number of Resident members was increased to 1,700.)

The number of Trustees was increased to ten, two retiring each year. The offices of Corresponding and Historical Secretary were abolished, although the latter made a report for the year 1926.

Whenever a candidate's name had been before the Committee on Admissions for eighteen months without action, it was to be removed from the list and his endorsers so notified, but it could be put up again. These were the main changes in the Constitution as printed.

Much time and thought was given to improving the character of, and attendance at, the Stated Meetings. In January, 1925, the Council voted:

1) All papers to be limited to 30 minutes. If longer time is needed for protocols, or experiments, summaries only shall be read;
2) All papers to be typewritten and a summary to be prepared;
3) The Academy reserves the right to publish the complete article, or

summary in the *Bulletin*. This regulation will be waived if other arrangements for publication are desired. The Academy does not wish this to be retro-active;

4) Announcement of these requirements to be sent to each speaker.

The Trustees authorized the payment of transportation for speakers at Academy meetings, as had been recommended by Dr. Stewart.

The Council authorized publication of programs in *Medical Week* at a monthly cost of $10. This was only continued one year.

The Program Committee now consisted of the three Vice-Presidents and the Director. They did their work well. The attendance and the condition of the weather was noted in the minutes of each meeting. At only a few was the attendance under a hundred. The highest attendance was 400, at 43d Street, too. At that overcrowded meeting in Hosack Hall papers were read by Sir Henry Gauvain, London, on the treatment of surgical tuberculosis; Dr. Edouard Rist, Paris, "Relations of Heart and Lung in diseased Conditions as observed by the Fluoroscope"; and Professor Francis Harbitz, Oslo, on "Periarteritis Nodosa."

Dr. Ernst Friedrich Müller spoke twice before the Academy; in 1925 on the "Mechanism of Insulin Action," and in October, 1926, on "Observations during the Period of Undernutrition in Germany."

Meetings were devoted to colloid chemistry and to alkalosis. The surgical relief of cardiac pain was discussed, and the rather discouraging results of operations in mitral stenosis, by incision of the schlerosed and stenosed cusps, were described in papers by Drs. S. A. Levine of Boston, C. S. Beck of Cleveland, and W. G. Penfield.

Three meetings were held on various modern conceptions of the functions and diseases of the liver, and one on rheumatic disease in children. The Sections on Medicine and Orthopedic Surgery held a joint meeting on poliomyelitis.

The Staff of Massachusetts General Hospital and the Faculty of the Albany Medical College each provided a program. The Department of Health presented studies on the recent epidemic of typhoid fever in New York City.

An effort had been made to start a Section on Gastro-Enterology.

The Council did not approve, but instructed the Program Committee to try to satisfy those interested. A meeting was arranged in cooperation with the New York Gastro-Enterological Association, at which 125 were present. The Section on Ophthalmology presented a symposium on headache. Dr. Ross Hall Skillern, Philadelphia, spoke on those of nasal origin, Dr. de Schweinitz, Philadelphia, of ocular headaches, Dr. Foster Kennedy on headaches from the viewpoint of a neurologist, and Dr. Ludwig Kast, from the viewpoint of an internist. The attendance, on a "clear night," was 375.

Dr. Max A. Goldstein gave a demonstration of modern methods of training of the deaf child, with teachers and pupils of the Central Institution for the Deaf, of St. Louis. Dr. Sachs discussed the mental and moral training of the child. Two hundred and twenty-five attended his lecture.

The Sections were very active and at eight of the twelve stated meetings in 1926 provided the programs. The average attendance varied from 58 at Obstetrics and Gynecology, to 135 at Dermatology and Syphilis, and 117 at Medicine and Genito-Urinary Surgery.

The Academy was cooperating in every way possible with the societies holding meetings there. In March, 1925, the old form of the Folder was changed, and notices of important meetings at the Academy, other than those of the Academy itself and the Harvey Society, were often printed. A "National Child Health Day" meeting, under the auspices of the Public Health Committee, the Section on Pediatrics, and the Health Department Bureau of Child Hygiene was thus announced; another on convalescent care, under the auspices of the Public Health Committee and Hospital Information Bureau of the United Hospital Fund. The Academy was interested in these meetings; but one held under the auspices of the Association of Italian Physicians of America and the Italian Brooklyn Medical Society, to hear an address on the "University of Bologna in the History of Medicine" (address in English), was far afield. Quite a contrast to the attitude of the Council some ten or fifteen years before, when the New York Pathological Society was refused the use of the Folder for its meetings.

The meeting of January 7, 1926, was an interesting one. The

Academy expected to be in its new building by the end of the year. This was the last annual meeting which would be held at 17 West 43d Street. Three papers were read. One, by Dr. Delavan, recounted the Academy's history from its first conception in 1846 up till 1890, and outlined very clearly its first conflicts and gradual development.

Dr. S. W. Lambert told interestingly of its life at 43d Street. When the Academy moved there in November, 1890, "New York still had many of the characteristics of a provincial town, limited, theoretically, to Manhattan Island but actually still bounded on the North by Central Park and the belt line of horse cars on 59th Street. Transportation in the city was exclusively by horse power except for the elevated steam car lines running to Manhattanville on the West and Harlem on the East side of the island. This was six years before Dr. F. P. Kinnicutt resigned from St. Luke's Hospital because that institution had removed so far from his home to its new location at 113th Street."

Dr. Lambert also described how scientific medicine had been advanced by the keen analysis of symptoms of disease and their relation to pathology of Delafield, by the diagnostic power of E. G. Janeway and the therapeutic insight of A. L. Loomis; he spoke, further, of the clinical contributions of A. A. Smith, G. L. Peabody, W. H. Draper, F. P. Kinnicutt, Jacobi and T. A. McBride in medicine, and of R. F. Weir, Charles McBurney, W. T. Bull, J. D. Bryant and L. A. Stimson in surgery. All of these papers had been presented at the Academy. It was an interesting story.

Dr. L. R. Williams, the Director, then spoke of the *Future* of the Academy. He said many of the suggestions and propositions he would offer came from the Fellows and from himself. They had not as yet been decided by the Council, but were merely suggestions subject to discussion. Many, he felt, were outside both the proper functions and the means of the Academy, and belonged to other organizations. Otherwise duplication of effort and waste of money would result. To this group belonged the proposals for a research laboratory; a museum of anatomy and pathology; a collection of instruments similar to the Hunterian Collection at the College of

Surgeons in London; an anatomical collection like that at the College of Physicians in Philadelphia.

He had many suggestions as to the organization and activities and functions of the Sections, the development of the Library by the accumulation of incunabula, and the establishment of a bibliographic and photostat service. Dr. Williams was looking into the future, preparing for it and warning against overoptimism.

The Carpenter Lecture of 1925, "Practical Management of Neurotic Patients," was given by Dr. L. F. Barker of Baltimore, and Dr. George E. Vincent of the Rockefeller Foundation gave the Anniversary Discourse, "The Doctor and the Changing Order."

So many requests were made for use of the building for fund raising that in 1925 the Council voted that no matter how worthy the cause, Stated Meetings of the Academy or Sections should not be used for the purpose of fund raising or for presentation of requests for funds from societies or agencies.

In November, 1925, the centennial of the birth of Charcot was celebrated. At a meeting of the Section on Historical and Cultural Medicine, Dr. F. H. Garrison presented an illustrated paper on "Mementos of Charcot and the Salpêtrière." In December at a joint meeting of the Section on Neurology and Psychiatry and the New York Neurological Society, Dr. Garrison again read his paper, Dr. Starr described the recent Centennial Celebration at Paris and described scenes at Charcot's clinic as he had seen them, Dr. Dana spoke on "Charcot and the Arts," and Dr. Sachs of Charcot as a "hypnotist and diagnostician." The Library gave an interesting exhibit of mementos, photographs, and literature dealing with Charcot.

Another exhibition was given on the 320th anniversary of the birth of Sir Thomas Browne. His works, especially "Religio Medici," and other interesting matter were shown, from the Library collection and also from those of Drs. Hellman and Moschcowitz, and the Union Theological Seminary.

In January, 1926, Dr. Robert T. Morris read a paper before the Section on Historical and Cultural Medicine, on "The Evolution of the Subject of Appendicitis," and the Library arranged an exhibit thereon.

So great was the interest in these exhibits, that the Council appointed a Committee on Exhibits, consisting of Dr. C. N. B. Camac, chairman, Rufus Cole, Karl Vogel, and John Wyckoff.

In the legislative aspects of public health, the Academy played a minor role in these years, except in one instance. There had been a fight for years between the anatomical departments of medical schools and the pathologists of hospitals in regard to autopsies. A compromise was finally reached and a bill, known as the "Autopsy Bill," was introduced. The Academy was instrumental in its adoption.

In February, 1925, it was voted

that the Council of the New York Academy of Medicine hereby appoint Drs. Dana, William Browning, Dever S. Byard, Louis I. Harris, Howard H. Mason, William H. Park, Frederick Tilney, Edwin G. Zabriskie and E. H. L. Corwin as members of a committee for the study of communicable diseases of the central nervous system and authorize this committee to cooperate with the Commissioner of Health of New York City, who has already appointed a commission for this purpose whose personnel is identical to that of this committee.

The Director and Public Health Committee were to estimate the expenses which might be needed and to solicit funds. If outside funds were not available the Council recommended that from any available balance, a small sum should be appropriated to the Public Health Committee for the specific use of this Committee.

In May, 1926, it was voted that in view of the anticipated recurrence of poliomyelitis this year, the Committee on Public Health Relations be asked to express an opinion as to whether the serum of persons who have recovered from an attack of the disease is of curative value, and secondly if the first answer should be in the affirmative, whether the Academy should take steps to secure before the occurrence of an epidemic a list of such persons who would consent to donate blood.

The Public Health Relations Committee was very busy. Numbers of questions were referred to it by the city departments and a few by the national government. It is impossible here to enumerate all these activities, valuable though they were.

In April, 1926, the Committee gave a dinner to Dr. Dana, its Chairman for the fifteen years of its existence. A marble bust from Athens, dating from the fourth century B.C., was presented to him.

The speaking program, arranged to simulate a meeting of the Committee, was carried out as follows:

1. Introductory remarks. *Dr. George David Stewart,* TOASTMASTER.
2. Reading of the Minutes.
3. Report of the Executive Secretary. *Dr. E. H. L. Corwin.*
4. "The Role of Neurology in Public Health." *Report by Dr. J. A. Miller.*
5. "The Doctor Peeps at a Fellow Practitioner." *Report by Dr. Joseph Collins.*
6. "Some of the Recreations of Dr. Dana in Art and Literature." *Report by Dr. F. Peterson.*
7. "How It Strikes a Junior Contemporary." *Report by Dr. Foster Kennedy.*
8. Rebuttal by Dr. Dana.

The Committee on Medical Education was also very active. A Bureau of Clinical Information on the ground floor was of increasing service; 520 consulted it in 1925, and 551 in 1926.

A daily bulletin was issued, citing surgical operations at 29 hospitals in 1925 and at 75 in 1926. A weekly bulletin of "Non-operative Clinics and Conferences" was published in *Medical Week*, on eight special subjects at 12 hospitals in 1925 and on thirty or more special subjects at 41 hospitals in 1926.

A booklet on "Opportunities for Clinical Study in New York Hospitals" was published and met with much favorable comment, including an editorial in the *Journal of the American Medical Association.*

During 1925, six societies had offices in the Academy, and forty-three held meetings there. The Statistical Secretary reported also that five "were given accommodations free of charge." In 1926, eight had offices there, forty-six held their meetings in the Academy, and seven were accommodated "free of charge."

In 1926 a group of Fellows subscribed $650 to buy rare books for the Library. Four were bought, and the bulletin, after announcing them, regretted the inability to buy a recently offered copy of Rabanus Maurus, "the first printed medical book," which was priced at $1,200.

Another very valuable gift was announced in June, 1926. An anonymous donor had promised the Academy $10,000 a year for five years, beginning January, 1927. The Trustees' minutes state "it is hoped that if this money is satisfactorily expended this income will be later capitalized."

In 1925 the Academy lost a very valuable Fellow by the death of Dr. Nathan E. Brill. The resolutions state: "Dr. Brill was elected a Fellow of the Academy in 1887, and was appointed a member of the Public Health Committee and served actively, regularly and intelligently as a member of this Committee until his last illness. He was appointed a Trustee in December, 1915, and has regularly attended the meetings of that Board since that time. He was a judicious counselor and always conscientious in his endeavors to work for the best interests of the Academy." It may be remembered that Dr. Brill was the only Trustee who voted against buying the 60th Street site.

Another old and most valuable Fellow died, Dr. Arthur M. Jacobus. He had served the Academy as Assistant Secretary and Recording Secretary from 1883 through 1891, and as Trustee from 1893 through 1912. As a Trustee he served on almost all the Board's Committees to investigate matters before them. He was seventy-two years old when he died, and had been a Fellow forty-seven years.

The moving of the Academy was of course an event of events. The actual moving of the Library was a triumph of planning. None of the furniture and fixtures was taken from the old building, which made it easier. The Library was closed to the public from July 15, but the periodical room was open to Fellows until two weeks before the new building was opened. On August 2, the moving of

133,000 books—134 truck loads—was begun. The contents of each case was plainly marked and its ultimate destination indicated. By September 7 the work was completed, every book in its proper place, and this in spite of the fact that the elevator for the nine floors of stacks was not in running order. The official account comments: "Nothing but praise can be said for the way in which the movers and the members of the library staff, especially Mr. Place and Mr. Smith, worked under the very trying conditions of August weather. Practically no damage was done to the books, and, as far as known, none were lost."

On November 4, 8,000 volumes of bound periodicals from the journal room, 2,013 volumes of "classics and incunabula," current journals, together with portraits and office furniture, were moved. Everything was in place by November 18 for the opening of the new building.

When it came to the sorting out and disposing of useless triplicate books and unbound periodicals, the library faced a problem. It had been so overcrowded and so understaffed that the very presence of many was not known. There was no time for the overworked staff to prepare lists to be offered for sale. A great number were chosen by representatives of other libraries and by the Medical Library Exchange. But after all the selections had been made, seven and a half tons remained to be sold as *old paper*, book dealers not being interested. This "old paper" brought just $75.50, a trifle over ten dollars a ton.

Section meetings were held at 43d Street through November 16, the last being that of Genito-Urinary Surgery.

The opening of the new building was a great event, carefully considered for over a year. It had been hoped that all would be ready immediately after the summer recess, but there were unexpected and unavoidable delays, and the date was postponed until November 18. That Academy affairs continued undisturbed was a triumph for the Director. To him had been left all matters, including publicity and even of expenses.

The Council had approved the Director's selection of the following twenty-two distinguished physicians, surgeons, and scientists to be elected Honorary Fellows:

Robert Bárány, M.D., Professor of Otology, Rhinology, and Laryngology, Upsala University, Sweden.

Edward William Archibald, M.D., Surgeon, Professor of Surgery, Director of the Department, McGill University, Montreal.

Charles James Martin, M.D., C.M.G., F.R.S., F.R.C.P., Director, Lister Institute, London.

Sir George Newman, M.D., K.C.B., F.R.S.E., D.P.H., F.R.C.P., Chief Medical Officer, Ministry of Health, London.

Sir Charles Sherrington, M.D., O.M., G.B.E., F.R.C.P., F.R.C.S., LL.D., F.R.S., Waynflete Professor of Physiology, Oxford.

Henry Head, M.D., F.R.S., F.R.C.P., M.R.C.S., LL.D, London.

Marin T. Tuffier, M.D., Commander Légion D'Honneur, Croix de Guerre, Surgeon, Paris.

Georges F. I. Widal, M.D., Hôpital Cochin, Paris.

Josef Jadassohn, M.D., Professor of Dermatology and Syphilology, University of Breslau.

Friedrich Müller, M.D., Professor and Director II, Medical Clinic, Munich.

Friedrich Neufeld, M.D., G.M.R., Director, Prussian Institute for Infectious Diseases, Berlin.

Vittorio Putti, M.D., Professor of Orthopedics, Instituto Rizzoli, Bologna.

Carlos Chagas, M.D., Director, Oswaldo Cruz Institute, Rio de Janeiro, Brazil.

John Jacob Abel, Sc.D., LL.D., Professor of Pharmacology, Johns Hopkins University, Baltimore.

Frank Billings, M.D., Sc.D., D.S.M., Chicago.

Harvey W. Cushing, M.D., Sc.D., LL.D., F.R.C.S., D.S.M., Surgeon in Chief, Peter Bent Brigham Hospital.

George E. de Schweinitz, M.D., LL.D., Professor of Ophthalmology, University of Pennsylvania, Philadelphia.

George Dock, M.D., Sc.D., Physician to Los Angeles General Hospital.

John M. T. Finney, M.D., F.R.C.S., D.S.M., Professor of Clinical Surgery, Johns Hopkins University, Baltimore.

Chevalier Jackson, M.D., Sc.D., Professor of Laryngology, Jefferson

Medical College; Professor of Esophagoscopy and Bronchoscopy, University of Pennsylvania, Philadelphia.

Theobald Smith, M.D., Sc.D., Director, Department Animal Pathology, Rockefeller Institute.

William Sidney Thayer, M.D., LL.D., D.S.M., Professor of Medicine, Johns Hopkins University, Baltimore.

It will be noticed that nine were from the United States, four from England, three from Germany, two from France (Paris), and one each from Canada, Sweden, Italy, and Brazil. On November 17 a dinner was given in their honor at the Waldorf-Astoria. The table list names 581 Fellows, many "with guests."

Dr. Brown, President, presided and made a brief address of welcome. Dr. George David Stewart was Toastmaster, introducing each speaker as only he could do. As a Toastmaster he was inimitable.

Dr. Harvey Cushing spoke on "Books and the Doctor," responding for the Boston Medical Library. It was a very amusing address, full of humor and banter.

The Toastmaster then altered the order of ceremonies and introduced the announced last speaker, "because he had to leave," "The Mayor—our Mayor, His Honor, Mayor Jimmy Walker." "His Honor" spoke lightly, as usual, without saying much, but acknowledged his own indebtedness to the Academy for its advice, at his request, on the candidates for Health Commissioner. Once he got rather mixed up, and spoke of the "Academy of Music," but after the laughter subsided he passed it off with "Well, after all it is not without its harmony."

Dr. George de Schweinitz, College of Physicians of Philadelphia, gave an interesting account of the founding and development of the College, its relations with the Academy and expressed the hope that the *entente* which had always existed between the two would forever remain unbroken.

Dr. W. S. Thayer delivered the real address of the evening. He spoke of the development of medicine when all was based on the authority of the "Master," up to the time of Laënnec, of whose death this year was the centenary. After briefly discussing Laënnec and his work, he amusingly described his being sent by the Angel

Ithuriel, who was "disturbed by the reports of the press and Sinclair Lewis's novels" to inspect medical circles in New York. He described what might have surprised him, delighted him, disturbed him, in a most humorous and yet serious way. His address is good reading today (*Bulletin of the New York Academy of Medicine*, Vol. III, 2d series, p. 78).

He closed by saying that when Laënnec made his report to Ithuriel he might have expressed the hope that after another century he be sent again to the New York Academy of Medicine, and suggested, if it was not too much trouble, that George Stewart be sent with him to preside at the dinner.

Although he was not on the program, Sir John McLean, of the University of Wales, was then called on. He was apparently the only distinguished foreigner present. After referring to an old Arabian proverb which said "four things come not back; the past life, the spent arrow, the spoken word, the neglected opportunity," he presented the greetings from the Chief Magistrate of Cardiff, and the ceremonies were concluded.

The next afternoon, November 18, 1926, at 3.30 the opening ceremonies were held at 2 East 103d Street, and were opened with a short dedicatory prayer by the Rev. Henry Sloane Coffin, D.D., President of the Union Theological Seminary. It consisted of just 248 words including the Amen. The last 178 are worth again recording, and might well be inscribed on the walls of the Academy. They were:

Foster here both the science and art of physical well being. May those who meet within these walls help each other to understand the causes and cure of disease, to be skilled in safeguarding and increasing public health, and to aid mankind to attain greater vigor for their work and play.

Grant that this Academy of Medicine, rich with the memories of physicians and surgeons honored and loved in their generations, may uphold the standards and traditions of a high calling, and inspire its members with open-mindedness to truth, diligence in study, courage in the discharge of duty, reverence for those they serve, and unselfish devotion to their welfare. In the midst of this wealthy city, enable these servants of humanity to remain untainted by sordid ideals, and, by their life and work, to assist in leavening the community with the spirit of the Son of Man who came not to be ministered unto but to minister, and who set men free from ills of the flesh and spirit that they might share His own abundant life.

Amen.

Dr. Brown spoke briefly of the development of the Academy, and of the services it had given and was giving to the profession and the community. Dr. Duel, Chairman of the Building Committee, told the story of the building of the Academy, from its origin. He paid his compliments to the Library Committee for their long fight for larger and better equipped quarters, to the Trustees and Fellows for their patience with long, long delays, and to Dr. Linsly R. Williams "to whom perhaps more than to all others the credit of the working efficiency of this building should be given."

Fellows and guests were then shown over the building, and refreshments were served.

In the evening the first scientific meeting was held. The Director presented the name and qualifications of each of the twenty-two Honorary Fellows, and they were unanimously elected.

Professor M. I. Pupin of Columbia delivered the Carpenter Lecture, "Ionization and Chemical Reactions," and the strenuous day closed. It is to be hoped the Director got a good night's sleep. He deserved it.

The Section on Orthopedic Surgery held its regular meeting the following evening. The move was certainly made without disturbing Academy routine, except for the library, which was unavoidable.

The Library held an excellent exhibition, in connection with the opening, of "Early and Later Medical Americana."

The Academy received much publicity in connection with the occasion. *The Medical Journal and Record* printed all the speeches at the dinner and opening, and the daily press printed extensive notices.

The Anniversary Oration was delivered by Dr. Nicholas Murray Butler, President of Columbia University, on "The Physician and the Larger View."

Dr. Brown was a most competent President. He gave much time to the Academy. He presided at two thirds of the Stated Meetings, and was very regular in attending meetings of the Council and Trustees.

1927–1928

Samuel Waldron Lambert

Dr. Brown was prevented by illness from personally delivering his address as retiring President, but it was read by retiring Vice-President H. S. Carter. The address defended the action of the Public Health Relations Committee in advising the newly elected Mayor on the choice of his Commissioner of Health. The Committee proposed no candidate of its own; it merely investigated the records of the twenty-five candidates for the office, with regard to their experience in public health. On the basis of this investigation, it endorsed four as particularly qualified, and the Mayor appointed one of them.

Dr. Brown also discussed the dangers of a "Director" of the Academy—the tendency to delegate to one man arbitrary powers. He showed how Dr. Williams had suggested changes in organization which gave responsibility to more Fellows, and made its administration even more democratic.

Dr. Lambert, as incoming President, said: "The New York Academy of Medicine is not a local medical group. It has become a national institution. . . . This building is an asset of which we may be proud, but it is also a liability which calls for more expenditures now and in the future. . . . This Academy, like every educational institution, must go on to new fields of work or retrograde from its position of prominence." The Fellows had taxed themselves by doubled dues, but must be ready to "expand into the unknown and compelling activities of the future." He stressed the importance of the work of the Committees on Public Health Relations and Medical Education, which in recent years had "linked this institution to visiting physicians from distant cities and to the general public and government of the city." In conclusion he stated that the recent decision of the Supreme Court on the legality of the Volstead Act threatened to bring the medical profession under a centralized governmental power, whereas during the entire existence of the United States the profession had flourished under state control, and the Academy might become involved in the controversy.

Dr. Samuel W. Lambert, thirty-second President, was sixty-six years old when he assumed office. A man of great personal force and charm, he had a very large practice, had been Dean of the College of Physicians and Surgeons from 1904 to 1919, was now Dean Emeritus, and Attending Physician to St. Luke's Hospital, Consulting Physician to New York Hospital (after fifteen years as Attending Physician there) and also to the French, Fifth Avenue, St. Vincent's, Ruptured and Crippled, and New York Orthopedic hospitals. When Dr. Osler called together a group to form the Interurban Clinical Club, Dr. Lambert was one of those invited and was elected the Club's first President.

Dr. Lambert was utterly opposed to the Volstead Act as interfering with the rights of the physician, and had brought suit to test its constitutionality in the Supreme Court of the United States. He lost his case by a vote of five to four.

In January the Director called the attention of the Council to the fact that the Supreme Court in its decision in April, 1925, had stated that Congress could not regulate the practice of medicine by means of the Harrison Narcotic Law, but in November, 1926, it had handed down a decision that that part of the Volstead Act which limited the right of physicians to prescribe was constitutional. The President was authorized to appoint a special committee to consider this matter.

In May the Academy adopted the following:

Whereas, The Federal Law, known as the Volstead Act, in the provisions of Section 7, the constitutionality of which has been upheld in a recent decision of the Supreme Court of the United States, limits the freedom of the physician in prescribing for his patients and

Whereas, This Congressional assumption of power belonging to the States takes away from the States their right to regulate the practice of medicine within their own borders, and

Whereas, This power may be extended so as to limit the use of other drugs for the satisfactory and scientific practice of medicine and to the discomfiture of the States, be it

Resolved, That the New York Academy of Medicine hereby records its opinion that Section 7 of the Volstead Act is a serious infringement upon the legitimate practice of medicine, and that the Council of the Academy is hereby authorized to take such steps as it may deem necessary to secure a modification of this Section so that there will be no limitation in the time during which one pint of spirituous liquor may be administered under due regulations to prevent the illegal use of spirituous liquor for beverage purposes.

Of course the Academy could do nothing, but the Council voted to print the resolutions and send them to every County Medical Society in the state and to all members of Congress.

These two years, the first at 103d Street, were very busy ones in getting settled and adjusted. A Committee was appointed to draw up House Rules, the most important of which was that in conformity with the Volstead Act, no alcoholic beverages could be served in the building, and smoking was prohibited in Hosack Hall and in the Library. Fellows and guests were "requested not to smoke during meetings" (including Section Meetings?), and presiding officers were asked to call attention to this request. In January, 1928, the House Committee was authorized to install ash receptacles on the backs of Section room seats, "if the expense is reasonable."

In 1927 the arrangement of programs was put in the hands of the Committee on Medical Education, which still performs that valuable function.

For some little time the question of closer relations between the Academy and the Harvey Society had been under discussion. The latter had been holding meetings every Saturday evening from October to May. An agreement was reached whereby the Harvey Society, retaining its autonomy as to administration, control of membership, dues, and selection of lecturers, should hold a meeting on the third Thursday of each month from October to May, replacing the Stated Meeting of the Academy on those days. This was a very wise decision. The Harvey Society conducted the first third Thursday meeting in October, 1928, and has continued to give regular meetings on those days ever since, as "affiliated with the New York Academy of Medicine." In June, 1928, the Trustees voted $300 for honorariums for lecturers for the Harvey Society and announced that $100 per meeting would be granted for 1929. The Academy still contributes something toward paying for Harvey lecturers.

Efforts were also made to bring about closer relations with the New York Pathological Society, the New York Roentgen Society and the Society for Experimental Biology and Medicine. During the next year they all became "affiliated with the New York Academy of Medicine" or gave their meetings under the auspices of the Academy.

The Academy's "Friday afternoon Lectures" were started in January, 1927. The first was given by Dr. Riesman of Philadelphia on "The Treatment of Pneumonia." Sixteen lectures were announced, and were at first called "Lectures of the Practical Lecture Series." The Council had approved paying the traveling expenses of out-of-town lecturers, but Dr. Riesman was the only "out-of-towner." A most excellent series of subjects and speakers were selected. The average attendance in 1928 was 150. The lectures have been continued with great success.

The Section on Historical and Cultural Medicine held a meeting in 1927, with Dr. Osborn speaking on "The Influence of Habit on the Evolution of Man and the Great Apes." Special cards of invitation were printed for this meeting. The Section also held a meeting when Dr. Aleš Hrdlička, of the Smithsonian Institution, spoke on "Origin and Antiquity of Man in America." Dr. Bernard Sachs was chairman of the Section.

Sections combined to hold meetings: Neurology and Psychiatry joined with Obstetrics and Gynecology, and the Section on Medicine had a joint meeting with the American Diebetic Association.

In 1927 the first "Exhibition of Works in the Plastic and Graphic Arts by American Physicians" was held in the Academy for two weeks. Dr. I. Seth Hirsch was the prime mover for the exhibit. The catalogue contained 545 items, shown by 78 exhibitors. It included etchings, dry points, lithographs, sketches and photographs; oils, water colors, pastels, aquatints and crayon pictures; sculpture, metal handicrafts and marquetry, bookplates, illustrations and a model of the U.S. Frigate Constitution, scale 1/8 inch to the foot, by Dr. Karl Vogel. Most exhibits were from New York, naturally, but others came from Philadelphia, Boston, Mt. McGregor, N.Y., Hyannis, Mass., Omaha, Neb., Superior, Wis., and Seattle. Three thousand persons attended. This was the first of several such exhibits held at the Academy.

A meeting of the Section on Historical and Cultural Medicine was held January 20, 1928, in memory of Dr. George S. Huntington, Professor of Anatomy at the College of Physicians and Surgeons. He was never a Fellow of the Academy, his whole life having been devoted to anatomy. He was one of the greatest anatomists of his day—or any day. Drs. C. F. W. McClure, Frederick Tilney and S. W. Lambert made addresses, all of which were published in the *Bulletin* of 1928.

In 1928 the Academy inaugurated the Graduate Fortnight, a two-week series of lectures, round tables, demonstrations, clinics, and exhibits on some special subject in medical science. The idea was suggested by Dr. Ludwig Kast. These "Fortnights" have gone on continuously ever since; the first was on "The Problem of Aging and Old Age." The Annual Meeting of October was included in this program, and Sir Farquhar Buzzard, Regius Professor of Medicine, Oxford, spoke on "The Pains, Penalties and Prohibitions of Old Age," Dr. B. P. Watson on "Menopausal and Post Menopausal Conditions in Women," and Dr. William Engelbach, on "Relations of Endocrine Disorders of Senescence." Seven hundred and fifty attended this meeting; the registration for the Fortnight series was 445. The Carpenter Lecture was given as part of the series: "The Pathology of the Aging Process," by Dr. A. S. Warthin, of the University of Michigan.

A dinner given by the Committees of Public Health Relations and Medical Education to Dr. Norris, Medical Examiner, was attended by sixty Fellows. Dr. Lambert was toastmaster, and speeches were made by Drs. James Ewing, Magrath, Medical Examiner of Boston, Professor Hektoen, Judge Corrigan, and Justice McCook.

Almost all the Stated Meetings were symposia, dealing with various aspects of a subject. They were well selected and mostly were well attended. "The Evolution of the Mind," with papers by Professor Henry Fairfield Osborn, Drs. Frederick Tilney and W. A. White of Washington, had a recorded attendance of 930.

The Anniversary Address on "Mind and Body" was delivered by Professor John Dewey of Columbia in 1927 and drew an audience of 700. In 1928 Chief Justice Benjamin Cardozo, of the Court of Appeals, drew 460 to hear a learned discourse on "What Medicine Can Do for Law." It made such an impression it was printed as a book.

The Carpenter Lecture in 1927 was delivered by Dr. Alonzo E. Taylor, of Stanford University, on "The Present and Future Food Supply of the United States."

A special meeting was held to consider outdoor cleanliness and street conditions. Dr. Sachs, who was intensely interested in the subject, discussed "The Viewpoint of a Physician and Citizen." Dr. Finley of New York University spoke of the public's interest in a clean city, and Drs. Harlow Brooks and W. E. Lambert on the effects of dust on respiratory and eye conditions, and so on. Resolutions were offered by the Vice-President of the Fifth Avenue Association, and the preamble was discussed by the Commissioner of Health.

The Council allowed the Italian Medical Society and the International Medical Association of Spanish Speaking Physicians to hold meetings in the Academy. Forty-nine societies held meetings in 1927 and forty in 1928.

At the meetings of the twelve Sections the average attendance for 1927 was 108; it was highest at Historical and Cultural Medicine, 246; for five Sections it was over 100, and for Orthopedic Surgery it was the lowest, 68. In 1928 seven Sections averaged over 100, Pediatrics having the highest, 193, and Orthopedic Surgery the lowest again, 55; the over-all average was 114.

The Library was very busy. Bibliographical and Photostat Departments had been organized and were very active. The former compiled lists of articles on subjects varying from "the influence of sex on the incidence of disease" to "color schemes for hospital rooms." The latter, beside making photostats, was also able to make photographic reproductions, and lantern slides were also produced.

A messenger service was added in 1928 and in that year the hours the Library was open to the public were extended to 5 P.M. A luncheon service was provided at the Academy.

In 1927 Columbia University deposited on permanent loan 21,000 theses from European Universities. This was a valuable addition.

A "Committee on Curiosities" studied the material on hand, and on its recommendation, it was voted the present collection be kept; that it be placed under the care of the Librarian and Library Committee; that a curator be employed to catalogue and classify it; that permanent cases be placed in the basement room to protect the present material; that additional material be collected, and that exhibitions of this material be held from time to time.

In 1928 the celebrated E. C. Streeter collection of medical classics and incunabula was sold to the Rosenbach Company, which asked $185,000 for it. Dr. Lambert was very anxious to have the Academy acquire it, and he was authorized to appoint a special committee to handle the matter. In three months $10,377 had been subscribed by the Fellows and the entire Library Staff. The President and the Director worked very hard. Outside contributions brought the total to $153,727, and the balance was underwritten by another "friend." Dr. Rosenbach added some items from his large stock. The Rockefeller Foundation contributed $85,000, and Mr. E. S. Harkness $25,000. The final payment was made in June. The Academy acquired a wonderful collection of some 1,200 volumes.

The Library arranged a number of exhibitions which in 1927 included interesting ones on Laënnec and auscultation; the centenary of the publication of Richard Bright's *Reports of Medical Cases;* centenary of the publication of Macmichael's *The Gold Headed Cane;* centennial of the birth of Lord Lister; Dr. Dana's collection of the School of Salerno; and his collection of portraits of medical men.

In 1928 there was an exhibition of books illustrating the history of Dentistry, in celebration of the bicentenary of Pierre Fauchard, and another of 164 items pertaining to William Harvey, on the tercentenary of the publication of *De Motu Cordis*. In December an exhibition was held of some of the early medical manuscripts and incunabula in the Academy. Many came from the recently purchased Streeter Collection. Dr. Streeter helped select those shown.

Apart from the contributions for the purchase of the Streeter Collection, several Fellows contributed money to buy rare books; Dr. L. Duncan Bulkley, a Fellow since 1874, left his library on cancer and $5,000, the income of which was to maintain and augment the collection. A rare book fund was established and Mrs. Walter G. Ladd contributed $10,589.67 to it.

The Public Health Relations Committee was as usual very busy. It made many studies and presented many reports, dealing with needs for greater laboratory facilities for the Department of Health and the administration of contagious disease hospitals; consolidation of municipal hospitals, "open hospitals," and the dangers of ambulance service during long transportation of patients. Recommendations were made to the Health Department regarding control of blood donors. A study made in 1928 of the usefulness of convalescent serum in the treatment of poliomyelitis was far from conclusive; it was voted to continue it in 1929, and $7,600 was donated for the purpose. Other studies and reports included ventilation of school buildings, hospital organization in its relation to Attending Staffs, asphyxia and resuscitation, school medical inspection, and maternal mortality. A contribution of $2,000 was made by Messrs. Samuel and Harry Sachs for the Committee's support.

In 1927 the Committee on Medical Education took on the publication of the *Bulletin*, greatly improving its scope and usefulness. The volume for 1927 contained 782 pages; in 1928 it was a ponderous tome of 1,320 pages. It published many important papers read at Stated and Section Meetings, Presidential and Anniversary Addresses, the Carpenter Lecture, and actions of the Council, Trustees, and the Academy, together with reports presented at the Anniversary Meeting. It is a very excellent sketchy history of the Academy for the year. Two dollars from dues was allowed for the *Bulletin* and the Trustees voted $4,000 for it in 1928.

The Committee continued to publish the daily bulletin of Surgical Clinics in 76 hospitals (almost all of them approved by the American College of Surgeons). It had a paid circulation of 220. The bulletin of Non-operative Clinics and Conferences held in 50 teaching hospitals was still published in *Medical Week*.

A revised edition of "Opportunities for Graduate Medical Study in Hospitals in New York City" was published. The Bureau of Clinical Information had become recognized as headquarters for visiting physicians, and as a source of information for opportunities for postgraduate instruction in New York and other cities in this country and abroad. In 1928, 735 out-of-town physicians registered in the Bureau, of whom 177 came from 35 foreign countries.

A Committee on International Medical Relations was appointed, a letter was ordered sent to various organizations in Europe inviting them to refer visitors in this country to the Committee and informing them that American physicians visiting Europe would present letters of introduction from it.

In 1927 the Academy lost four Fellows who had played important parts in its life. Dr. Robert F. Weir, a Fellow since 1866, President 1901–2, died at the age of eighty-nine. He had not been active for many years. Dr. Charles H. Peck, a very active and progressive surgeon, contributed much to the scientific program. A Fellow since 1898, he had been a vigorous chairman of the Surgical Section and was Vice-President in 1918–20.

Dr. Walter B. James had been a Fellow since 1889, an active chairman of the Library Committee, and had taken an important part in securing the financial aid of the Foundations. A generous contributor to the support of the Academy, and its President from 1915, he also served as a Trustee and member of the Council, giving freely of his sound advice and valuable opinion. Although his health had been very poor during the last few years of his life, he never lost interest in the Academy. His loss was keenly felt. "In view of the unusual services rendered," he was named a Benefactor of the Academy, to which he left $25,000 for the Endowment Fund. After his death, Mrs. James gave the Library some fifty valuable books, among them several early editions of the works of Sir Thomas

Browne, to supplement Dr. James's copy of the first edition of Harvey's *De Motu Cordis.*

Dr. W. Gilman Thompson, a Fellow since 1885, had contributed many papers at Stated Meetings, and as Chairman of the Library Committee in 1894 emphasized its needs, in season and out. He was Vice President, 1904–6, and Trustee 1909–24. Several times he was offered the nomination for President, but always said he was too busy to accept. When he became seventy years old (1926), he gave up all committee work—and he was on many committees—as he had said he would do. On his death in 1927 the Council passed suitable resolutions. He left the Academy $10,000.

Portraits of the late Dr. Stephen Smith and Dr. W. H. Park were presented to the Academy.

Financially the Academy did pretty well in 1927 and 1928. It lived within its income.

The Rockefeller Foundation was paying 5 percent interest on its promise of $1,250,000 for endowment, and announced its intention of paying $500,000 of the principal in 1928 and in 1929, and the balance in 1930. This would be considerable money to invest wisely. The Trustees appointed a Committee of Five on Finance, and an advisory finance committee, composed of the President of the Bank of New York and Trust Company, Messrs. George Blagden of Clark, Dodge and Co., J. B. Mabon, G. H. Milliken, and Dr. Edward Peaslee, formerly President of the Fidelity Bank. All were genuinely interested in the Academy and gave good advice as to investments for several years.

An Assistant Treasurer was appointed by the Trustees. In April, 1928, the Trustees appropriated $760 for lighting the Fellows' (now Hartwell) room. There evidently was trouble with lighting that room from the beginning.

In June, 1928, $1,700 was appropriated for laying a Terrazzo Floor in the Collation Room, and cutting the carpet into rugs.

Dr. Samuel McCullagh, a Fellow since 1904, presented the Academy with a die and $3,000 for a fund to establish a medal for Distinguished Service in Medicine. His ideas of the administration of the fund were interesting:

My wish is that no restrictions shall be placed upon the judgment of the Council as to the manner in which the income of this fund may be dispensed, so long as it carries out the original intent of the gift. By this I mean that decisions as to the choice of the recipient, the frequency of its award, the metal of which it shall be made, the award of accrued income in addition to the medal itself, the simultaneous award of multiple medals where collaboration has existed, and all similar questions shall be left entirely in the hands of the Council.

Lastly, in case that circumstances should arise in the future under which it seemed advisable that the giving of such a medal be abolished, I should like the fund diverted to such purpose as seemed best at the time.

A number of bequests were refused by the Trustees, among them one from Dr. L. D. Mason of $5,000, the income to be devoted to a lecture on Alcohol and other narcotics, the special topic to be selected annually by the American Medical Association. Notice was also received of a proposed bequest of $250,000 for the advancement of medical research, no grant to be made to any individual of a certain religious faith, nor to one working in an institution under control of that faith.

York and Sawyer, the architects of the new building, who had drawn many plans for 43d Street and 60th Street, were voted "an appreciation of their services, for their patience and consideration as architects over a period of sixteen years," and the Council expressed its entire satisfaction with the present building.

Dr. Lambert was a very active and interested President. He presided at over 70 percent of the twenty-nine meetings held, and was very regular in his attendance at Council and Trustees' meetings. His interest in, and efforts for, the Library and Public Health Relations Committee were very valuable. He was instrumental in forming the Rare Book Fund and in raising money for its endowment. He continued his interest in both these committees for a number of years. He was made a Benefactor in 1941.

1929–1932

John Augustus Hartwell

DR. SAMUEL W. LAMBERT, in turning over the presidency to Dr. Hartwell, emphasized the Academy's activities in medical education and his great interest in the development of the Library.

Dr. Hartwell made a long and very thoughtful address, in which he spoke of the Academy's efforts to elevate the standards of scientific and ethical medicine, and pledged his full support to those ends. He warned the Fellows there was much to be done to make the Academy the leader it should be in the professional life of the city, and one essential was that every Fellow should be of unblemished character.

Dr. Hartwell, thirty-third President, was just sixty years old, and had had an interesting and strenuous career. He lost his mother when he was twelve and his father, who had maintained a small school, the following year. With small means he entered the Yale Sheffield Scientific School at the age of sixteen. An excellent athlete, he played football and rowed on the crew all through his three years, and graduated "with Honors," later receiving his degree "cum laude" from the Yale Medical School. After some postgraduate work there, he served as Surgical Interne at Presbyterian Hospital and began a long connection with Cornell Medical College, holding many positions of ever-increasing responsibility. When elected President of the Academy he was Associate Professor of Surgery, Consulting Surgeon to Bellevue, Presbyterian, Memorial, New York Infirmary for Women and Children, and a number of other hospitals. He had served through the First World War, making some important investigations and studies of the A.E.F.

Elected a Fellow in 1901, he was Vice President, 1918–20, and later a Trustee. All through his four years as President he and the ceaselessly active Director worked hand in hand. The first two years at 103d Street had been spent in getting settled, developing a competent staff, and feeling out its strength. Now it was ready to go forward. But going forward was not an easy matter, and it is not surprising that Dr. Hartwell was reelected to a second term.

To give in detail and chronologically all the actions taken would require too much space; they can only be discussed very briefly.

Applications for Fellowship were far in excess of the vacancies. Each year there were from 150 to 160 applications. As in the four previous years, the Committee on Admissions sent out an appeal to the entire Fellowship, urging their cooperation in providing "complete information, whether favorable or unfavorable" about every candidate. The Committee on Admissions was very particular in recommending names, as was the Academy in accepting them. A three-fourths vote was necessary for election, and in 1930 a name was returned to the Committee for further consideration. It was re-presented, and the Academy refused election.

At the close of 1928 the Academy had authorized the President to appoint committees on the By Laws; Sections and Societies; Honorary Fellowships and Honors; International Medical Relations; and Discipline. The last-named was later called the Committee on Professional Standards. It had existed since 1926; its duties were to investigate every complaint by a Fellow, other physician or layman, against a Fellow, and to take action on its own initiative on any breach of professional conduct, such as objectionable newspaper and magazine notoriety. This committee originally consisted of seven, but was later increased to ten. It was kept pretty busy, especially after the first year. Complaints were of the most varied kinds: from laymen of overcharging and of negligence; undue publicity; and use of a Fellow's name in connection with the sale of stock for a patent process.

Most of the charges were trivial or groundless. Others were more serious. One Fellow posted notices in a factory that he would treat compensation cases. His defense was that because the State Society forbade such advertisement, there was no reason why the Academy should be subservient to the State Society! He was reprimanded, and, as he continued the practice, was forced to resign.

Signed testimonials were officially frowned on. The Council voted

"The use of a Fellow's name in the form of a testimonial for advertising purposes is contrary to the traditions and best interests of the medical profession and should under no circumstances be granted."

A serious case was presented in 1930. Advertisements appeared in various newspapers carrying the picture of Dr. Shirley W. Wynne, a Fellow of the Academy and also Health Commissioner of New York. The advertisement in question was issued by the Colgate Company for its toothpaste. The statement first issued over the name of Dr. Wynne pointed out the simple fact that toothpaste was never more then a cleansing agent. Later, however, Dr. Wynne was quoted to the effect that Colgate's was a better cleansing agent than others, which statement was based on evidence submitted to Dr. Wynne by chemists in dental laboratories.

At his own request, Dr. Wynne appeared before the Committee. He pointed out that his motive in granting the testimonial was that he felt that advertising agents had gone a great deal too far in making extravagant and fraudulent claims in the fields of dentifrices and cosmetics. The Bureau of Food and Drugs had been able to control a certain amount of these advertisements when the product contained substances actually deleterious to health, but he had not found any means to curb various toothpaste advertisements. The possibility of counteradvertising had been suggested to him, but the Department did not have funds to carry on an activity of this kind. The further suggestion was then made that if the Commissioner of Health would recognize commercial concerns which did not engage in extravagant and fraudulent claims this would have a useful influence on the character of the advertisements.

Dr. Wynne then stated his conviction that the testimonials had not brought about the effect which he had hoped for and that the advertisement would be discontinued.

The Council wrote Dr. Wynne that it still believed its resolution (quoted) was for the best interests of the profession.

A few cases of paid-for testimonials were reported—one offender was reprimanded, another suspended for six months and later forced to resign.

The ever present problem of fee splitting came up again—and the following resolutions were passed:

Resolved, That the secret division of a fee or fees with any person or persons, who may be instrumental in influencing a patient, or patients, to apply for operative care or professional advice is unworthy of any member of the medical profession.

Resolved, That if such a division of fee is made by a member of the New York Academy of Medicine, it should be counted as a sufficient ground for the expulsion of the member.

Resolved, That the Council may either reprimand the person, or permit his resignation, or recommend him to the Academy for expulsion, and be it further

Resolved, That a copy of this resolution be printed on the form of application for fellowship.

Another matter referred to this Committee concerned the practice of competing ambulance companies to pay commissions to physicians on calls for private patients. The practice was condemned, a statement ordered published in the *Bulletin*, and the matter was called to the attention of the County Society.

The Library had by now a large collection of manuscripts, incunabula, and early medical books. The Rare Book Room occupied the space on the main library floor now comprising the reference room, beyond the Fellows' room and including the circular stairway to the present Rare Book Room. An expanded passageway rather than a room, it was unsuitable for any proper arrangement or maintenance of these books. The Librarian's office was the room now occupied by Miss Doe. Moreover, the Rare Book Room housed the great number of old instruments and so on, the future (*in spe*) museum.

Mrs. Laura E. Smith, Assistant Librarian, resigned after thirty-eight years of invaluable service. A fund was raised among the Fellows, which was presented to her, and she was retired on a modest pension. In 1930 she was made Librarian Emeritus.

Gifts of instruments and pictures continued to pour in. The collection of photographs and engravings was greatly in need of attention; although it numbered 2,300, only 99 Fellows were included!

Miss Martha Lambert (Mrs. J. Ogden Bulkley) gave much time to mounting and arranging the items. Dr. Dana's collection of 2,000 medical prints was purchased by a group of Fellows. A valuable portrait of Hippocrates on porcelain was presented by Dr. Lambert. Portraits of Dr. Biggs and Dr. S. W. Lambert were also accepted.

A small collection of caricature busts of physicians of note in the 1840s, by Dr. James de Berty Trudeau, a Founder of the Academy, were presented by Miss Sayre.

Dr. Margaret Wilson gave a very valuable collection of more than 4,000 books on Food and Cookery, said to be the most complete collection in the world. She continued to add to it. Dr. Wilson was later made a Benefactor.

The Permanent Library Fund was enriched by an anonymous gift of $10,000. Dr. S. W. Lambert gave the first volume of the new *General Catalogue of Printed Books* in the British Museum, and promised to pay for the remainder as published.

The Library organized several valuable exhibits: incunabula; Dr. Wilson's collection on foods and cookery; alcohol—its uses and abuses; bindings; medical and surgical aspects of acute bacteremia, in connection with the 1930 Graduate Fortnight; and several others.

Repairing of books, long neglected, was started. In 1929 alone, 5,000 volumes were rebound or repaired, and the enormous number of duplicates was reduced by gifts to other libraries, including over 4,000 volumes to the newly organized Queens County Medical Library.

The Library issued the "*De Contagione*" of Fracastorius, with a translation, the first of its "History of Medicine" series to appear.

The users of the Library increased steadily from 31,800 in 1929 to 47,042 in 1932.

A few years earlier, the Academy had asked Fellows to send in reprints of articles published elsewhere than in the *Bulletin.* By 1930 some 20,000 of such reprints were on hand. To catalogue them by author would cost $6,000, so that was stopped, except in special cases.

The Stated Meetings were well planned, and mostly well attended. The New York Pathological Society gave two, and the

Sections organized most of the rest. They were all symposia on definite subjects and many speakers came from out of town.

The Sections were also holding important and well-attended meetings. There was an advisory committee of five for each Section with one of the Vice Presidents as chairman. They did good work both as to the individual Sections and in arranging the Stated Meeting programs. The attendance rose each year for all Sections and for most of them individually. In 1931 the largest average attendance was 338 for Medicine. In all four years the average attendance was below 100 in very few Sections and in 1932 in only one.

The Anniversary Addresses were given by Dr. Simon Flexner. in 1929, on "The Infinitely Small in Medicine"; in 1930 by Prof. F. J. E. Woodbridge, Professor of Philosophy at Columbia, "The Preface to Morals"; Dr. James Ewing in 1931 on "The University and the Medical Profession"; and Dr. W. B. Cannon of Harvard on "Enemies of Society" in 1932. The attendance varied from 325 to 463.

The Carpenter Lectures were all given as part of the Graduate Fortnights.

In 1931 the Biggs Memorial Lecture (started in 1925) was taken over by the Academy. Dr. Williams remarked, "It was a strange arrangement that the New York Tuberculosis and Health Association should hold the money and provide the speaker, the County Society furnish the audience, and the Academy of Medicine loan the use of its Hall." The memorial fund was increased by Mrs. Biggs to $4,000.

Dr. Thomas W. Salmon, a most brilliant and distinguished psychiatrist, died in 1927. A group of his friends and admirers raised a fund of $100,000 to give, annually, a series of Lectures on Psychiatry. The first series was given in 1932 by Dr. Adolf Meyer of Baltimore.

Over thirty other organizations were holding their meetings in the Academy. Beside these, a special notice was issued for an afternoon lecture on public welfare work in Vienna by Professor Julius Tandler, Commissioner of Health, Hospitals and Public Welfare in that city.

On April 4, 1930, the entire Fellowship was invited to attend a dinner given by the Academy in honor of Dr. William H. Welch, who had reached his eightieth birthday. Dr. Lambert acted as Toastmaster, and the speakers were Drs. Theobald Smith, C. N. B. Camac, James Ewing, and Rufus Cole. Dr. Cole read a poem to this "Scientist, teacher, leader, sage, custodian of knowledge gained through the ages."

Dr. Welch remarked that he had dodged a dinner tendered him in Baltimore, but when Dr. Williams telegraphed an invitation to come to New York and meet his old friends, that was just "coming home." He made a very interesting speech about early experiences, admitting that he had reached his "anecdotage."

A letter was sent out announcing that another celebration would be held at 12 noon, Tuesday, April 8, in Memorial Continental Hall, Washington. Dr. Livingston Farrand was to preside, President Hoover, Dr. Simon Flexner, and Dr. Welch would make addresses, and the procedure could be heard over the radio in Hosack Hall. At the same time a limited number of portrait etchings of Dr. Welch would be presented to important medical organizations, and these speeches would also be heard over the radio. The Academy would receive one etching and it would be on exhibition in Hosack Hall.

The following letter is of interest.

I take pleasure in informing you that my contribution to the endowment fund which is now to be raised will be $10,000. You will find enclosed a check for $5,000. The remainder will be forthcoming on or before January 10th, 1931, with interest from April 1st.

It is my desire that this contribution be named for the late Dr. William S. Halsted and that as far as possible the income be utilized for (in order of preference), (1) books on the history of medicine; (2) books on surgery; (3) any other purpose of the Academy.

As I do not want to hamper the Trustees in any way I leave it entirely to them to use the income for any ordinary or extraordinary function of the Academy. I might suggest, however, in order that the name of so great a man and surgeon be kept alive, the income be occasionally used to pay for lecturers (at ordinary stated or section meetings) or for their traveling expenses. On such occasions the name of the fund might well be printed on the folder announcing the meeting.

I am making this offer to the Academy on the occasion of the 80th anniversary of the birthday of Dr. William H. Welch because I know the news will please him very much. As I understand him and his reverence for Dr. Halsted this fund will give him much more happiness than were it named for himself. It is my desire that at least for the present my name be not mentioned in connection with the fund.

Dr. Emanuel Libman was the donor.

Another dinner was given by the Committee on International Medical Relations to fifty-three delegates to the International Hospital Congress. At least ten were laymen and only one was an Honorary Fellow of the Academy, Professor Chagas of Brazil. Thirteen speeches are listed on the program!

The Committee on Public Health Relations was, as always, very active. In 1929 the Police Department raided the office of a private physician who was giving advice on birth control and seized her records. This caused a great deal of newspaper notoriety. The whole matter was seriously discussed and the Academy, on the report of the Committee, published a very guarded statement, protesting against the seizure of confidential records as a dangerous precedent, but withheld final judgment until all the facts were ascertained.

A number of reports were made to the various city departments. Action was taken on bills on animal experimentation, chiropractic, privileges for osteopaths, housing, and workmen's compensation. Administration of the Veterans Relief, housing laws, school ventilation, food handlers, work permits for children are only a few of the subjects taken up. In 1929, the Committee published a book called *Preventive Medicine;* it received such universal approval that a second, revised edition was published the next year.

The Committee was also instrumental in the formation of a special committee to revise and reclassify the nomenclature of disease. Under the direction of Dr. H. B. Logie this study lasted several years and was supported by outside agencies, notably the Commonwealth Fund. That Fund also financed a three-year study of maternal mortality, which was also started in 1930.

Another committee was formed to investigate the effect of convalescent serum in cases of poliomyelitis. This study and the provision of such serum, financed by outside sources, was continued for three years.

A joint committee with the Pathological Society met with a committee of the Metropolitan Funeral Directors Association and smoothed out many difficulties in regard to obtaining autopsies. Its results were published in the *Bulletin.*

The Committee on Medical Education organized four very successful Graduate Fortnights, the attendance at which remained high. At several of the evening sessions the attendance was over 1,000. The demand for tickets to the clinics exceeded the number available, and one visitor wrote of the 1931 session: "I do not believe that so much about an important subject has ever been taught in so short a time. It is something new in the history of medicine." The same Committee was responsible for organizing the Stated Meetings and assisting in the Section programs. The plan was working out very well. The Friday afternoon lectures were also well attended, and well arranged.

The Bureau of Clinical Information was still serving a large number of physicians, many from out of town. A committee investigated its activities and reported it as one of the most useful in the Academy. Its bulletins of operative clinics were in considerable demand, and its non-operative clinics, published in *Medical Week*, were much used. The use of these bulletins was strong evidence of the efforts of physicians, without much opportunity for hospital or dispensary experience, to try to keep up with the times. That is what the Academy was working for.

The Committee arranged with a local group of the American College of Surgeons to give a series of clinics on fractures, with attendance limited to fifty. The series was oversubscribed.

A committee appointed to study the value of the *Bulletin* reported that, instead of being more or less of a "house organ," it could and should become a real journal of medical information. In 1932 advertisements were accepted for the first time, but even so, because of financial difficulties, the *Bulletin* had to be cut to half its size that year. In 1930 it had an exchange list of 577, and its subscriptions had increased threefold.

The Committee was authorized by the Council to publish a list of foreign clinicians for distribution to Fellows and interested physicians, and did so. It also investigated the training of specialists, and published a valuable report on that. A new and enlarged edition of opportunities for postgraduate education was published. The Committee also investigated interneships in 15 hospitals, to find out how much the hospitals were contributing to the medical education of internes. In 1929 Mrs. Alexander Cochran Bowen announced she would provide funds to give two young internes just finishing their service a chance to study abroad. She continued to do so until 1942 when, on her death, she left $100,000 to establish a fund. Two young doctors were granted this scholarship in 1931 and 1932.

A Committee on International Medical Relations, established a few years earlier, was merged, as a subcommittee, with the Committee on Medical Education. It made an elaborate investigation of facilities for foreign physicians who wished to acquire hospital training in this country, with a view to an interchange with foreign universities. The plan did not get very far.

At the request of the State Commission on Saratoga Springs, the Academy appointed a committee to study spas, and it made an extended tour of various European establishments in 1929. With the approval of the Committee on Public Health Relations and the Council this report was published, and was of great service in developing Saratoga Springs.

The Medical Information Bureau, with Dr. Iago Galdston as Executive Secretary, was very active. It was at first a joint Bureau with the County Society, and handled matters of publicity for both organizations. For a short time it was called the Press Relations Bureau. Its purpose was to control medical information in the lay press within reasonable and accurate bounds. It tried to advise on medical news and claims received by the daily press, the value and soundness of which the press had no way of judging. It also established a sort of supervision of radio addresses on health matters. Through an arrangement with the Associated Press, it furnished a daily Health Column which was published in several hundred papers. This activity was maintained for a number of years.

In a very short time its position was recognized, and hundreds of specific requests for an opinion were received from various newspapers as to the value of articles submitted to them, the advisability of certain advertising, and so on. The Bureau also worked with the broadcasting companies, and nearly 400 radio addresses were supervised. The Council ruled that proposed addresses by Fellows should go through this Bureau. The National Tuberculosis Association and the Red Cross used its services in broadcasting programs, as did the Society for the Control of Cancer, Children's Welfare Federation, League for the Hard of Hearing, National Society for Prevention of Blindness, and many others.

In 1932 the Bureau organized and directed the "Academy Hour" over WABC, with weekly broadcasts for thirty-six weeks reaching practically every part of the country. It was doing a fine piece of work. From 1929, under the guidance of Dr. Orrin S. Wightman, it gave an annual dinner for representatives of the press, which did a great deal to bring about closer cooperation.

The Bureau was partly supported by grants from the Milbank Fund.

A Committee on Medical Jurisprudence, under its enthusiastic chairman Dr. Israel Strauss, was active all through these four years. It held many conferences with committees of the Bar Association, the New York County Lawyers' Association and at times the Columbia Law School. It gradually worked out modifications of criminal procedure, and four bills were prepared, which were discussed with the Department of Correction and with judges of the Court of General Sessions. These bills dealt with the qualifications of certified psychiatrists, the procedure regarding mental condition of defendant at a trial, the employment of experts when defendant is unable to pay for one, and procedure when a person in confinement appears insane or mentally defective. The Committee had most cordial cooperation from everyone concerned.

In 1928 a Committee on Honorary Fellowship and Honors had been appointed. In 1929 it recommended for Honorary Fellowship Drs. R. H. Chittenden (Yale), Jules Bordet (Brussels), Sir Thomas Lewis (London), Ernst Fuchs (Vienna), Sir Frederick G. Hopkins

(Cambridge University), Mme. Curie (Faculty of the Sorbonne, Paris), and René Leriche (University of Strassburg). All were elected.

In 1929 the Academy Medal was awarded to Dr. Carl Koller, a Fellow, discoverer of cocaine as an anaesthetic in eye conditions, and in 1931 to Dr. David Marine, a non-resident Fellow, for his work on the thyroid.

The Committee on Modification of the Volstead Act was also active. Dr. Coleman had presented a preamble and resolution in 1929, charging that the law making the diagnosis available to any prohibition inspector whenever liquor was prescribed violated the confidential relations of patient and physician. This inviolability had been protected from earliest times, just as the relations of priest and penitent, lawyer and client had been. The resolution expressed the opposition of the Academy to this forced betrayal of confidential communication.

The resolution was tabled for some time, but in May, 1931, a long preamble outlining Dr. Coleman's complaint, the action of the Legislature in freeing the medical profession from the authority of Congress over medical practice (Hastings Act), the recommendations of the Wickersham Commission, which unanimously voted the removal of this cause of complaint, was followed by resolutions condemning the provisions interfering with medical practice and urging each Fellow to demand of his Senators and Congressmen the repeal of these portions of the Volstead Act, and ordering that a copy be sent to the members from New York in the Senate and in the House of Representatives.

In 1929 the Constitution and By Laws were amended, mostly as to wording for the sake of clarity, but a few changes were incorporated. The important ones were as follows: Corresponding Fellows were reestablished after many years. Members of the teaching staff of a medical school outside of New York and physicians of unusual eminence were eligible. The Committee on Sections was made a standing committee, and the Committee on Admissions was enlarged from nine to twelve members, one-third retiring each year. One of the Vice Presidents was to be chairman of the Committee on

Sections, and the Recording Secretary was now no longer an ex-officio member of all standing committees.

All through Dr. Hartwell's administration the tremendous increase in "specialism" caused a great deal of concern. A physician, just graduated from a medical college, was accepted in a special hospital and after a year, or less, without any general experience became a full-fledged specialist. The ophthalmologists were the first to organize a National Board to try to regulate the so-called specialists. In 1924 a Board of Otolaryngology was formed, and from 1930 to 1933 Boards were organized and functioning for Obstetrics and Gynecology, Dermatology, and Pediatrics.

It was proposed in 1930 that the Academy should elect *members* instead of Fellows. The qualifications for membership were to be the same as then in force for Fellowship. When elected, a "member" joined whatever Section he chose and had all the privileges of the Section except that of holding office.

The Advisory Committees of the various Sections were to determine just what should constitute the requirements for eligibility for "promotion" from Member to Fellow. A Fellowship Committee was to be formed, composed of one member from each Section, to serve three years. When a member submitted evidence of his qualifications to become a Fellow, the Advisory Committee of the Section would recommend his name to the Fellowship Committee who could then recommend his name to the Council for promotion to Fellow in a specialty, for example, Otolaryngology. The present Fellows were to retain their status and could apply to be made Fellow in any specialty.

This was a very complicated matter, and was under discussion for three years before the Committees of Admissions and Medical Education, Section Advisory Committees, Officers of Sections and the Council. The plan was finally submitted to the Academy in December, 1932, and was voted to be in force the next year, but all Fellows and Associate Fellows elected prior to 1933 were to retain the title of "Fellow," and all who had applied for Fellowship or Associate Fellowship prior to 1933, if approved, were to be voted on for Fellowship.

The requirements were as follows:

1) Certification by the American Board of Ophthalmology, American Board of Otolaryngology, American Board of Obstetrics and Gynecology, or other national board maintaining equal standards; *or*
2) Award by an approved university of an advanced degree in the specialty together with a period of special practice to make up a total of at least five years work in the specialty, *or*
3) An approved residency or special internship of a minimum of 2 years duration, with a satisfactory amount of basic science work and a period of special practice to make up a total of at least five years work in the specialty; *or*
4) Five years of experience and training in special practice of a character which has met the approval of the section concerned; *or*
5) Qualification by reason of distinguished professional service and standing and at least 10 years in practice; *or*
6) For those not engaged in clinical practice, an equivalent experience and training in a teaching, research or other non-clinical medical field.

Considerable opposition to many phases of the plan cropped up, and in December, 1933, the Council voted the whole matter in abeyance, until after further study.

The finances of the Academy were a source of constant worry to the Trustees and the Director. The years 1929 to 1932 were bad business years, everywhere. At the end of 1929 the endowment showed a market value loss of $14,000 in stocks and $5,500 in bonds. The Academy had a very able lay Committee on Finance and it gave good advice. By the strictest economy, the year ended with a balance of only $504.94. This was made possible by an anonymous gift of $10,000, received through Dr. Hartwell, for general purposes, and $7,500 from Mrs. Harriman and $1,000 from the Altman Foundation for the Public Health Relations Committee. There were a few other smaller general gifts.

In November, 1929, the President sent out a circular letter to all Fellows, explaining the allocation of their dues and the needs of the Academy. He drew attention to the importance of gifts and bequests and urged the Fellows to do what they could to get their patients to leave money to the Academy, if possible without restrictions and, if they could, to bequeath something themselves. A Committee on Gifts and Bequests prepared a booklet outlining the Academy's needs and asking Fellows to tell the Director of anybody who might be willing to give financial aid. In 1930 another statement of the need for an additional endowment of $2,200,000 for new activities was prepared and sent on request.

In 1930, thanks to contributions of $33,500 for current expenses, the Academy finished the year with a balance of $5,120.84, and in 1931 a balance of $2,652.54. In 1932, however, the financial depression was at its height. Reduced income from investments indicated in March that a deficit of $5,000 would be incurred by the end of the year. The Trustees recommended that vacancies occurring on the staff be not filled, unless absolutely necessary, and that all higher salaries be cut 8 percent and other salaries down to $1,500, 5 percent. That this reduction was accepted by the Staff should be recorded. In spite of the fact that extra donations were discouragingly small, the Academy managed to close the year with a surplus of $1,274.00.

The original plans for 103d Street had had to be cut somewhat, as the gift from the Carnegie Corporation was only increased by $530,000. But the Trustees had thought it wise to buy the adjoining lot on 103d Street. In 1929 they also bought three lots at 10, 12, and 14 East 103d Street, for possible future needs. The properties returned sufficient income to pay for themselves for a number of years, until it was necessary to use them for the overflow of the stack rooms and museum material.

In 1930 the Council realized that the building was already inadequate for its purposes and aspirations. Accordingly the Committee on Gifts and Bequests was instructed to try to secure funds for an addition to the building, and also additional endowment. Mr. E. S. Harkness agreed to donate $350,000 for the building, if $400,000 for endowment could be received before July 1, 1931. During the year it was felt that the addition to the building should be greater than originally planned, and an attempt to raise $100,000 more was planned; the subsequent reduction in building costs, however, made only $50,000 more necessary. Mr. Harkness consented to extend the time limit on his gift to December 31, 1931. The Council, Trustees, Fellows, and the Director made tremendous efforts to raise the money. By November 24, 1931, the endowment of $400,-000 was secured or pledged and only $32,000 of the $50,000 was still needed for building. By the end of the year this had been pledged.

Long before the money was raised or pledged, a building committee was appointed and Dr. A. B. Duel was again made chairman.

Excavations were started in the spring of 1932. York and Sawyer were again the architects and Mark Eidlitz & Son the contractors. Unexpected difficulties were encountered and matters were further delayed by a strike, so that completion was delayed until the spring of 1933. The original building had been constructed in three separate parts, the main building, the stacks and the Hosack Hall Annex. It had also been built so that additions in height were possible. The alterations were completed without serious interference with Academy functions.

In 1929 the Academy faced another problem. Dr. Williams, who had been Deputy Commissioner of Health for the State under Dr. Biggs, was offered the Commissionership by Governor F. D. Roosevelt. The pressure brought to bear upon him to accept was very strong. Dr. Williams decided to ask the advice of the Council. The Council then passed the following at its meeting January 22, 1930:

In view of the fact that the services of the Director are now being sought for a position of the highest importance in the public health field, and that such urgent pressure has been brought to bear upon him that he has felt compelled to seek the advice of the Council and ask its opinion as to the decision he should make, the Council deems it proper at this time to record upon its minutes an appreciation of the services rendered by the Director.

The pledge of a considerable increase to the Academy's endowment obtained in 1923 made possible the inauguration of a new program of activities. These were undertaken in 1924 under the leadership of the Director. The work of the various new committees was stimulated by his leadership and expanded after the Academy was installed in its new building in the autumn of 1926.

The routine activities in the field of clinical information, library maintenance and public health and hospital survey, have now been in full operation for three years. During the last year the activities of the Academy were studied anew by an important committee which recommended that they be continued and that several new projects of primary importance be undertaken. The Council believes that these projects are of such fundamental importance for the community and the medical profession, that funds must be obtained and studies launched as soon as possible. These undertakings will undoubtedly lead ultimately to sweeping changes of method in the medical administration of hospitals, the Post Graduate training of physicians, and will promote better medical care for the sick and the prevention of disease.

During his tenure of office the Director has displayed ability for organization leadership and cooperation in the highest degree. The Council feel that without him the Academy would have fallen far short of its present position; It also feels that without his leadership it will fail to achieve the further developments which promise so much for the welfare of the medical profession, City and State. As heretofore the Academy is anxious to cooperate in every movement which will further the interest of public health.

Be it therefore resolved, That the Council has carefully weighed the relative importance of the important public health position of limited duration with the advantages offered for leadership in the promotion of the Academy's activities, and although it recognizes the fact that the health position will seem to offer a wider field in the eyes of the public and press, the Council is of the firm belief that it would be wiser in the interests of the public of the City and State of New York, and of the Director himself, for him to remain in his present position.

Dr. Williams declined the appointment.

In 1932 the Academy established the custom of presenting diplomas to newly elected Fellows at the next Stated Meeting. In April, Dr. Hartwell presented the certificate with these words:

Having fulfilled the required qualifications for fellowship in the New York Academy of Medicine, and having been elected thereto by the vote of its Fellows, you are hereby declared to be Fellows of the Academy in good standing.

In token of this the President is authorized to present to you the diploma of the New York Academy of Medicine bearing its seal and the signatures of its Officers, which admits you to all the rights and privileges of fellowship. On behalf of the Council, the Officers and the Fellows of this Academy, I would call to your attention that these rights and privileges are of no mean order. The Academy holds a position of honor in the community and nation.

I would ask that, in enjoying these privileges, you also recognize the responsibility inherent to them and do your utmost to further the interests of the New York Academy of Medicine in Medical Education, Public Health and the Practice of Medicine.

In the fall it was decided this presentation should only be made at the Annual and May meetings.

At the December elections in 1932, Dr. Bernard Sachs was elected President. Dr. Hartwell had been one of the really hard-working Presidents.

1933–1934

Bernard Sachs

DR. SACHS, elected thirty-seventh President, was a very distinguished neurologist. Having received his M.D. in Germany, after several years' study under Charcot and others he had rapidly made a name for himself. At the age of thirty he had been made Professor of Nervous and Mental Diseases at the New York Polyclinic. He had been President of the American Neurological Association in 1894 and 1932, and was elected President of the first International Neurological Congress held at Bonn in 1931.

He was a very public-spirited citizen, proud of his city and anxious to have even greater reason for pride. He had been a Fellow since 1887, an active member of the Committee on Public Health Relations since 1914, and a Trustee since 1926. Like Dr. Hartwell, he was insistent on high standards of professional ethics and on improving the status of medical education. His Presidential Address was along these lines.

Three very important events occurred during his Presidency. The first was the publication of the report on maternal mortality.

In 1930, the Public Health Relations Committee, with the backing of the New York Obstetrical Society and with funds provided by the Commonwealth Fund, had started an investigation of all deaths in childbirth in the City of New York. Dr. R. S. Hooker was made the Director of the study, and gave full time to it. A Subcommittee on Maternal Mortality, consisting of Drs. Frederic E. Sondern, chairman, B. P. Watson, Philip Van Ingen, and R. S. Hooker, and an Obstetrical Advisory Committee of Drs. B. P. Watson, chairman, John O. Polak, George W. Kosmak, and Harry Aranow, were appointed. Dr. Polak died in 1931 and Dr. Charles A. Gordon was appointed in his place.

A photostat copy of every death certificate which even mentioned the condition of pregnancy was forwarded each week by the Health

Department to the Academy. Every physician connected with a case was interviewed by an investigator within a month after the death. In every hospital death, the institution was inspected and its routine studied. Each month the Obstetrical Advisory Committee studied the individual reports and determined the "responsibility" for death. The main work, outside of collecting, tabulating, and analyzing the 2,041 individual reports, fell on this Advisory Committee. It worked hard and long. The investigation received the most complete cooperation from all physicians and hospitals contacted. It covered the years 1930–32.

The report was finished in the summer of 1933. The Subcommittee was authorized by the Executive Committee of the Public Health Relations Committee to go ahead with the editing of the report, and arrange for its publication, which the Commonwealth Fund was anxious to do, and do promptly.

A conference was held between the Subcommittee on Maternal Mortality, the Bureau of Medical Information, and the Commonwealth Fund. It was decided that the Subcommittee should prepare a review for the *Health Examiner*, published by the Academy. Dr. Hooker had it ready by November 13. A review for the *American Journal of Obstetrics* or the *Journal of the American Medical Association* was proposed, but it was decided it would be more desirable that publicity in the medical journals should follow, rather than precede, any possible reviews of the report in the public press. The Bureau of Medical Information was to deliver a copy of the report to representatives of the press and to review any reports prepared by them. The Commonwealth Fund was to have no active responsibility in the matter.

Dr. Galdston did better. With the copy of the report he submitted to the press a full, sensible and accurate statement. It was carefully worded and summarized the findings in a complete and honest manner. It was to be released November 20, and was headed "Why Women Die in Childbirth."

The report received a tremendous response from the press. Most of the articles were brief, and had various headlines, but none of them were objectionable. The New York *Times* and New York

Herald Tribune reviewed it quite extensively. It is noticeable in reading the 300-odd notices from 39 states and Canada, how serious and unspectacular they were. And a surprising thing was that the papers kept referring to it for several months. It was a news item.

But, as was doubtless expected, with the appearance of the press comments, the storm broke. A number of letters from Fellows were received, protesting at the Academy's *method* of publicity. At the meeting of the Academy, December 7, 1933, three Fellows, all officers of the County Society, presented resolutions stating that the press release by the Academy "left the impression upon the lay public of questionable practices on the part of the profession, and such publicity not only failed to bring about any remedial measures but has caused a reaction of distrust and fear upon the part of the public." The Academy was urged to condemn the action of the Council in authorizing publicity of the report before the members had expressed their wishes. The resolutions were later withdrawn. Several other letters were received from Fellows and non-Fellows.

The New York Obstetrical Society later protested in the public press. The *Bronx County Medical Bulletin* (organ of the Bronx County Medical Society) published a scathing article accusing the Academy of serving "as the tool of certain interests to the detriment of the physician and to no benefit to the public." The Queens County Society and the Medical Society of the County of Albany also sent in protests. All were on the *methods of publicity*.

On the other hand, letters are on file applauding the report. The Science Editor of the *Literary Digest* wrote:

> . . . I wish to be numbered among the many who feel grateful to the New York Academy of Medicine for its frank and forthright announcement of the results of the Survey on Maternal Mortality.
>
> I can imagine that an organization of lesser integrity might have been tempted to keep secret findings such as this, when they appeared to reflect upon some portion of the medical profession.
>
> You undoubtedly have done medicine and the general public a great service in making all the facts public immediately in such a courageous, thorough, and competent manner.

The Chairman of the Committee on Maternal Welfare of the Philadelphia County Medical Society wrote: "You have done a splendid piece of work and I congratulate you and the Advisory Committee on your courageous presentation." The Federal Children's Bureau, which was making a study of its own, also wrote in appreciative approval.

The Council immediately appointed a Subcommittee on Publicity of Maternal Mortality Report, consisting of Dr. S. W. Lambert and Dr. J. A. Hartwell, last two Presidents of the Academy. Everybody who complained was invited to meet this Committee. Every letter of complaint was answered by the President, and the whole matter was handled in a most statesmanlike manner. To the tact, frankness, and courtesy of these two gentlemen and Dr. Sachs the Academy owes much. They made a careful study of the whole matter and presented a report which was sent to all critics and the whole Fellowship. The report may be summarized as follows:

The intention of the Council was that there should always be cooperation between Fellows, Academy Committees, and the Medical Information Bureau on all matters which might be of publicity value to the lay press.

The Public Health Committee was authorized to issue statements in the name of the Academy when approved by the Executive Committee, by three-fourths of the members of the full Committee present and voting, and with the approval of the President. This had been done.

The Medical Information Bureau was charged with guiding and advising on all matters of publicity affecting medical practice and procedure in so far as it might exert its influence upon publicity agencies. Definite regulations for Fellows as to publicity had been adopted by the Council, May 27, 1931, and by the County Society's Comitia Minora, October 9, 1931. In the present case, cooperation had been obtained by repeated conferences between Drs. Hooker and Galdston and Mr. Taylor of the Commonwealth Fund. The question of a review of the report in the medical press had been considered, and, on the advice of a member of the Obstetrical Advisory Committee, it was decided to postpone this until after the publication of the Report.

This answered the criticism of unauthorized methods of publicity.

The proposed releases (by the press) were submitted to the Bureau, which did a fine job in persuading the press to accept a prepared statement which summarized the views of the Committee. The statement was appropriately and accurately captioned "Why Women Die in Childbirth."

The startling nature of the findings caused fears that the story would react harmfully on the profession. This was not the fault of the Committee on Maternal Mortality. Facts must be stated freely but accurately if the labor and expense of the investigation was to be justified. To minimize would have justly caused a charge that the profession was shielding itself against attack. It was now up to the profession to correct the evils disclosed.

As to future publicity, the Subcommittee recommended:

that whenever any study which may have publicity value is undertaken by the Academy or its committees, the advice of the Medical Information Bureau Committee shall be sought in reference to its publicity aspect; and to facilitate this, that the minutes of all committees other than those held confidential (namely Fellowship, Admissions, and Professional Standards) shall be made available to the Medical Information Bureau, but no publicity thereon shall emanate except upon the written authority of the Council or the Committee on Public Health Relations, in accordance with its powers under the By-Laws.

And your Subcommittee further recommends:

That this report be approved by the Council and that those Fellows who have protested as to the manner of publicity be invited to appear before your Subcommittee to hear the evidence upon which it is based, and that all Fellows and Members be furnished with a copy.

This report in full (three and a half legal cap pages), mimeographed, signed by John A. Hartwell and Samuel W. Lambert: "approved by the Subcommittee of Maternal Mortality and their Obstetrical Advisory Committee, Frederic E. Sondern, Chairman; approved unanimously by the Council at its regular meeting on

December 13, 1933, B. Sachs, President, Foster Kennedy, Secretary" was sent broadcast.

The document concludes:

> The Council of the New York Academy of Medicine desires to express complete faith in the Report on Maternal Mortality in New York City, and considers it an outstanding piece of thorough medico-statistical research, done by an eminent committee of conservative and socially-minded men.
>
> The Council would emphasize that such important facts which have a bearing on the improvement of medical practice and welfare of society must not be suppressed.
>
> The Council takes this opportunity to express to the members of the Obstetrical Advisory Committee, namely Dr. Benjamin P. Watson, Dr. John O. Polak,* Dr. George W. Kosmak, Dr. Harry Aranow and Dr. Charles A. Gordon, full appreciation of their arduous labors and successful achievement, and to Dr. Ransom S. Hooker, the Director of the Study, thanks for his fidelity and wisdom.
>
> The Council also wishes to tender the thanks of the Academy to the Commonwealth Fund for the generous support of the undertaking and the publication of the Report.
>
> (Signed) *Foster Kennedy*

* Deceased

The Report and the action of the Council in supporting the Committee made a profound impression, both here and abroad. It received several most complimentary notices from the British medical press for its honesty and straightforwardness.

March 7, 1934, a joint meeting was held by the Academy, the New York Obstetrical Society, and the County Medical Society on the *constructive* aspects of the Report on Maternal Mortality. It was a frank facing of the situation, the accuracy and importance of which no one questioned. Dr. Aranow, prominent obstetrician in the Bronx and member of the Advisory Committee, gave a résumé of the findings. Dr. George L. Brodhead discussed the conclusions and recommendations, and Dr. George W. Kosmak spoke on the significance of the Report and the measures suggested for carrying out its recommendations. Drs. A. W. Bingham of East Orange, C. B.

Lull of Philadelphia, Edward C. Podvin of New York, S. S. Goldwater, New York City Commissioner of Hospitals, J. L. Rice, Commissioner of Health, and Thomas Parran, New York State Commissioner of Health, took part in the discussion which followed.

Many requests were made for a "popular edition," and after much hesitation a brief summary for the nonprofessional reader was authorized and was prepared by Dr. Galdston. "Maternal Deaths, the Ways of Prevention" was published, again by the Commonwealth Fund. Within the year the edition of 1,500 was exhausted and a second edition was published in 1938. Dr. Bundesen, Health Commissioner of Chicago, ordered 1,300 copies for "distribution where it would do the most good."

That a great reduction in maternal mortality has occurred since the Report came out is unquestioned. How much of this is traceable to the Report, it is impossible to say, but from the immediate activities of lay and professional groups, it is fair to say it had considerable influence. That the Report has not been forgotten is evident from two articles from which we quote:

Ten years ago, almost to the day, the New York Academy of Medicine published the findings of its Committee on Public Health Relations based on a study of more than two thousand deaths from diseases and conditions associated with childbirth. In introducing this courageous report, the Committee observed that "the spectacular progress of the last years in the reductions of many death rates has not been paralleled by any drop in the rate of death from puerperal causes." Its unequivocal conclusion was that as a conservative estimate almost two thirds of the deaths were preventable. . . . The disclosures made by this distinguished body of specialists, their concrete recommendations, the probing activities by other medical groups throughout the State, which brought about radical changes in obstetrical practice and hospital procedures, and the coincident developments in chemotherapy have produced astonishing results. Now the sentence quoted above may be justly inverted: "the spectacular progress of the last years in the reduction of the death rate from puerperal causes has not been paralleled by the drop in the rates of death from most of the other important causes." The Committee considered that it should have been possible to prevent 65.8 per cent of the maternal deaths. In 1933 the New York State rate was 63 per 10,000 live and still births;

in 1942 the rate was 22, a reduction of 65.1 per cent! This almost perfect correspondence between scientific hypothesis and actuality, while striking, would be unimportant did not the present favorable condition represent a stage in an uninterrupted downward trend. (*Health News*, New York State Department of Health, October 18, 1943.)

And again:

The Annual Report of the New York City Commissioner of Health shows that in 1946 the maternal death rate was 1.2 per thousand live births. . . .

The death rate from causes associated with pregnancy and childbirth for New York City is now very substantially below one-third of the rate for the year 1932 when the Academy of Medicine published its report on the maternal mortality in New York City. Thus, the medical profession in New York City has now far more than achieved the goal set by the Academy report which stated, in 1933, that "two-thirds of these deaths are preventable." Nevertheless, even today the causes to which the 1946 maternal mortality is attributed indicate that a considerable number of these maternal deaths are preventable. (*N.Y. Medicine*, March 5, 1947.)

The second matter that occupied the attention of the Academy, and particularly that of the Council, was that of Fellowship as distinguished from membership. In 1933 the Committee on Fellowship was made a standing Committee of the Academy. It consisted of twelve members, one from each Section of the Academy, proposed by the Nominating Committee and elected by the Academy on March 2, 1933. Three meetings were given over to classifying the present Fellowship and an application form was drawn up. In April, with the approval of the Council, the Committee sent out a notice it was ready to receive applications for designation as Fellows, in various Sections. From May to the end of 1933, the Committee considered 474 applications for special designation and recommended 281 to the Council. The Council approved all but 39, which were held up temporarily because of objections that had been coming in as to the method of selection. The Council voted in December that no more names would be considered until a satisfactory plan had been worked out. None was evolved.

That was all that happened in the matter during Dr. Sachs' presidency. It was not until March 7, 1935, that everyone was satisfied. Each Section was to form its own standards. Although these were not uniform, they were considered adequate. The By Laws were also amended to allow those Fellows elected before 1933 to be designated Fellows of a particular Section upon their own application. This made things very much simpler for the Committee. During the year only three applications to be admitted as Fellows and three for "promotion" to Fellow were received and all were approved.

In 1936 only seven applications for "promotion" were received and approved, and in 1937 the Committee reported it had been inactive. "Few" applications for "promotion" were received (two), and none were presented to the Council. The Committee raised the question whether it was necessary longer to continue the election of "Members" and possible later "promotion" to Fellowship. The National Boards had increased to such an extent as to make continuance of the plan very questionable. The Council decided the experiment had been tried for too short a time to decide. The Committee report ended: "The Committee on Fellowship will begin to function again in 1938."

In 1938 it reported only seven applications for "promotion," four of which were rejected. The membership seemed to be "very apathetic." In 1939 the Committee was abolished and the plan abandoned.

The third event of importance was the opening of the new extension of the Academy in the fall of 1933. It was all done smoothly and with little discomfort and no interference with the activities of the Library itself. No formal ceremonies were held. One reason, perhaps, was the fact that the Director was ill.

In January, 1934, the Academy suffered a terrible blow in the death of its Director, Dr. Linsly R. Williams. He was stricken with pneumonia October 7, 1933, and was taken to the Hospital of the Rockefeller Institute, where everything that up-to-date science knew was resorted to, while the entire staff devoted their best energies in his behalf. Complication after complication set in and, after a long fight, Dr. Williams died January 8, 1934, in his fifty-ninth year.

His death called forth editorials from the New York *Times* and *Herald-Tribune.* One rarely sees such evidence of personal appreciation, respect, and regret as was expressed in those editorials. Strong appreciation was also expressed in the *American Review of Tuberculosis, Journal of the Outdoor Life, New York Medical Week,* and *New York State Journal of Medicine.*

Dr. Williams was also well known and appreciated abroad. He had been made, during a period of eleven years, a Chevalier, Officer and Commander of the Legion of Honor, and also a Knight of the Order of Dannebrog of Denmark. A fine tribute appeared in *La Presse Médicale.*

What Dr. Williams had done for the Academy will never be fully known. His ambition was to make it the place to which anybody and everybody in search of information and advice on all matters which had a medical angle, however slight, would instinctively turn. To that end he accepted positions on endless committees and gave, without complaint, of his time and thought to their problems. A firm believer in hearty cooperation, he smoothed out many a difficult situation. He felt that organized medicine had its own distinct field, and that the Academy should never intrude into that field; also that the Academy had its field, and organized medicine should never interfere with it. Relations between the two organizations were none too cordial in 1924. In the ten years of Dr. Williams's Directorship he revolutionized that situation. The clearing up of the trouble over the Maternal Mortality publicity, in which all the County Societies were involved, is largely an example of his personal influence.

The continued support of the Academy's ever-increasing program, from the Foundations, was largely due to his record. They knew if he asked their support for something, he thought it really worth while. They knew they only had to decide that point for themselves; that if support was granted, it would be wisely and economically administered. And it always was.

Everything he suggested to the Academy was not always at once accepted. He knew how to bide his time. He quietly kept the matter before them and usually the Trustees and the Council came to see it as he did. His patience was extraordinary; it was only exceeded by his fairness in seeing another's point of view. He never wasted words. He would sit in silence through a controversial meeting, and when everything seemed to be hopelessly bogged, he would offer some logical and well-expressed method of handling the matter, which was usually promptly accepted.

He secured the utmost cooperation of the entire staff of the Academy. Not too particular over trivial details, he demanded a great deal of work from each, and they did it willingly, because they knew he was himself working twice as hard as any of them.

Special resolutions of a most personal and appreciative character were passed by the Committees on Public Health Relations, Library, Admissions, Medical Education and Medical Information Bureau, and, at the meeting February 1, the Academy passed, by a silent rising vote, the following:

The Trustees, Council and Fellowship of The New York Academy of Medicine record with deep sorrow the death of the Director of the Academy Dr. Linsly Rudd Williams.

Ten years ago, the Academy began, through the generous support of numerous friends, greatly to extend its sphere of influence. Its efforts at this time resulted in the fulfillment of a long cherished hope for this new building with all of its beautiful and modern equipment. A liberal endowment made it possible to place the activities of the Academy upon a sound and permanent basis, worthy of its best traditions and devoted to the high ideals of the medical profession.

Dr. Williams, as the first full-time Director of the Academy, at this crucial period of its history, was largely instrumental in securing this generous support and was a guiding influence in selecting the site and determining the Byzantine-Romanesque type of architecture of the building. The notable success which has attended this development is due in the largest measure to the statesmanlike leadership, the sound judgment, and the extraordinary qualities of mind and heart which characterized Dr. Williams' administration of the affairs of the Academy.

Dr. Williams brought to the Academy a training in the service of the Department of Health of the State of New York, and of the Army in France after the War, and later in the United States as Director of the National Tuberculosis Association.

While Dr. Williams gave the Academy, which he served with such distinguished success, the benefit of the ten best years of his long and brilliant career, his influence was felt far beyond the activities of the Academy itself.

In the field of public health, preventive medicine and social welfare he was pre-eminent, serving the community in ways that were extraordinary in their variety and importance. For a number of years and up to the time of his death, he was President of the New York Tuberculosis and Health Association, and served a term as President of the National Tuberculosis Association. He was a director of the Milbank Memorial Fund and of the Bellevue Yorkville Health Demonstration. He was a member of the Board of Managers of the Association for Improving the Condition of the Poor and of the State Charities Aid Association. His wise counsel was continually sought by practically all public and private agencies in the field, whether in City, State or Nation.

In the sphere of medical education, he was a great power for good. This was evidenced not only through the Academy activities, but also throughout the community, and particularly in Columbia University which he served for several years as Trustee representing the College of Physicians and Surgeons.

These numerous outside interests, however, in no way ever detracted from his main interest and devotion to the Academy of Medicine, but on the contrary did much to enhance its influence and prestige in the community.

It is obvious that such a brilliant career was only possible because of ability of a very high order, but at this time, the hearts of his numerous associates are moved rather by the memory of Dr. Williams' rare personal qualities. A quiet manner, a quick response to human needs and interests, a logical but sympathetic judgment, a rare sense of humor, a devotion to the highest ideals of honor and of service, these qualities endeared him to all with whom he came in contact. A beloved friend has been lost as well as an outstanding public servant.

Therefore, be it resolved: That the New York Academy of Medicine hereby records its profound sorrow in the death of Dr. Linsly Rudd Williams, its deep appreciation of his notable services to the Academy, and to the community; and as a token of the affection and honor in which his memory will ever be held by the Academy of Medicine,

Be it further resolved: That this memorial be inscribed in the minutes of the Academy, and a copy sent to Dr. Williams' family.

The Trustees and Council on January 24 held a joint meeting. Dr. Hartwell being asked to leave the room, the Trustees and Council unanimously elected him to the position of Director, at the same salary as Dr. Williams had received. Dr. Hartwell was then recalled and on being informed of their action said:

In accepting this appointment, I hope you appreciate that it will be utterly impossible for anyone to fill the place of Dr. Williams. My only advantage is that I have had an opportunity to serve with him rather closely over a very considerable period so that I have imbibed a good many of his viewpoints and methods of work. I shall try to follow in his footsteps as nearly as one can whose temperament and training are quite different from Dr. Williams'. I feel it an ad interim appointment and I shall try to build up an organization so that when it comes time, either at your discretion or my own, for me to retire, there will be some provision so that we won't be caught in the same unfortunate predicament that we have at the present time. I may have to ask your indulgence in one matter. I am no longer young and have not been well for some years though I am now, but if the affairs of the Academy will allow me to be absent for a few days occasionally, I might like to ask your permission to do so with the understanding that it will be without pay. If this meets with your pleasure I shall be glad to accept and conduct the affairs of the Academy.

The Trustees had of course continued Dr. Williams's salary during his long illness, and voted to do so until February 1, 1934. In the meantime, December 15, 1933, Dr. Hartwell had been appointed Director ad interim. A special meeting of the Council was held February 14, 1934, at which a letter was read from Mrs. Williams, thanking the Academy for its action in continuing Dr. Williams's salary, and enclosing a check for $1,622.40, which she asked be paid to Dr. Hartwell in accordance with what she knew to be Dr. Williams's wishes.

A memorial meeting was held April 26, 1934. Dr. John H. Finley spoke of Dr. Williams as a citizen, Dr. Livingston Farrand of his contributions to public health, and Dr. Hartwell of him as "Friend of the Academy and its Fellows." It was a very impressive and well-attended meeting. The addresses, the editorial tributes, and the more personal resolutions passed by various organizations were published in a small volume, *In Memoriam—Linsly R. Williams.*

The death of Dr. Williams was a severe blow to the Academy. Things slowed up a little, not much indeed, and it is not strange that it should have been so. Dr. Hartwell shouldered his responsibilities manfully, and served the Academy well for five long, hard years. The established work was carried out faithfully and successfully, in spite of financial troubles. Many projects that had been considered were never fully developed. In fact it is doubtful if much that was planned or hoped for could ever have been carried out.

The Committee on Public Health Relations was very busy. Its outstanding contribution was the report on Maternal Mortality already described. It made a valuable study of diabetes, resulting in the establishment of an Association of Diabetic Clinics.

The increase in amoebic dysentery, and the preventive and curative measures suggested were studied and submitted to the Health Department. "The policy pursued by the Health Commissioner was in accordance with the recommendations made in the report."

The overcrowded condition of the city hospitals was studied, and the Committee urged the Mayor and Board of Estimate to make arrangements whereby patients could be referred to volunteer hospitals and recognized as "city charges." The Committee protested at the ruling that "indigent" maternity cases could not be accepted by private hospitals as "emergency cases" under city charge if they had received prenatal instruction.

The necessity of regulating cosmetics, many containing poisonous drugs, was considered and the "Tugwell Bill" dealing with the matter was endorsed. The amendment to the State Constitution in regard to preferment for veterans in Civil Service appointments was opposed.

The Committee again studied the indiscriminate sale of barbituric acid compounds, and recommended the Code be altered to forbid their sale except on prescription. At the request of the Health Commissioner it reported on the value of Vitamin D reinforced milk, and on the use of Grade B milk in Baby Health Stations. It also recommended to him that fumigation after cases of typhus and smallpox be continued because "(1) there is likelihood that not all of the possible vectors of transmission of these diseases are definitely known; (2) there is no harm done by fumigation; and (3) the expense involved is negligible."

The Committee made extensive reports on the Psychiatric Service at Bellevue, care of the chronically ill, and ambulance service, "with recommendations." At the request of the Commissioner of Hospitals, the problem of tonsil and adenoid operations was studied and recommendations were made which the Commissioner promptly put into effect.

At the request of the Borough President of Manhattan, the Committee selected a list of twenty-nine names to be carved on the façade of the new building for the Departments of Health, Hospitals, and Sanitation. In December, Mayor-elect LaGuardia wrote asking the Academy's opinion concerning the essential qualifications for heads of the Departments of Health and Hospitals. The Committee gave its opinion. These are just a few of the matters mentioned in the annual reports of the Committee for 1933 and 1934.

The new addition gave the Academy three "exhibition rooms" and more much needed space for workrooms, and of course the beautiful Rare Book and Historical rooms. Practically all of the addition up to and including Mezzanine floor was devoted to the Library, except a small part of the floor to the east of Hosack Hall. The Academy had accumulated during the years a considerable amount of material of historical interest. This was all supposed to be in the care of the Committee on Library. Dr. Williams had been much interested in the possibility of developing a museum illustrating medical development, but he realized the Academy had not the financial or physical equipment for it. He never gave up the idea. In 1934 the Council set aside "the upper of the three exhibit rooms" in the addition for a permanent museum, and among the numerous committees listed that year is one on Museum. It disappears from the list in 1942, and its activities never appeared in the printed Annual Reports. Gifts continued to be reported by the Library Committee each year.

The Library Fund was increased by the gift of $26,250 from the Carnegie Corporation, $10,000 from the estate of Dr. Frederic Kammerer, a Fellow. Mrs. McLean donated $13,500 toward a library fund in memory of her husband, Dr. Stafford McLean, also a Fellow; this fund subsequently amounted to $20,000. The New York Neurological Society contributed $1,000 to buy books on neurology and psychiatry.

In 1932 a "publication fund" was established, thanks to Dr. S. W. Lambert's interest, and through his efforts was increased by $8,250. It was made a "revolving fund" expended for reproduction of classics, and the income from the sale of the publications accrued to the fund. Its management was placed in the hands of a Committee composed of the President, the Director, the Librarian, the Chairman of the Library Committee and one Trustee selected by the other four members. Dr. Lambert had discovered that the original woodblocks for the first issue of Vesalius' *Anatomy* were stored in the basement of the Munich University Library. Arrangements were made to have them struck off, and a new edition of Vesalius, a wonderful piece of press work, was produced in 1935. An exhibition of the woodcuts was held in the fall of 1934.

The work done by the Library staff was much helped by the services of volunteers, who worked part time, some only for a few weeks, others for a period of several months. They helped in keeping the card catalogue up to date, checking up on the receipt of current journals and reports, and in countless other small, but valuable ways. Nine volunteers worked in 1933, and nineteen in 1934.

Exhibits were arranged commemorating the 100th anniversary of the publication of Beaumont's book on gastric digestion and another on "Metabolism" during the Graduate Fortnight in 1933. Little was done in 1934 except for a few small exhibits by Fellows who brought and showed their own collections on subjects which interested them.

Two thousand fewer readers used the Library in 1933, but in 1934 there were 51,703, an increase of 6,762. In the months of March and October over 5,000 readers signed the Register.

The Committee on Medical Education continued to be very active, carrying out its usual activities with energy. It continued lists of operative and non-operative clinics as before.

The Friday afternoon lectures continued to draw an attendance of from 200 to 250.

The Graduate Fortnight was continued with ever increasing attendance. In 1933, as the expense was considerable, it was decided to charge a fee of $2.00 for registration to all but Fellows and those taking part in the program. Complimentary tickets were also issued to hospital internes and residents, approved hospital fourth-year medical students, medical officers of the government service, and a few others. Six hundred and forty-three physicians paid the $2.00 fee in 1933 and in 1934, the "registration fee" having been raised to $3.00, the issuance of tickets was stopped when the paid enrollment reached 700. The average attendance at the evening lectures in 1933 was 650, the smallest attendance, 448. In 1934 the average attendance during the first week of evening lectures was over 900 and the second week 840. As part of the 1933 Fortnight, a meeting was arranged in cooperation with the County Medical Society. Nearly 1,800 attempted to hear the papers presented and loud speakers were installed in two Section rooms to accommodate the overflow.

The afternoon Hospital Clinics were all well attended.

The Committee continued to publish the *Bulletin* regularly. Lack of funds prevented its enlargement as planned, but it contained approximately sixty-four pages in each issue.

The Bureau of Medical Information was very active. Practically every newspaper in New York kept calling on it for information and for advice in articles received on doubtful subjects. Its daily Health Column for the Associated Press was continued, 313 appearing in 1933 and 1934. It arranged about 350 radio programs, many for other organizations. In 1933 it inaugurated the Academy Radio Hour, addresses being delivered every week throughout the year by Fellows of the Academy. In this connection, the Bureau published a booklet, entitled *On The Air* and giving instructions to doctors on the preparation of radio talks, which was reprinted by the

American Medical Association and National Tuberculosis Association.

In 1933 the Bureau took on a new activity. In 1929, the New York County Society organized a group of physicians from the five County Societies in Greater New York, led by the enthusiastic Dr. A. J. Rongy, as "The Greater New York Committee on Health Examinations." Dr. Iago Galdston was its Secretary. They planned an intensive campaign to popularize periodic health examinations. A budget of $25,000 was provided by the Metropolitan Life Insurance Company, the Milbank Memorial Fund, Altman Foundation, Life Extension Institute, the New York, Brooklyn, and Queens Tuberculosis and Health associations, and the New York County Medical Society. It carried on a whirlwind campaign from October 15 through December 31, 1929. The story of that campaign published under the title, *For Health*, by the Greater New York Committee on Health Examinations, is interesting reading. It had the support of Dr. Williams from the start. He was, as a member of the Medical Society of the County of New York, one of the original committee. Two meetings, one a public one, were held at the Academy. As a result a small magazine, *Health Examiner*, was started in 1929 and Drs. Williams and Galdston were on its editorial board of six. It was published by the Committee until 1933, when the Academy took over publication. The Editorial Board was increased to eleven and the format was greatly improved.

It was in the *Health Examiner* that the first professional review of the Report on Maternal Mortality appeared. This very useful little publication gradually broadened its scope from urging periodic health examinations to covering the whole subject of preventive medicine. In 1936, at the end of Volume V, the name was changed to *Preventive Medicine*, beginning with Vol. VI. The first issue announced "with this issue *Preventive Medicine* is initiating the publication of an inclusive review of the practice of preventive medicine by the general practitioner. The review will cover all periods from conception to senescence." Publication ceased abruptly in August, 1939, the last article ending "to be continued in September."

The annual dinner to the press was continued, thanks to Dr. O. S. Wightman.

The Committee on Professional Standards were busy. Rumors, at any rate, of fee-splitting were frequent. At the request of several Fellows, in March, 1933, the Committee presented a statement. It recalled that the County Society had discussed the subject at great length in 1932 and that "some action" had been taken that same year by the State Medical Society. It stated that the American Medical Association's "Principles of Medical Ethics" forbade the division of fees or the giving of rebates and that the "Principles of Professional Conduct of the Medical Society of the State of New York," adopted in 1905, also forbade the giving, directly or indirectly, of any "gifts, gratuity, commission or bonus in consideration of or return for the referring or procuring of any patient for medical, surgical or other treatment," or receiving from any person gratuities for referring patients for pathological examination.

It quoted at length the action of the Academy in 1911, which strongly condemned the practice of fee-splitting, calling it a sufficient cause for expulsion. This action had been reaffirmed in 1930, and every effort had been made to make known the Academy's attitude.

The Council accepted the report and reaffirmed the Academy's stand.

Several trivial complaints were received, but one matter occupied much time and caused much trouble. A Fellow was accused of being responsible for the appearance of handbills and of menus of the Seaboard Air Line advertising the Florida Medical Center, which he ran. The Committee felt the publicity was objectionable, in itself contrary to the best interests of the Academy, and that it reflected adversely upon the doctor and the medical profession.

In refutation, it was claimed that the information about the Center had been given to the agent of the air line only in an attempt to procure better train service for it. The doctor was ignorant of the nature of the publicity, and when he heard of it ordered it discontinued. Although it was continued for three months, he had, after his first protest, allowed the matter to lapse. He was considered guilty and was suspended by the Council for one year. He then took the matter to the State Court of Appeals, which decided in the Academy's favor.

In 1933 the Academy elected thirteen Honorary Fellows, as follows:

Charles Achard, Professor of Clinical Medicine, Faculté de Médecine, Paris

Roberto Alessandri, Professor of Clinical Surgery, University of Rome.

Sir Charles (Alfred) Ballance, K.C.M.G., C.B., M.V.O., LL.D., M.S., F.R.C.S., Herts, England

Frederick Grant Banting, MC., M.D., F.R.C.S., D.Sc., LL.D., Professor of Medical Research, University of Toronto

Sir Henry Hallett Dale, C.B.E., M.A., M.D., F.R.S., F.R.C.P., Director of the National Institute for Medical Research, London

Otfried Foerster, Professor of Psychiatry and Neurology, Schlesische Friedrich-Wilhelme-Universitat, Breslau

Carl G. Forssell, Professor of Radiology, Karolinska Mediko Kirurgiska Institutet, Stockholm

James Bryan Herrick, M.D., Emeritus Professor of Medicine, Rush Medical College, Chicago

Cornelius Ubbo Ariëns Kappers, Professor of Comparative Anatomy of the Nervous System, University of Amsterdam

George Richards Minot, M.D., Professor of Medicine, Harvard

William Gibson Spiller, M.D., Professor of Neurology, University of Pennsylvania, Philadelphia

Alfred Vogt, Professor of Ophthalmology, University of Zurich

Karel Frederik Wenckebach, Professor of Medical Pathology and Therapy, University of Vienna.

In 1934 the following five were elected:

William H. Howell, formerly Professor of Physiology, Johns Hopkins University

August Krogh, Professor of Animal Pathology, University of Copenhagen

Frederick George Novy, Professor of Bacteriology, University of Michigan

Claude Regaud, Director of Pasteur Laboratory of the Radium Institute, University of Paris

Sir Humphry D. Rolleston, Bt., formerly Regius Professor of Physic, University of Cambridge.

The third Academy Medal was awarded in 1934 to Dr. Charles Norris, Chief Medical Examiner, a Fellow of the Academy.

The stated meetings were interesting. A symposium on the effects of tobacco in man drew an attendance of 411. The Biggs Memorial Lecture in 1933 was given by Dr. Herman Mosenthal on "Diabetes Mellitus; Problems of Present-Day Treatment," and was listened to by 726. ("Weather rainy.") On the other hand, in 1934, the Biggs Lecture by Dr. Bedell of Albany, on "Causes and Prevention of Blindness," weather also "rainy," drew only 77.

The Carpenter Lecture in 1933 on "The Influence of the Diencephelon and Hypophysis upon the General Autonomic Functions," by Dr. Wilder Penfield, Professor of Neuro-Surgery at McGill, was listened to by 594. In 1934 the Lecture was delivered by Dr. A .C. Ivy, Professor of Physiology and Pharmacology, Northwestern University, on "The Applied Physiology of the Gastro-Intestinal Tract Innervation."

The Anniversary Address in 1933 was delivered by the Hon. Joseph V. McKee, late temporary Mayor, on "Medicine and Modern Sociological Trends," and in 1934 by His Honor the Mayor, Fiorello H. LaGuardia, on "The Medical Profession in the New Age." Mr. McKee drew an audience of 251 and Mayor LaGuardia, 363.

All the meetings were well arranged and mostly well attended.

The Section Meetings were, on the whole, well attended. In 1933 only three had an average attendance of under 100, the lowest being that of Historical and Cultural Medicine, with 71; in 1934, it was the only one under 100. Medicine ranked highest in 1933 with an average of 173, but in 1934 Neurology and Psychiatry had the high average of 248, Pediatrics 227, and the others well over 100.

The Academy had been interested in the administration of workmen's compensation and in January, 1933, a letter was read at a meeting of the Council from former Governor, then President, Roosevelt, asking the Academy to make suggestions regarding the report of a committee (the Cullman Committee) appointed by him to consider the matter.

The State Medical Society was rather disturbed that it had not been consulted. The Council agreed that it should be, and the following letter was sent to Governor Lehman:

On December 29, 1932, the New York Academy of Medicine received a communication from the Honorable Franklin D. Roosevelt, requesting the Academy to study the report of his committee which had investigated the medical abuses of the Workmen's Compensation Law, and to make recommendations and suggestions for correcting these abuses.

We appreciate the confidence which has been placed in us by Governor Roosevelt and we desire to do everything in our power to aid in the solution of the present difficulties.

We desire to point out to your Excellency, however, that a matter of this kind involves the entire medical profession of the State of New York; that although the Academy has been deeply interested and much concerned in the operation of this Act for the past twelve years, and has made a number of studies and reports on the subject, we feel that any recommendations and suggestions which we might make will not have the full support of the medical profession of the State unless the study be made by representatives of the Medical Society of the State of New York in cooperation with representatives of our own organization.

We feel convinced that if you would be willing to appoint a committee, consisting of five representatives of the Medical Society of the State of New York and five representatives of the New York Academy of Medicine, it is practically certain that such a Committee would work in complete harmony and would make recommendations and suggestions that would have the full support of the medical profession of the State.

Governor Lehman accepted the suggestion in a personal letter to Dr. Sachs. The Committee, of which Dr. Eugene H. Pool was the chairman, worked very hard and presented a valuable report in 1934. It confirmed the findings of the Cullman Committee—that medical care and treatment of injured workmen had in many cases degenerated into a commercialized venture, with rebating, fee-splitting, organized solicitation and "lifting" of cases, in which so-called medical clinics and unscrupulous people exploited the injured worker. Certain changes in the law, recommended by the Committee, were introduced into both branches of the Legislature and endorsed by the Academy.

The Committee on Medical Jurisprudence presented several bills about to be introduced to the Legislature. The Council approved of all.

Mayor O'Brien called on the Academy for suggestions for members of the "local beer board," and Mrs. José M. Ferrer, Mr. Barklie Henry, Gen. John F. O'Ryan and Mr. John McKim Minton, Jr., were recommended.

Dr. Goldwater, Commissioner, requested the appointment of three Fellows on the Advisory Council for the Department of Hospitals. They were appointed.

The Milbank Fund asked the Academy to cooperate in a study, at its expense, of physicians' incomes. The Council decided this was impossible.

December 3, 1933, is a famous date. The Prohibition Racket was declared over. On December 15 the Council celebrated by revoking the House rule prohibiting the serving of alcoholic drinks in the building. In anticipation of the revocation, the Volstead Committee had been discharged October 25, with a vote of thanks for its efficiency.

Dr. Walter Mendelson presented the Academy with a cap and gown, and the Council voted, March 28, 1934, that hereafter the President and Secretary should appear at Stated Meetings in academic regalia.

In 1934 Dr. I. S. Hirsch, a Fellow, reported that he had seen the statue of Dr. J. Marion Sims, which used to stand in lonely isolation in Bryant Park and which the Academy had unsuccessfully asked to have moved to its neighborhood, standing, neglected, in a Park Department Storage Yard. Dr. Sachs and the Director approached Commissioner Moses and asked that it be placed in a niche in the Park wall opposite 103d Street. The Commissioner at once promised to do so, had the statue overhauled, built a proper pedestal, and it was unveiled with proper ceremonies on its new and appropriate site October 20, 1934. Dr. John H. Finley spoke of Dr. Sims as a citizen, and Dr. George Gray Ward, Chief Surgeon of the Woman's Hospital, as a surgeon.

Dr. Stewart died in March, 1933, in his seventy-first year. The Academy adopted the following resolutions:

The New York Academy of Medicine records with sincere feeling its deep sense of sorrow and loss in the death of its greatly beloved Fellow, George David Stewart, which took place at his home on March ninth.

Dr. Stewart was elected to Fellowship in 1895 and for nearly forty years devoted much of his effort and abundant energy to furthering the interests of the Academy. In 1916 he became Vice-President and three years later was elected to the Presidency. He received the unusual honor of being asked to hold this office for three successive terms, until 1925, as the Academy refused to relieve him from leadership at that critical time.

It was during this period that the long-considered plans for the new Academy building were brought to completion and to no one belongs greater credit for this accomplishment than to George Stewart. His broad vision made it easy for him to grasp the opportunity for unusual service which lay before us, were we provided with adequate facilities. His power of persuasion was a chief factor in convincing our many benefactors that we should be accorded their support. His active interest in, and work for, the Academy were not lessened by his retirement from the Presidency. He continued as a Trustee until the time of his death and devoted much thought to the work of the Committee on Public Health Relations of which he remained a member until 1929.

With his magnetic personality, his rare gift of humorous expression and his wisdom acquired through wide experience, he was a dominant figure among his fellows.

Dr. Stewart was unusually well endowed by nature to become such a figure. Untiring energy applied to the enlargement of this endowment made of him a man of great insight, rare force, fine tact and a lover of culture and the beautiful. His leadership was kindly and his followers found it easy to become his disciples.

It is known that he was influenced by a strong religious feeling and he brought to every decision a sense of fairness which made his counsel much sought. As a surgeon and teacher he has left the world his debtor. His writings testify to the breadth of his training and he exerted great influence in keeping the role of general surgery equally broad.

In his death we have lost a forceful leader and teacher, a wise counselor, a kindly man and a dear friend. The Academy desires to express its great appreciation of these qualities and enter upon the Minutes this testimony to the memory of one we can ill afford to lose.

These were very troublesome years for the Academy financially. The years of depression had not been kind to the value of the endowment fund. In 1933, the book assets from invested funds were $2,881,293, of which $1,652,988 was in bonds and stocks, the then market value of which was $992,247 at the end of the year. The estimated income for 1933 was $238,650 and the budget had been made out for $236,296. The actual income was $231,550, from all sources, including gifts. The expenditures had been cut to $230,835, so the Academy closed the year with a balance of $715.29.

The Advisory Finance Committee had been consulted freely and their advice was probably taken. Many investments were sold and at the end of 1934 the investments, outside of mortgages, were listed at $1,626,197, the market value of which at the end of the year was $1,369,965. Sale of stocks and bonds, which was advised by the Advisory Committee had netted a loss of $308,999.90, which was written off. The Academy therefore started the new year with invested assets (stocks and bonds) of $1,626,198. With the aid of gifts it went through the year 1934 with a deficit of only $652.92, although one of $4,000 had been expected.

The Trustees and Council were doing everything possible to cut down expenses and increase revenue. For a number of years the list of non-operative clinics was published by the Committee on Medical Education in *Medical Week*. In 1933, at the suggestion of that Committee, it was voted to publish the list "at least twice a year, in *Medical Week*, provided funds were available." In 1934 the Committee's bulletin was mimeographed and sent out direct from the Academy.

In 1934 the announcement published since 1927 in the Directory of the American Medical Association, calling attention to the Academy's facilities and inviting visiting physicians to make use of them, was discontinued.

The Treasurer sent out the following letter:

November 17, 1933

Dear Doctor:

In receiving the announcement of your election to the Academy, you will note that you have been classified as a Research Member which entitles you to full utilization of the Academy without initiation fee and with the nominal dues of $10 annually.

This class of membership was created in order to admit to the Academy that considerable group of most desirable men who are engaged in full time activity of a research or administrative or teaching nature, generally on a rather limited salary. However, at the present time, many of these men are receiving very generous salaries. Some of them in recognition of the privileges which the Academy affords to them make a practice of supplementing the nominal dues with an additional annual donation to the Academy. If you find yourself in a position to do this, it would be very greatly appreciated by the Trustees and would help them in the difficult task of meeting the mounting expenses of the operation of the Academy.

Sincerely yours,

Seth M. Milliken
TREASURER

For bibliographical service the Library Committee was authorized to charge $1.50 an hour instead of $1.00, Fellows to be charged half rates. This was to be tried for one year or less "at the discretion of the Librarian."

At the annual election in December, Dr. Eugene H. Pool was elected President and Dr. Sachs a Trustee. Dr. Sachs presided at every Stated Meeting of the Academy, and was absent only once each year from the meetings of the Council and Trustees. He was a dignified, active, and devoted servant of the Academy.

1935–1936

Eugene H. Pool

DR. EUGENE H. POOL, thirty-fifth President, was sixty-one years old when he assumed office. He was a very distinguished surgeon and had contributed much to the advancement of Surgery. Elected a Fellow in 1904, he had been Chairman of the Section on Surgery, a Trustee since 1925, and had long experience with the Academy's affairs.

The Stated Meetings were mostly well attended. The Hermann M. Biggs Memorial Lectures were given in May, and attracted varying audiences, 148 in 1935, while that delivered by the Rt. Hon. Lord Horder, of London, in 1936 had an attendance of 525.

The Carpenter Lectures had become part of the Graduate Fortnight, and the Anniversary Addresses—delivered by Walter Lippmann in 1935 and by James G. Rogers, Master of Timothy Dwight College, Yale, in 1936—were attended by 700 and 151, respectively.

The Section meetings all drew an average attendance of well over 100, except Historical and Cultural Medicine and, in 1936, Genito-Urinary Surgery.

The Medical Information Bureau inaugurated a series of lectures to the laity on the "Art and Romance of Medicine," as they were called until 1943. The second in the series, November 14, 1935, was on "Medicine in the Days of the Grand Monarch." The attendance is recorded as 1,400. The lectures were all well attended and were published by the D. Appleton-Century Company in 1936.

In 1936 Dr. Joseph Collins offered $6,000 a year to establish a Lectureship on Neurology, Psychiatry and Allied Subjects. His offer was accepted and the lectures were started in 1937, but we hear no more of them.

In November, 1934, a meeting had been given over to the problem of acute appendicitis. Dr. Krech read a very careful report on the records of fourteen private hospitals. A committee was appointed to make a report on the subject and the preliminary report was of such importance that the Council authorized the Public Health Relations Committee to attempt to raise funds for an exhaustive study. Unfortunately funds could not be raised.

The Walter M. Brickner fund of $10,000, the income to be expended on books, was established in 1935, and in 1936 Dr. Lambert on behalf of an anonymous friend presented a check for $50,000 to be known as the "Nemo Library Fund," income to be spent for the general uses of the Library. Mr. and Mrs. Carll Tucker also promised $2,170 a year for three years to pay certain salaries. This gift was also received "through Dr. S. W. Lambert."

The Library attendance in 1935 was 55,607. One day in October, 265 persons registered. In 1936 the total attendance increased to 58,523. The record day's attendance was 292. The report for 1936 states "It was noticed one afternoon during the Christmas holidays that every one of 107 seats in the Reading Room and the Periodical Room was occupied whilst numerous other readers were busy at the catalogue tables and the delivery desk."

In 1936 the Library Committee appointed two subcommittees to study the work done in the Library and to calculate its future needs. Membership was made up from the general Fellowship. They presented long reports which were combined and illustrated with graphs. The situation was summarized as follows: (1) the number of readers had more than doubled in ten years; (2) the budget of the Library had decreased, resulting in decrease in the purchase of books, decrease in the number of the Staff and underpayment of several; (3) the provision for housing the collection of books and periodicals, now numbering over 218,000, not counting duplicates, would soon be exhausted.

Probably due to lack of help, there were only two important exhibits in 1935, one on "Development of the Stethoscope" and the second in connection with the Graduate Fortnight, illustrating "the growth of our knowledge of the respiratory tract and its diseases." The latter was a very interesting exhibit and consisted of eighty-two books, from 1525 to 1927.

In 1936 there was an exhibit in connection with the Fortnight, on "Trauma: Occupational Diseases and Hazards."

An effort was made to do something about the museum. A volunteer curator was attempting to arrange and identify the miscellaneous collection, and two large exhibition cases were bought to contain some of them. Unfortunately he had to give up his work.

In 1935 and 1936 the Public Health Relations Committee spent much time in studies bearing upon revision of the city charter, and made valuable suggestions, a number of which were accepted and incorporated in the new charter, which was adopted by popular vote in November 1936, and went into force January 1, 1938.

Studies were also made at the request of Magistrate Anna Kross on the Women's Court and the control of prostitutes, and a continuing study of the whole subject of the control of venereal diseases. Twelve suggestions were submitted to the health authorities. The Committee reported on the grading of milk and recommended the existing Grades "A" and "B" be continued.

In 1936 the Committee had completed twenty-five years of service. No formal action was taken, but the report of the Committee for that year outlined very briefly its development. In *Neighborhood Health*, a publication of the Department of Health, appeared, on the first page, this statement:

A QUARTER CENTURY OF SERVICE

By *John L. Rice*, M.D.

I know from personal experience during the past two years of what great help the Committee on Public Health Relations of the New York Academy of Medicine has been not only to the Department of Health, but to the City as a whole. The Committee now in its twenty-fifth year of service to the community has achieved through this long period of continuity of well-directed effort a definite and unique position of usefulness. Its activities reveal the practical idealism of the leaders of the medical profession and demonstrate the applicability of objective inquiry to the several domains of public health and administrative and educational medicine. Each annual report of the Committee has been a valuable review of current health problems.

Several of the original group of physicians who have voluntarily given their services for these many years are still active on the Committee which has changed its chairman but once in the course of its existence and has employed the same executive secretary from the beginning. Thus there has developed a tradition, a philosophy and policy of action based on knowledge and experience which is perhaps unequalled in the annals of voluntary public health work.

The Committee, composed of a group of physicians chosen from among the members of the Academy of Medicine and appointed annually by its President with the approval of the Council, is authorized to voice the opinion of the Academy in matters to which it has given consideration. All the members are outstanding figures in the various fields of medicine, with extensive experience in clinical practice, in hospital work, in teaching or public health administration. The demands made upon the Committee on the part of numerous governmental and civic agencies have led the Committee to study a wide range of subjects and to express their collective, impartial, unbiased and expert judgment on a great variety of matters. During the past year alone the Committee concerned itself with the control of the milk supply; control of the sale of harmful drugs and cosmetics; problem of venereal diseases; child delinquency; care of the chronically afflicted; home medical and nursing care of the indigent; occupational diseases; city budget for health and hospital services; revision of the city charter, and many other matters of similar character.

The City is to be congratulated on being able to turn to such a body for advice and guidance.

No matters of importance were brought before the Committee on Professional Standards. Its campaign of previous years seemed to have produced results.

The problem of the relations between the public and the medical profession had already become an acute one. The Council appointed a committee "to Investigate Problems Relating to Medical Practice," whose function was "to study matters related to medical practice, health insurance and allied problems." This Committee did not attempt to offer solutions, but gathered valuable information as a basis of future action. Later it yielded the field to the Committee on

Medicine and the Changing Order, appointed at the end of 1942, and was discontinued in 1946.

During the last few years there had been an ever-increasing influx of foreign physicians, who, because of conditions in Europe, sought asylum in America. The greater part sought recognition in New York, and many applied for membership in the Academy. Some were distinguished physicians, but the vacancies in the membership were few. To grant them admission to the exclusion of New Yorkers seemed unfair, and the Council voted that a five-year residence in the United States was necessary before applicants could be considered as eligible.

Finances were a constant source of concern to the Trustees, who were faced with a choice of operating on a budget considerably in excess of expected income, trusting to gifts to make up a deficit, or of seriously curtailing established and valuable services. They chose the former course of action. A committee was appointed to raise funds with Dr. Shepard Krech as Chairman. It was divided into four subcommitees:

1) to secure endowment from wealthy individuals;
2) to secure annual donations;
3) to interest individual members in the problem;
4) to prepare a booklet for raising funds.

In 1935 the Academy received for new endowment $69,127.55; to meet the deficit, $20,125; and an additional $11,000 for specific expenses. It closed the year with a deficit of only $1,973.35.

In 1936 the endowment was increased by $105,000 and gifts for current expenses totaled $27,000, resulting in a balance in the Treasury of $1,242.38.

Dr. Emanuel Libman and the late Dr. Walter Brickner were elected Benefactors.

The Academy Medal was presented to Dr. A. N. Richards of the University of Pennsylvania.

Dr. Leo Mayer suggested that the Academy offer an annual "award of distinction" for the most significant contribution to surgery of the bones, joints, and tendons, the contribution to be presented at some regular meeting of the Section on Orthopedic Surgery. A special committee decided that such awards were not successful, judging by experiences at the Presbyterian Hospital and elsewhere, and the matter was dropped.

The Council voted that all candidates for the receipt of Academy diplomas must appear for the presentation in academic dress, and the expense of procuring the gowns must be borne by the candidates.

The use of the Loomis Entertainment Fund, started in 1895, for serving a collation to the Fellows after each Stated Meeting was discontinued. The income from the fund was to be used for entertainment of distinguished guest speakers.

Dr. Foster Kennedy presented the Academy with a beautiful pair of silver candelabra for formal occasions.

At the end of July, 1935, a long familiar figure in the Academy retired—Felix Wesstrom. He had come to the Academy in 1893 as an elevator boy, became janitor, and had done almost every kind of service in the forty-two years he served the Academy, including a brief period of collecting dues. He lived in the Academy for several years, and at one time answered night calls for the Nurses' Bureau. He knew practically every Fellow by name, and won the regard of all. In 1928, when he completed thirty-five years of service, resolutions of appreciation had been passed by the Council. He was retired on a pension in 1935.

In December, 1935, Dr. Charles L. Dana died. Elected a Fellow in 1886, he had been very active in the Academy's affairs and development. In 1894 he had been Anniversary Orator, and was elected Vice-President in 1901 and President in 1905. From 1907 to 1933, he had served as a Trustee, resigning the latter year on account of ill health.

After graduating from Dartmouth, Dr. Dana had become secretary to Senator Morrill of Vermont and spent four years in Washington, studying medicine on the side. It was probably his political experience which prompted him in 1926 to write Dr. S. A. Brown, the President, suggesting that the newspapers of New York be communicated with and an advisory service be proffered them by the Academy. He conceived the idea of a Public Health Committee, and was its Chairman from 1911 till 1928, and continued to serve on its Executive Committee through 1932.

The Council adopted the following resolutions, which were read before the Academy:

RESOLVED THAT:

The Council of the New York Academy of Medicine desires to record its deep sense of loss in the death of Dr. Charles L. Dana, a former President of the Academy.

Among the many very great services that Dr. Dana rendered to the public and the medical profession, the influence which he exerted upon the policies of the Academy was of paramount importance and the work which he did for the Academy was an outstanding contribution.

His devotion to our institution was practically co-existent with his professional career. Very early he recognized that under wise guidance the Academy of Medicine was destined to take a leading position in all those things whereby the medical profession comes in contact with and serves its community. His contributions naturally led to his becoming the President of the Academy, a position which he filled with unusual devotion and success.

He served as a member of the Council for term after term. Not satisfied with such contributions, he finally conceived the idea of the creation of a Committee on Public Health and became its first Chairman which offices he held over a period of twenty years, until his retirement from active work. It is well recognized that this Committee under his wise guidance has been an unusually faithful servant to the City of New York, and the credit therefor belongs to Dr. Dana.

Dr. Dana, in whatever capacity, was wise in counsel, constructive in thought and resourceful in effort. The Academy is greatly his debtor and the Council thus testifies as to the regard in which he was held.

In April, 1936, Dr. Arthur B. Duel died. He had been a Fellow since 1899 and had been a valuable worker for the development and interests of the Academy. It was he who first interested the Carnegie Corporation in the Academy and who suggested Dr. Linsly R. Williams as Director. He had been Chairman of the Building Committee in charge of the original building at 103d Street, and in 1931 became Chairman for the Extension, completed in 1933. A distinguished otolaryngologist, well known abroad as well as at home, he had been of great value to the Academy.

Two days after Dr. Duel's death, Dr. Harlow Brooks died. He was a very prominent physician in New York, and had been a Fellow of the Academy since 1904. He was a member of the Committee on Medical Education and was its very efficient Chairman from 1932 through 1934. He was Vice-President, 1932–34. He had a very large following and was also prominent in the County Medical Society.

Dr. Pool was a very valuable President. He presided at all but four Stated Meetings and was very regular in his attendance at Council and Trustees' meetings.

1937–1938

James Alexander Miller

DR. J. A. MILLER was sixty-three years old when he became thirty-sixth President of the Academy.

After graduating from Princeton, he received his M.D. from the College of Physicians and Surgeons in 1899. He had been on the Attending Staff at Bellevue since 1903 and, when elected, was "Visiting Physician in Charge of Tuberculosis" and Professor of Clinical Medicine at the College of Physicians and Surgeons. He had been very prominent in the whole field of tuberculosis, was Consulting Physician and President of the Board of Trustees of the Trudeau Sanatorium and Consulting Physician to several other hospitals.

Elected a Fellow in 1904, he had been very active in Academy affairs, especially in connection with its Public Health Relations Committee, of which he had been Secretary from its foundation in 1911 until he became Chairman in 1928, serving as such up to the time of his election as President. He had also been a Trustee since 1925, and had served for a number of years on the Committees on Budget, Gifts and Bequests, and to Investigate Problems Relating to Medical Practice. He was thoroughly acquainted with Academy affairs.

In his Presidential address he emphasized the financial difficulties of the Academy and urged every Fellow to participate in Academy activities.

In May a Stated Meeting was held on "Academy Policies and Finances." The President and Director spoke, as did also the Chairmen of the Standing Committees on Library, Public Health Relations, Medical Education, the Medical Information Bureau, and Committee on Fund Raising Campaign. The attendance was 311. The Academy learned a great deal about its problems.

As a result of suggestions of Dr. Baehr's Reviewing Committee on Academy Activities, the character of the Stated Meetings was changed and improved, and a closer relation between Sections and the Council was established. A Stated Meeting on Hypertension was attended by 647, one on Evaluation of Sulfanilamide Therapy by 725, and a symposium on Serum Therapy in Pneumonia by 654.

An important event in public health matters occurred in 1937. The Public Health Relations Committee had been of great assistance in the preparation of "A Standard Classified Nomenclature of Disease" which was completed in 1935. It was at the instigation of this Committee that the National Conference on Nomenclature started work in 1928. The Academy had provided it with an office for eight years without expense and had aided in obtaining financial support, and in receiving and expending funds for the conference, amounting to over $100,000, chiefly provided by the Commonwealth Fund, Carnegie Corporation, Metropolitan Life Insurance Company, Prudential Insurance Company, Connecticut General Insurance Company, and the Rockefeller Foundation. The report was already being extensively used by medical colleges and hospitals, and this year the Council on Medical Education of the American Medical Association assumed a permanent responsibility for its further introduction and revision.

A very valuable study was made by the Committee on Hospital Interneships. The Municipal Civil Service Commission sought to place under its own supervision the examination for appointments. As a result of the Committee's detailed study and report, the Civil Service Commission was denied supervision. The Department of Hospitals adopted rules which were substantially those recommended by the Committee.

Many other valuable reports were published. The relations with the Departments of Health and Education during these two years were particularly close, and an opinion was asked for and given on many important matters.

The Medical Information Bureau in 1937 appointed a special committee to investigate advertising material put out over the seal of the State of New York, by the Department of Agriculture, in an effort to increase the consumption of milk. This advertising was paid for by a special tax imposed upon producers and distributors of milk. The Bureau requested the Director of the Bureau of Milk Publicity to cooperate in eliminating undesirable material. He replied that "the authority of the scientific authorities which have been used as sources of the statements made" could be easily verified, and suggested that a representative of the advertising agency be consulted. One was invited to appear but failed to do so.

Some of the statements published were so absurd that a few are worth quoting:

> Clear up your complexion with milk.
> Milk gives you a lovely smooth skin.
> Milk for a glamorous complexion.
> To keep keen, keep up your Alkaline Reserve.
> Milk has a definite Alkaline effect.
> The minute you begin to feel below par—alkalize with milk.
> Milk is one of the finest natural things in the world to help keep your nerves, muscles, and brain clicking with hair-trigger sureness. Milk will help you think faster and act faster.

The subcommittee urged the Public Health Relations Committee to protest forcefully to the Bureau of Milk Publicity and request the Governor to suppress these exaggerated and often false statements. This was ordered by the Council.

The Library continued to be overcrowded. Over 61,000 readers were recorded in both years. A small but insistent group of Fellows complained about the ever-growing number of lay readers and demanded better accommodations for Fellows. A critical review of Library functions and activities was made, and the Council restated the Academy's responsibility for general service to the public without increased restrictions in favor of the Fellows.

The staff was too constantly overworked to arrange many exhibits; but a small collection of "Books on Public Health" was assembled at the time of the meeting of the American Public Health Association in 1937, and a small exhibit was arranged for each of the Graduate Fortnights.

In 1938 the Council ordered an exhibition of the portraits of the Presidents of the Academy. It attracted a good deal of attention and the Council changed the name of the "Collation Room," to "the Presidents' Gallery." The Academy has, or has been promised, oil portraits of all its past Presidents except Drs. Isaac Wood, Cock, Batchelder, Post, and Parker.

Many gifts of historical interest were presented for the dormant museum and were safely stored and catalogued.

The Library Publication Fund brought out three additional volumes, making six altogether in the "History of Medicine Series, Issued under the Auspices of the Library of the New York Academy of Medicine."

In 1937, Dr. F. P. Reynolds reached the age of retirement. He had been connected with the Academy since 1925, when he became its salaried Assistant Secretary, and served also as Medical Secretary of the Committee on Medical Education from 1931. Dr. Mahlon Ashford was appointed Executive Secretary to succeed him.

Beginning with 1938, after careful study of the subject, the Academy's *Bulletin* was changed in format and made a more strictly professional journal. It no longer gave over its April number to the Annual Reports; these were now published as separate documents. Finances unfortunately prevented the increase in size of the *Bulletin* as planned.

The Graduate Fortnight in 1937, on "Medical and Surgical Disorders of the Urinary Tract," had a paid registration of 620, and the evening lectures were attended by an average of 548. In 1938 registration increased to 787. The subject was "Diseases of the Blood and Blood-forming Organs," and the evening lectures drew an average of 859.

The Friday afternoon lectures, arranged by this Committee, were attended by an average of 300 in 1938. The attendance is not recorded for 1937. The Committee also collaborated with the New York Heart Association and with the New York Diabetes Association in a series of lectures.

In 1937, at the request of the Commissioner of Health, the Academy sponsored a series of lectures and hospital demonstrations on modern methods of diagnosis and treatment of syphilis. Seven lectures were given at the Academy and fourteen clinics in selected hospitals. It is interesting that the Council considered these lectures so important that the Academy held a Stated Meeting at 4.30 P.M., at which the lecture by Dr. A. B. Cannon, on "The Significance of Serological Tests in Syphilis," was read. It was the first time since 1847 that a Stated Meeting was held in the afternoon.

In 1938, with the County Society the Committee arranged a series of five lectures on Practical Obstetrics. It also, in cooperation with the Bureau of Medical Information, arranged a series of fifteen lectures for school teachers on the "Health of the Pupil," under the joint auspices of the Academy and the Board of Education. These lectures filled Hosack Hall to capacity.

The Physicians' Art Club gave an exhibition in both these years, but discontinued it the following year.

The Academy Medal was awarded to Dr. Béla Schick, just twenty-five years after the publication of his work on diphtheria.

In 1938 the Bureau of Medical Information became a Standing Committee. This was only after four rather stormy years. Originally started in 1928 as a joint Committee of the Academy and the County Medical Society, it was at first housed by the New York Tuberculosis and Health Association, and later transferred to the Academy. Its original purposes were: "To facilitate the dissemination of authentic information on medical and public health matters; to stem and curtail quackery and to promote better understanding between the public and organized medicine." Its services had been greatly expanded. To the press, it offered advice on the accuracy of statements of new "discoveries" in medicine and the propriety of advertisements of claimed "remedies," and on "feature" articles in various papers. It had prepared "releases" of the Biggs, Salmon and Carpenter Lectures, Lectures for the Laity and Presidential and Anniversary Addresses. It had done much to help the Graduate Fortnights.

The County Society had also profited by publicity of its important addresses and actions.

It had taken an active interest in the broadcasting of medical information, and had established an "Academy Hour" with weekly broadcast addresses by Fellows selected by the Sections, which were carefully edited and supervised. In 1937 these fifty-two talks resulted in requests from 7,295 persons for printed copies. In 1938 a number of them were reprinted in lay journals, such as *Hygeia*, *Talks*, *Radio Digest*, and *Radio Review*. The Director of Radio Talks of the Columbia Broadcasting System stated in 1937, "The wide response we receive indicates that it is serving a highly useful purpose in familiarizing the public in relatively simple terms, with the progress of medicine and with what is available to the public in the medical field."

It had arranged many radio hours for other organizations and prepared a leaflet of instructions for radio speakers. Its Executive Secretary wrote a short signed health article daily for the Associated Press, which was published as "authorized by the Academy." Three hundred and thirteen of these articles appeared each year in 400 papers all over the country.

Inquiries gradually increased, and commercial organizations, voluntary health groups, private individuals and physicians were constantly calling for advice and opinions. The Bureau had an advisory committee of 101 members, all specialists in their particular fields, to one or more of whom questions were referred.

The Executive Secretary had also attended to the publication of the *Health Examiner* and its successor, *Preventive Medicine*. It was a very busy, active, and useful Bureau.

The Laity Lectures, arranged by the Bureau, in 1937 drew an average attendance of 439 and in 1938 approximately 400. The first two series of lectures were published by the D. Appleton-Century Company, *Medicine and Mankind* and *Milestones in Medicine*. Royalties from these publications amounted to $223.33 and $136.50 during these two years.

Questions were raised, from time to time, as to whether the type of work carried on by the Bureau was really within the scope of Academy activity. The Council always felt that it was, and that it should be continued. Matters came to a head in 1935. An Omaha newspaper had heard of a baby born with a diaphragmatic hernia—or "upside-down stomach," as the newspaper termed it—and as an advertising project had arranged for the baby to be sent to The Truesdale Hospital in Fall River, Mass., for an operation. Dr. Truesdale was an eminently ethical surgeon and unsuspectingly accepted the case. It was extensively advertised in Omaha, and the Associated Press naturally heard of it. They insisted that the Executive Secretary of the Bureau of Medical Information should attend the operation, at their expense, and make a report. The Director agreed with apprehensions, for otherwise, the A.P. said, some less ethical person would probably be sent. The report was a very simple statement in which the Executive Secretary emphasized the fact that it was not an unusal operation.

Unfortunately the A.P. did not stick strictly to Dr. Galdston's report. The result was an inquiry from Boston, and several letters from Fellows including one from the then President, Dr. Pool.

A Committee was appointed to investigate the whole status of the Bureau of Medical Information, and to recommend as to its functions and activities. The Committee was apparently divided as to the wisdom of continuing the Bureau. The report was unsatisfactory to the Council, which appreciated what the Bureau was doing for the Academy and had approved its every activity.

A second Committee made an extended report, and the Director was instructed to investigate certain matters still further and report later. He announced that the State Society was making plans to take care of its own publicity, and the County Societies, now represented on the Bureau Committee, were inclined to do the same thing. The final decision was that the daily signed article for the Associated Press should no longer be published under the Academy's endorsement, and that the Bureau should be made a Standing Committee of the Academy with direct representation on the Council, to which it should report each month. This terminated the unsatisfactory dual authority over this activity.

Dr. Miller in his Valedictory Address announced this change, and spoke upon the work of the Bureau. The New York *Times* commented editorially on his address, and on Dr. Goodridge's Inaugural as follows:

For nearly a Century the New York Academy of Medicine has played a part in the city's life that should be better known. What that part is, both the outgoing president, Dr. James Alexander Miller, and the incoming president, Dr. Malcolm Goodridge, reviewed Thursday evening with scientific restraint, yet with understandable pride. . . .

The press of the city owes it especial thanks for maintaining a bureau of information which may be consulted by reporters and by editors who must comment upon advances in medicine and surgical practice. As a result, there is now less occasion than there was to complain of too enthusiastic accounts of new cancer "cures," "miracles" of surgery that have been well known to the profession for years, or hormones that promise to be fountains of youth and elixirs of life. Moreover, the general public has exactly the same privileges as writers and radio lecturers on medicine. In other words, it may ask any proper medical question with the assurance of receiving a proper and authoritative answer. . . .

Unlike most institutions of learning, the Academy has made it a special point to meet the requirements both of the medical profession and the public. In these days when organized medicine is charged with having failed to keep pace with social progress it is a pleasure to point to the Academy as an institution which has "socialized" medicine in the best sense of that bad term.

And the *World-Telegram* stated, also editorially:

Dr. James Alexander Miller, retiring president of the New York Academy of Medicine, enumerated among the Academy's services to the public, its Medical Information Bureau, which answers questions and explains abstruse professional lore for newspapers, the radio and inquirers generally.

The practice is entirely justified, for in the complicated mazes and rapid developments of medicine to-day any layman is bound to be confused. He is a perfect victim for impostors. If he speaks without a guide, he is almost certain to stray, thereby scattering misinformation. In the Academy's long career since 1847, the public service performed through this Bureau will rank high.

Leaning backward to avoid sensational publicity, medical men too often have blocked sensible discussion. The Information Bureau has reduced misunderstandings of this sort.

The *Herald-Tribune's* editorial, after mentioning a few of the services the Academy had rendered, closed with this sentence: "The

Academy is one of the best friends this community ever had."

Since then there has been no trouble about the Committee on Medical Information. The daily signed article by Dr. Galdston was given up in 1940, and the Academy Radio Hour in 1943.

The Committee today has little to do with commercial radio announcements, the programs extolling the value of various patented medicinal products being too profitable to the companies.

The Committee on Medical Information, which as a bureau was a problem child of the Academy, has become one of the most active and important departments of the Academy.

In 1937 the Treasury Department raised the question of the Academy's exemption from taxes under the new Social Security Act. Counsel prepared a comprehensive brief on the matter under the several Federal Statutes, setting forth the services being rendered to the laity, the several government agencies, and the medical profession generally. It was an impressive statement of Academy activities. After a hearing before Federal authorities, the Commissioner of Internal Revenue ruled that the Academy was entitled to exemption under the Federal Social Security Act, and also from income tax. It also was not subject to Federal Capital Stock tax, so long as the form of the organization, its purposes and method of operation remained unchanged. Contributions to the Academy could be deducted, according to prescribed limits, from individual income tax returns. This settled a very important matter for the Academy. The "form of organization, purposes and method of operation" have certainly remained unchanged.

During 1937 the general and library endowment funds were increased by $10,124,94. The Academy Fund Campaign Committee raised $23,700 to meet the deficit, and $1,565 more for general purposes. Nearly $5,000 for specific projects was given, and as a result the Academy had a balance of $4,675.55 at the end of the year.

The budget adopted for 1938 was $267,658.52 with an estimated income of $234,700. Again the Academy was running on an estimated deficit. But again, gifts and bequests came in and the year finished with a deficit of only $1,438.79. This was made possible only by the receipt of $24,372 through the Fund Campaign Committee and donations for special activities, amounting to $17,636.00. In 1938 the salary cuts made in 1930 were restored.

This was a thoroughly unsatisfactory method of financing, and in 1938 a Committee on Academy Activities was appointed, with Dr. George Baehr as Chairman. A similar committee had been appointed in 1929, and its report had served as a "charted course" for Academy work since. The Council each year had studied the matter but not in an intensive way. This Committee's report, which was not presented until 1939, stated that no activity of the Academy could be given up without a distinct loss of service to the profession and the public. It even felt some services should be increased.

Meanwhile the investment of Academy funds in mortgages was causing much worry. The depression had endangered many of them. The Comptroller, Mr. Eberle, showed rare judgment in handling the matter, and the Academy was extricated from what seemed like a very weak position to one of increased strength.

The Academy lost a valued member on the death of Dr. John H. Wyckoff. A Fellow since 1918, he had been an active and interested member of the Committee on Medical Education since 1928. He had been the Chairman of the New York Committee on the Study of Hospital Interneships and Residences which this Committee had been instrumental in organizing. His mature judgment, broad vision, and exceptional knowledge of the many problems connected with medical education, made him an invaluable councillor. He had not completed the first year of his Trusteeship.

In 1938 Dr. Samuel W. Lambert reached the age of eighty, and the Council sent this letter:

Dear Dr. Lambert:

Your friends in the Council of the New York Academy of Medicine salute you and extend congratulations upon the achievement of your eightieth birthday.

For many years you have been a leader in the medical profession of New York City, distinguished alike for your clinical wisdom and insight, by your contribution to medical education through the administration of a great medical school and, even more particularly, by your personal influence upon the development of medical students and young physicians.

In the midst of your unusually numerous professional activities you have found time to develop the cultural side of life in the promotion of both the arts and letters. This has been of peculiar value to the Academy as through it your great interest and devotion to the development of the library of the Academy was stimulated.

You have served with distinction as President of the Academy and for many years as one of its Trustees, but it will probably be by your extraordinarily valuable contributions to the development of the library that your services to the Academy will be especially remembered.

Your colleagues in the Council are in a position to especially appreciate how greatly the Academy has profited by your experience, wisdom and counsel and they will always remember your lively interest, incisive discussion and searching questions, as well as your keen sense of humor, by which our deliberations were for so many years both enriched and enlivened. Your personality has endeared you to us all and your abilities have placed us as well as the Academy greatly in your debt.

The members of the Council, therefore, join in wishing you continued health and happiness and send you this letter as a token of their esteem and deep affection.

1939–1942

Malcolm Goodridge

Dr. Goodridge, thirty-seventh President of the Academy, was sixty-six when he assumed office. At the end of his third year at P. and S. he contracted a mild tuberculosis but graduated and went immediately to Saranac and Lake Placid. He worked at the Saranac Laboratory and practiced in Lake Placid. Returning to New York in 1900, he started practice with everything against him. He had had no interneship and it was hard sledding, but he made his impression by hard work, and was appointed to the Attending Staff of Bellevue in 1909 and was now Consulting Physician to it, and also to New York Hospital. Connected with the teaching staff of Cornell from 1910, he was Professor of Clinical Medicine there at the time of his election. He had been a Fellow of the Academy since 1906 and a member of the Public Health Relations Committee since 1930.

No recent incumbent could have undertaken the duties of President under harder circumstances. Europe was in a turmoil and World War II broke out in September, 1939. While we did not declare war against Japan and Germany until 1941, we were practically at war from the start. In addition to that, Dr. Hartwell was to retire from the Directorship in April.

Dr. Goodridge's Inaugural was a frank statement of what the Academy was facing, and the very sketchy ideas many Fellows had of what it did and how it did it. He urged greater interest on the part of all, and participation by more Fellows.

Dr. Wilcox was selected by a special committee to fill the post of Director. An active and very successful practitioner in pediatrics, he had been selected to succeed Dr. L. Emmett Holt as Professor of Pediatrics at the College of Physicians and Surgeons in 1922, and succeeded, with rare tact and judgment, in a difficult and much needed reorganization of the department, which he had continued to direct, at great personal sacrifice until 1931, when

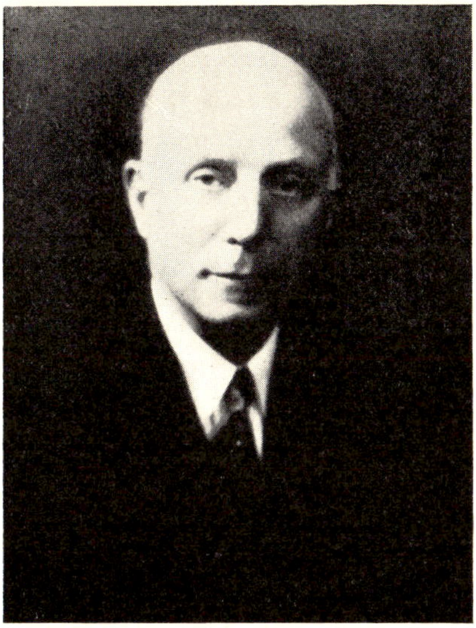

JOHN A. HARTWELL, 1869–1940
Thirty-third President, 1929–1932; Director, January 24, 1934, to April 1, 1939

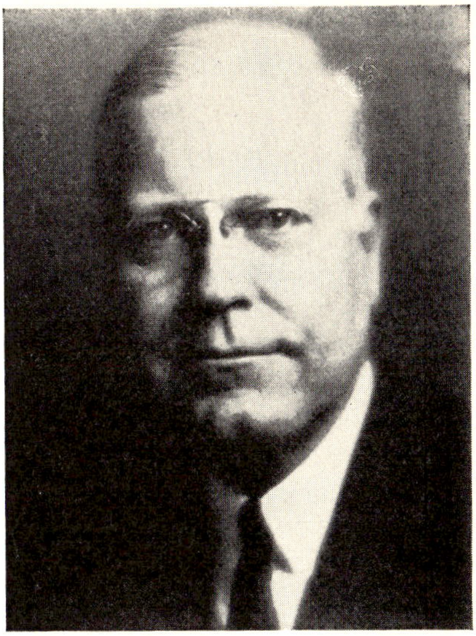

JAMES ALEXANDER MILLER
1874–1948
Thirty-sixth President, 1937

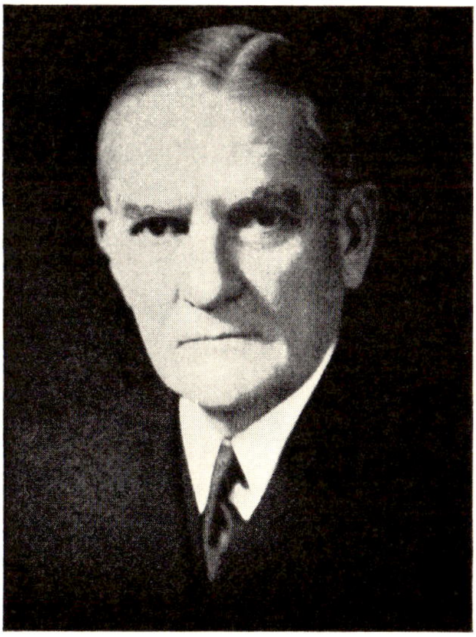

MALCOLM GOODRIDGE, 1873–
Thirty-seventh President, 1939–1942

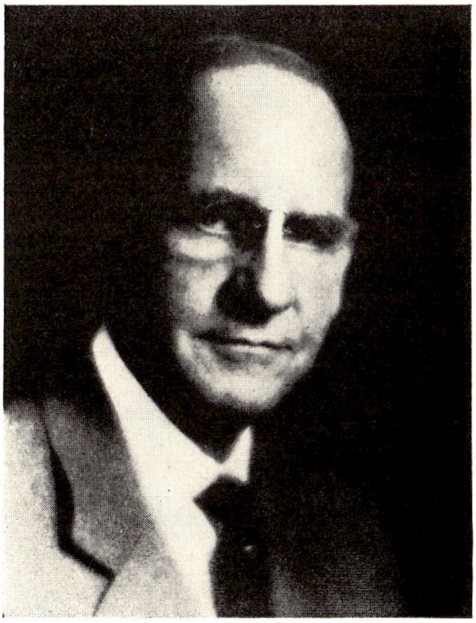

HERBERT B. WILCOX, 1874–
Director, April 1, 1939, to October 1, 1946

he retired. Elected a Fellow in 1907, he had been a fine chairman of the Section on Pediatrics, Vice-President, 1935–37, and had served on the Committee on Public Health Relations and the recently appointed Committee on Activities of the Academy. In accepting the Directorship, he gave up private practice and devoted his entire time to Academy affairs. His calm deliberation and judgment on early problems boded well for the Academy.

On Dr. Hartwell's retirement the Council voted:

. . . Dr. John A. Hartwell, for five years the Director of the New York Academy of Medicine, retired on April 1, 1939.

He served the Academy with great distinction in spite of physical handicaps that would have stopped the ordinary individual.

The Council of the Academy wishes to take this opportunity to record its keen appreciation of the courageous, vigorous and dignified manner in which he conducted the administration of Academy affairs.

During the year 1939, the Council made every effort to keep expenses within the appropriations. The Trustees had adopted a budget for 1939 of $257,280, with an estimated income of $235,900. That meant an expected deficit of $22,280, minus contributions. Every possible step was taken to reduce personnel and operative costs without too much curtailment. The Library was closed on Sundays to relieve the overworked staff as well as save expense. The assessment for room space and service was increased to approximate the general cost of office space elsewhere. The publication of *Preventive Medicine* was discontinued. The Annual Report was reduced by fifty-six pages, thus saving $280 for printing. The subscription price of the *Bulletin* for the United States, Canada, and Cuba was increased for 1940 to $3.00, and for foreign countries to $4.00. In 1940 the number of subscribers had increased 220.

The Fund Raising Committee, Dr. Krech chairman, was released with thanks for its efficient work in raising a total of $62,000, and a new and larger committee, Dr. Mixsell, chairman, was appointed. It succeeded in raising only $10,047.50 during the year, but many potential supporters were reached, and old ones were constantly informed of the Academy's work and needs. This was all done in a quiet, unobtrusive way. The expected deficit of $22,280 was reduced to $16,297.

At the annual meeting in 1940, the Academy's problems, plans and requirements were fully and frankly discussed by Dr. Goodridge, and they were given considerable publicity by the press. January 26, 1940, the following letter was received by Dr. Goodridge:

The other day I read that the Academy of Medicine had a deficit of $18,000.

For many generations my family has been identified with the medical profession and in our time, my father and brother were doctors. Because of these associations, and because of the many magnificent men in the profession whom it has been my good fortune to know, I am aware of the role that the Academy of Medicine has and is playing in holding up the standards of the medical profession. I know what it has stood for in my family, what it has done for me, and what it is doing for the community every minute of the day.

I am enclosing a check for $18,000 to take care of the deficit, which I hope you will make me happy by accepting.

Very truly yours,

Bernard M. Baruch.

Mr. Baruch was made a Benefactor.

In the first four months of 1940 subscriptions for augmenting the budget were received for $26,930. The Committee was enlarged by eleven members to create an Advisory Lay Council of eleven, who agreed to lend their aid in securing adequate support for the future. The members of the Lay Council were:

Walter S. Gifford, President American T. and T. Company, Chairman
Arthur M. Anderson, Vice-President J. P. Morgan and Company
George Blumenthal, President-Emeritus, Mount Sinai Hospital
Lewis Brown, President, Johns Manville Corporation
Clinton H. Crane, President, St. Joseph Lead Company
Marshall Field
Joseph M. Hartfield, Attorney
David M. Heyman, of Adolph Lewisohn and Sons
Philip W. Lennen, Lennen and Mitchell

George W. Merck, President, Merck and Company
Edward L. Shea, President, North American Company

The title was later changed to the "Steering Committee." (A name proposed for it was the "Committee on Public Relations," but this was likely to be confused with the long-established Committee on Public *Health* Relations and on the protest of that body the proposal was withdrawn.) The goal set by the Committee was to raise $300,000 for needed additions to the Library plant, $250,000 to provide $50,000 a year additional income for operating expenses over a period of five years and to lay the foundation for increase of endowment, so as to eliminate deficits as well as repeated requests for contributions.

In April, 1940, at a special joint meeting of the Council and Trustees Dr. Goodridge outlined the situation; the general opinion was that the Academy must procure professional services for fund raising. The Council approved the plan, and in May, the Harold F. Strong Corporation was engaged to manage the publicity. Mr. Price was assigned as its representative with the Academy. Mr. Price soon left the Strong Corporation, and was later appointed to carry on these activities for the Academy. He has continued to do so ever since.

The set-up for the financial management was changed. The New York Trust Company was appointed Investment Counsel. Changing of investments, except in mortgages, was discussed each month by the Executive Committee of the Trustees and the Investment Counsel, and approved by the Trustees at a later meeting. The management of mortgages was in the hands of the Comptroller, Mr. Eberle, who has done a fine piece of work, saving the Academy many thousands of dollars by his wise actions. This is the present form of handling Academy finances.

By the end of 1940, the Steering Committee had secured $14,000 toward the Library projects and pledges of $91,862 for operating costs during the next five years.

The Stated Meetings were well planned and the average attendance these years was 346 and 375.

The Biggs lectures were given in 1939 by Mr. Frederick Osborn of the American Museum of Natural History, on "The Significance to Medicine of Present Population Trends," and in 1940 by Dr. Paul D. White, Harvard Medical School, on "Heart Disease, a World Problem."

In 1939 the Academy arranged a two-day Round Table Discussion on Convalescent Care, under a grant from the Josiah Macy, Jr., Foundation. Fifteen hundred copies of this valuable report were printed and, so great was the continued demand for it, that three years later a second edition of three thousand copies was printed by the offset process.

Again in 1939, another series of lectures on practical obstetrics was given in cooperation with the County Medical Society. There was an average attendance of 128.

The Academy helped, in 1940, in furthering plans to meet war conditions. Meetings were held for the committee in charge of transportation and distribution of British child refugees and the State Committee for a Long-range Program for Medical Preparedness.

At the request of the Surgeon General of the Army, a meeting was held under the auspices of the Blood Transfusion Betterment Association, to consider all problems connected with acquiring plasma and sending it to Great Britain. From this resulted the establishment at the Academy of a Red Cross Central Station, where donors were seen and assigned to the six hospitals where the blood was to be taken.

In cooperation with the Bar Association and the County Society, a series of lectures on medico-legal aspects of actions for compensation for disability from personal injury was given.

In 1940 a series of five lectures were given on the care of mother and newborn child, replacing those formerly given on practical obstetrics only.

The Friday afternoon lectures were continued and drew an average attendance of 236 in 1939, and 217 in 1940.

The Lectures to the Laity continued to be popular and drew average audiences of 500 in 1939 and 779 in 1940. It was voted by the Council in 1940 that the first of these lectures each year should be called the "Linsly R. Williams Memorial Lecture."

The Graduate Fortnight in 1939 was on the subject of "The Endocrine Glands and Their Disorders." There was a paid registration of 753. The fee was now $5.00. The opening lecture was given jointly with the County Society, and the average attendance at the evening meetings was 1,024. For the first time the registration fees more than covered the expense incurred, and a donation for the Fortnight received from the Josiah Macy, Jr., Foundation was returned with thanks. The balance was included in the budget for the next year.

In 1940 the subject was "Infections." The registration was not as high and the attendance at the evening lectures was only 478, but the clinics at the various hospitals were well attended, as were the pathological demonstrations and the morning round tables. The first lecture was designated the "Ludwig Kast Lecture," in recognition of Dr. Kast's having first suggested the Fortnights.

The Bowen Scholarships, which had been established for foreign study after hospital interneship, could not be awarded in 1940 on account of the European War, and scholarships in American Medical Colleges were substituted.

The State Department in Washington was interested in seeking rapprochement with the republics of Central and South America, and the Academy was made its representative in New York to receive members of the medical profession and assist them in getting the experience they desired. This work was carried on by the Committee on Medical Education. In 1940 over sixty called, advance notice being given in many cases by the State Department through the Consular Service. In 1942 letters were received from the Department of State and the Pan American Union thanking the Academy for establishing this service. It is still functioning.

The Committee on Medical Information was ever growing in importance. In 1939 it prepared a simple statement regarding broadcasting, entitled "On the Air—A Few Notes on the Preparation and Delivery of Radio Talks." In 1940 a critical study of radio broadcasting of health information was proposed and a grant was obtained from the Rockefeller Foundation to establish a fellowship to study the matter. A committee of three supervised the study and Dr. Robert Schultz was appointed the "Fellow." He made a valuable report, which was referred to the Foundation. It showed, among other things, the excellent response to the Academy Hour, as shown by letters received after each broadcast.

One of the results was a Health Education Conference in October, 1940, composed chiefly of representatives of the medical profession, official health agencies, and voluntary health organizations. Messrs. Howard Blakeslee of the Associated Press and Sterling Fisher of the Columbia Broadcasting System made addresses and Dr. Alan Gregg and Mr. Frank Kiernan took part in the discussion.

The requests from the press for opinions on accuracy of material submitted were increasing and the most cordial relations were maintained. The annual Press and Radio dinner was still being given and was largely attended. The daily column for the Associated Press was discontinued in 1940.

The Library was working under great difficulties. In 1939 readers numbered 64,357. On one day in December, 127 were in the main reading room at the same time, and during that day 266 registered in the Library and Rare Book Room. The shelves were full and the card catalogue had little space left. Three and one-half extra workers were authorized by the Trustees the latter part of the year.

In 1940 the number of readers fell off after May, and the total was only 62,356. Failure to receive foreign periodicals may have accounted in part for this difference. The budget for operative costs was reduced from $29,500 to $18,300, the lowest figure since 1924. The extra workers allowed the previous year were discontinued, and a vacancy in the Bibliographical Department was not filled.

In spite of an insufficient and overworked staff, an exhibition of "Some Contributions to Our Knowledge of the Thyroid and Parathyroids" was prepared for the Graduate Fortnight in 1939, as well as a "Practitioner's Shelf" of books on endocrinology, arranged by Mr. Place.

In 1940 in connection with the 500th anniversary of printing, an exhibition of 78 items on "Printing and Medicine" was arranged by Miss Annan, the list of which was published in the *Bulletin of the Medical Library Association,* Vol. 28. In 1940, in connection with the Graduate Fortnight on "Infections," Miss Annan again collected an exhibition of "Books on the Discovery of Vaccination, Its early Advocates and Opponents," and there was a "Practitioner's Bookshelf of works on Infections," again arranged by Mr. Place.

The Committee on Public Health Relations continued its active cooperation with the City Departments. An exhaustive study of personnel and methods of increased usefulness was made for the Department of Health; recommendations were submitted for changes in the Sanitary Code regarding tuberculosis, all of which were adopted; and numerous other studies and reports, on the most varied subjects, were prepared, all of great value.

The duties of the Committee on Medical Jurisprudence were transferred to the Public Health Relations Committee, and the Committee, after twelve years of valuable service, was discharged, with appreciation of services rendered.

The alert Committees on Medical Education and Public Health Relations reported to the Council that a petition was before the Charter Committee of the Board of Regents for authority to initiate a new medical schoool to be called the "Gorgas Institute of Medical Science." The Council sent a memorandum to the Board, emphasizing the necessity of meeting four essential requirements before the new school should receive a charter, none of which obviously could be met. We hear no more of the Gorgas Institute.

In 1940 the Constitution and By Laws were amended and brought up to date, including all the changes made since 1933, the last published edition. The distinction between "Fellows" and "Members," which had been tried for five years, was abolished. Since 1935 only nineteen members had applied for advancement to Fellowship. All members elected during that time automatically became Fellows. The Standing Committee on Fellowship was therefore abolished.

The Committee on Revision of By Laws had recommended that graduates from hospital interneships be eligible for "Junior Fellowship." The Council, after long deliberation, did not give its sanction.

The hub of the radius of twenty-five miles as the limit for Resident Fellows was changed from the City Hall to the Academy Building, thus "eliminating a large part of the lower bay" and bringing in more of Westchester.

On proof of fee-splitting, authority was given to the Council to expel the guilty Fellow, without a vote of the Academy Fellowship.

An Executive Committee of the Trustees, consisting of *two or more* members of the Board, were given authority to act ad interim for the Board. The Committee, as organized, now consists of a majority of the Board, so their unanimous action can never be overridden by the Board.

Life membership was established. A Fellow could at any time after election become a life member exempt from annual dues, and retain all rights of Fellowship. This did not do away with the exemption from dues, on request, after thirty years of Fellowship.

All other changes were simply to clarify existing rules.

When the Academy had moved to 103d Street, the serving of a "collation" from the Loomis Fund after each Stated Meeting was suspended, and the income from the Fund was made available for entertainment of guests of the Academy. It was now utilized for paying for lunches and dinners which the various Executive Secretaries were required to attend.

The Budget for 1940, as adopted by the Trustees, was $231,605.89 and the expected income, including "Contributions $10,000," was $229,970, leaving another but smaller expected deficit. In May it was announced the receipt of an appropriation of $9,460 from the Carnegie Corporation would probably enable the Academy to close the year without a deficit. But, owing to unavoidable emergency expenditures and diminished income, the Academy actually closed its year with a deficit of $10,012.84.

At the close of 1940 one of the Academy's most devoted members passed away, Dr. John A. Hartwell. Few men had served it with greater devotion and loyalty; few had ever been called to fill so many positions. President for four years, on the death of Dr. Williams he had become the Director and served as such for five years. During two of those years he had suffered from a peripheral circulatory disturbance which at times crippled him. With rare courage he ran Academy affairs from his hospital bed, and ran them satisfactorily. His resignation was for some time in the hands of the Council, which was loath to accept it.

On retiring he had become Associate Director of the American Society for the Control of Cancer, which was not an exacting job. Devoted sportsman, he had always said he hoped to die with a rod or gun in his hand. He went to the South Side Club on Long Island for duck shooting. He had to be carried to his blind, and as his guide handed him his gun, he fell back dead.

The Council passed these resolutions:

The Trustees and Council of The New York Academy of Medicine, mindful of the long and devoted service rendered by Dr. John A. Hartwell, record with sorrow the great loss sustained by them in his recent death.

Dr. Hartwell has served the Academy for many years in many capacities—three years as Vice-President, four years as President, three years as a Trustee, and five years as Director. In all of these, the Academy benefited, in addition to his direct service, equally by the credit reflected from his contributions in the councils of the City and State.

Dr. Hartwell's ability to carry on in spite of the handicap of prolonged illness won for him the admiration of all his fellows. His capacity (rarely seen in members of our profession) for judicially considered expression earned for him the soubriquet of "medical statesman."

Beyond all this, his personal charm made for him innumerable friends.

It is the wish of the Trustees and Council that this note be made a part of the meeting and that a copy be sent to Mrs. Hartwell.

In 1941 Mrs. Hartwell established the John A. Hartwell Memorial, and the Fellows' Room was renamed the Hartwell Room. This fund keeps this room up and also contributes to the Rare Book Fund.

Although these two years had been difficult ones, and the financial program was in an experimental stage, the internal affairs of the Academy had never been more harmonious. Dr. Goodridge had given a great deal of time to its affairs. America's entrance into the war was imminent. His renomination was obvious and desired. At the time of the Civil War, Dr. Anderson had been reelected twice, and during the first World War, Dr. James had been reelected. Dr. Goodridge was reelected without opposition.

His second Inaugural Address was a forceful account of what the Academy had become, and what its obligations were. He felt keenly the ignorance of the public as to what the Academy was, and to a certain extent the ignorance on that subject on the part of the Fellows. They had a great aversion to advertising, and had carried this aversion into the administration of the Academy. He felt this philosophy was a mistake—that the public should know what the Academy was doing and what it stood for.

He quoted Dr. Lambert as saying in his Inaugural Address, delivered in 1927, a few weeks after the Academy had moved to its new quarters: "The New York Academy of Medicine is not a local medical group. It has become a national institution. . . . This Academy like every educational institution must go on to new fields of work or retrograde and slip from its position of prominence."

He called attention to the fact that the Library served more than six times as many readers as any other medical library in the country, and that 87 percent of its readers were not Fellows; that its bibliographical service was one of three such medical services in the country; that its catalogue of 86,000 portraits of 30,000 medical or scientific individuals was in constant use.

He emphasized the various great contributions to public health made by the Public Health Relations Committee in its completed thirty years of service; the continuous service of the Committee on Medical Education to the profession of this city, country and to foreign visitors; the great service rendered the public through the Committee on Medical Information, with its wide influence with the public press; and many other things, both of accomplishment and of only partial accomplishment.

In closing he said, "We have no delusions concerning our importance, and no illusions in regard to our accomplishments. What we have done in the past will give you some conception of what we are today. Our hope and our ambition in matters concerning public health and medical education are endless." It was an evening of mixed snow and rain, and the attendance was only 267, but the address was published in the *Bulletin* and so reached every Fellow, and it is hoped was read by each.

During 1941 and 1942 the Stated Meetings were carefully planned and always with able speakers. The attendance varied to an extent hard to understand. The condition of the weather and the attendance is recorded in the minutes; and there is no relation between bad weather and small attendance. The lowest in 1941 was 132 and the highest 504 in May, at which a memorial of Dr. Banting was read and the meeting given over to a discussion of diabetes and insulin.

In 1942 attendance naturally fell off. The lowest recorded was 85, when "Recent Developments in the Treatment of Pulmonary Tuberculosis" was discussed, and the largest at a joint meeting given by the Surgical Section and the New York Surgical Society, at which 525 were present. Another large meeting, attended by 465, was a discussion of "Special Therapeutic Agents in Infections—Gramicidin, Penicillin and the Sulfonamides."

The Sections were particularly hard hit by the war absences. A special committee—the Chairman of the Committee on Sections, and Dr. Miller for the Council—met with the Section Chairmen and Secretaries and reviewed the whole matter. Conditions were frankly discussed and criticized, and a much better understanding was reached on all sides.

The Biggs Lectures were given each year. In 1941 Dr. C. A. Mills, Professor of Experimental Medicine, University of Cincinnati, spoke on "The Relation of Climate and Geography to Health" before an audience of 462, and in 1942 Dr. J. S. McLester, Professor of Medicine, University of Alabama, discussed "Nutrition and the Nation at War." The attendance was 525.

The By Laws of 1920 stated "The Anniversary Discourse shall be delivered in November, at a meeting to which the public shall be invited." In 1926 this was changed to read: "At least one meeting shall be held annually to which the public shall be invited and at which an appropriate discourse or lecture shall be given." From 1938 through 1941 there is no notice in the *Bulletin* or in the announcements of Stated Meetings of any "Anniversary Address." In 1941, on recommendation of the Committee on Medical Information, it was voted that hereafter the January Lecture for the Laity be called the "Anniversary Discourse." In 1942 it was therefore officially resumed, and was delivered by Dr. A. A. Brill on "The Freudian Epoch."

On recommendation of the Public Health Relations Committee, the Council voted that the President and the chairman of that Committee and of the Committee on Medical Education appoint:

1) a Committee to study and formulate a statement as to the essential medical staffs of hospitals and medical schools;
2) a Committee to circularize Fellows of the Academy over forty-five years of age to ascertain the amount of time they would be willing to give to additional hospital work; and
3) for these two committees also to hold a meeting to discuss the subjects of malaria and quinine emergency and the cultivation of medicinal plants in the United States.

It was soon realized that the first of the matters was really not a function of the Academy. The hospitals and the medical schools worked out a plan with the Surgeon General. In regard to the second, the Academy was able to render service in bringing older men back into hospital service, and many responded gladly.

For the third project, the Committees arranged a meeting at which Dr. Marston T. Bogert, Emeritus Professor of Chemistry at Columbia, read a very valuable paper on "Malaria and Quinine as the Chemist Sees It," and Mr. R. H. Cheney, Chief of the Biological Department of the Long Island University and Curator of Medicinal Plants at the Brooklyn Botanical Garden, spoke on "Drug Production by Cultivation in the United States as the Biologist Sees It." This was an interesting and well attended meeting.

The Public Health Relations Committee published in 1942 its pamphlet, "Thirty Years in Community Service, 1911–1941." This condensed into 106 pages a brief outline of the work of the Committee, in all of its many-sided activities. It is a most interesting and impressive record.

In 1941 the Academy was cooperating in many war activities. It assisted in the Red Cross membership campaign and helped other organizations in their programs, notably the Medical and Surgical Aid to Britain, Bundles for Britain, and American Women's Volunteer Service. In addition all its facilities were made available to near-by stations of the Army and Navy.

The Council authorized five meetings on advanced first-aid and acute traumatic surgery, under joint auspices with the County Society, provided the program was approved by the Subcommittee on Lectures of the Committee on Medical Education, and the County Society attend to the circularization.

The Council also voted to extend invitations to Academy meetings to medical officers in near-by Army, Navy, and public health stations, through Commanding Officers, and to send the daily Surgical Bulletin to commands on request.

In response to the Treasury's request, the Council decided, against some opposition, to allow speakers to urge upon Academy audiences more widespread and greater purchase of defense bonds, to permit a sales booth in the Academy, and in the Academy folder to urge greater buying.

Dr. Robert L. Levy complained of the speech of the new President of the County Society, Dr. Ramirez. In January, 1942, the Council issued the following:

At a recent meeting of the Medical Society of the County of New York, statements were made to which publicity has been given concerning fee-splitting, a practice which has been disapproved by The New York Academy of Medicine.

The New York Academy of Medicine wishes to avoid any possibility of being considered as in sympathy with the statements made on that occasion. Its Council, the governing body, therefore considers it advisable and necessary to restate the Academy's position regarding this financial relation between the patient, his family physician and the consultant.

A prime motive in the original organization of the Academy was "The separation of the regular from irregular practitioners" and "The promotion of the character, interests and honor of the fraternity, by maintaining the union and harmony of the regular profession of the city and its vicinity."

In 1911, under the Presidency of Dr. William M. Polk, the following resolutions were adopted:

Resolved, That the secret division of a fee, or fees with any person, or persons, who may be instrumental in influencing a patient, or patients, to apply for operative care or professional advice, is unworthy of any member of the medical profession.

Resolved, That if such a division of fee is made by a member of The New York Academy of Medicine, it should be counted as of sufficient ground for the expulsion of the member.

Resolved, That the Council considers it its duty to investigate charges against members made on the basis of such division of fee, and on receipt of proof of offense the Council may either permit the resignation of the person or expel him from the Academy.

In 1933, the Academy reaffirmed this stand.

Finally in 1938, a prerequisite for admission to Fellowship in the Academy was established which requires each applicant for admission to sign the following statement:

If elected to membership, I hereby subscribe to the Constitution and By-Laws of The New York Academy of Medicine now in force and hereafter adopted and to the following resolutions:

Resolved, That the division of a fee or fees with any person or persons who may be instrumental in influencing a patient or patients to apply for operative care or professional advice is detrimental to the interests of the community and unworthy of any member of the medical profession.

Resolved, That if such a division of a fee is made by a member of The New York Academy of Medicine, whether *secretly or known to the patient,* the member shall be liable to expulsion from the Academy by a three-fourths vote of the Council.

This, therefore, is and will continue to be the attitude of The New York Academy of Medicine on the question of fee splitting.

The problem of émigré physicians was a troublesome one. Some of the Fellows took the stand that the Academy should do all in its power for them, and lower its barriers; others felt as strongly the danger of this rush of unassimilated and perhaps unassimilable groups. A special subcommittee was appointed to study the matter. It was composed of Drs. J. A. Miller, A. E. Cohn, Goodridge, the Director and Mr. F. L. Polk, Counsel of the Academy, and reported as follows:

Introduction. Your Committee begs leave to submit the following report, which is based upon a careful study of the whole émigré physician situation, and in support of this report begs leave to submit the accompanying memorandum, which sets forth the facts which constitute the basis for their report.

Report and Recommendations. (1) The concentration of the large number of émigré physicians in New York City is most unfortunate and is harmful to their own interests, to the interest of the medical profession, and to the best interests of the community.

(2) The main predisposing causes of this situation are found in the liberal action of the New York State Licensing Board and of the local county medical societies in New York State, and secondly in the contrasting resistance to their acceptance by other states and other county societies. The legal difficulties to their employment in either army or defense service is another important factor, and lastly, personal difficulties such as those of language, age and lack of adaptability to American methods and surroundings.

(3) It would appear that the difficulties are largely legal and political and partly social, humanitarian and economic, and are not the responsibility of the Academy of Medicine either in fact or in principle, but rather that this responsibility belongs to the local New York City county medical societies, the New York State Medical Society, the Federation of State Medical Boards, and the American Medical Association, working in conjunction with such voluntary organizations as the National Committee for the Resettlement of Foreign Physicians, and with governmental agencies which might with propriety be consulted.

(4) Inasmuch as the Academy through this Committee has recognized the scope and nature of this problem, we recommend that the following resolution be adopted by the Council.

Resolved: That an expression of the intention of The New York Academy of Medicine toward men and women at a disadvantage either because of race or religion or because of exile be spread upon the minutes of the Council to the effect that The New York Academy of Medicine has always been sympathetic to the misfortune of its professional brethren and this is and has been its fixed policy.

In connection with the relations with Latin American visitors, Room 60 was assigned as a reception room for them, and the Committee having charge was authorized to attend to details of arrangement and the possibility of securing a full-time Spanish-speaking receptionist, provided it cost the Academy nothing.

This duty was assigned to the Committee on Medical Education, which established an "Inter-America Division." The question of the "receptionist" was arranged by Dr. Ashford. A journal called *America Clinica* and printed in Spanish and Portuguese was published in New York for circulation in South and Central America. It was invited to move its editorial office to the Academy. The invitation was accepted and the staff acted as interpreters as occasion arose. But the arrangement was of short duration; within a few months all relations were severed with *America Clinica.* In 1946, however, they were reestablished by the Council and *America Clinica* is again published with the Academy's "collaboration."

In 1941 the Committee on Museum was discharged, with thanks, and the Committee on Medical Education was instructed to consider the establishment of a permanent Medical Museum. It recommended the material be "organized" to be possibly located in 10 East 103d Street. Most of it was transferred a little later to that building, and lay there undisturbed accumulating dust and dirt until it was almost excavated by the Library Staff in preparation for the Centennial Celebration.

In response to a request from the United Hospital Fund, the Committee on Medical Education was authorized to appoint a committee of seven to act in an advisory capacity on research projects contemplated by the hospital membership. This has continued in operation ever since.

The award of the Bowen Scholarships was suspended for the duration of the War.

The Library Committee during these two hard years continued "as usual." As was to be expected, attendance fell off considerably. Only 56,953 readers signed the register in 1941, and in 1942, the number fell to 48,972. This was perhaps fortunate as many of the experienced staff left for war positions.

The Library personnel established a rotating exhibit of "War in Medical Literature." Each month a collection of current books, pamphlets, and magazine articles on a special subject were arranged in the lobby of the Library, where they were accessible to all and attracted wide attention.

In anticipation of a possible complimentary "token bomb" from Germany, the Library was authorized to microfilm the "shelf list," and although the risk was considered slight, the rare books were boxed and stored in an inside area on one of the lower floors. This of course increased the daily labors of the staff for there seemed an unusual demand for those books stored far away.

In November, 1941, the *Bulletin* published a "progress report" of the Steering Committee, which stated "When the Budget Committee meets, the specter of a deficit will be absent for the first time in several years." The Steering Committee announced that it had raised $181,519 in cash or pledges for the "five-year plan" and was hopeful of obtaining the remainder (total $250,000). At the end of the year 1941, the Academy's books showed a balance of $8,597. Encouraged by this showing, the Budget Committee adopted a program for 1942 calling for expenditures of $262,215, some $6,000 more than in 1941. But things did not go well. Two hundred and fifteen Fellows were in active service with the armed forces. Before we went into the war, it had been voted that they be classed as Army and Navy Fellows, paying $10 dues. But, actually at war, dues were remitted for the period of service.

In 1942 the Constitution was amended to increase the number of Fellows from 1,700 to 1,800. This did not help much, for many promptly went into the armed forces.

By April the Treasurer estimated a deficit of $6,000 to $7,000, and the Council voted the establishment of a "public relations Counsel." Mr. Donald Price, until then on temporary appointment, was continued in that position.

Income from investments was nearly $15,000 less than the previous year. As a result the year closed with a deficit of $20,293.77, although expenditures were some $6,000 within the budget. The cost of professional financial advice had been just one half that of the previous six years, and $461,854 were added to the endowment. Of this,

$100,000 was from the estate of Mrs. Bowen, to establish foreign scholarships; Mrs. Bowen had paid the interest on the amount since 1929.

In 1941 the Council recommended, and the Academy subsequently elected, thirty-five distinguished physicians from Latin American republics as Corresponding Members.

Dr. F. P. Reynolds, former Assistant Secretary and Medical Secretary of the Committee on Medical Education, was elected an Honorary Fellow, and Dr. S. W. Lambert a Benefactor.

Dr. Ashford presented the Academy with a bust supposed to be of Dr. S. S. Purple by the American sculptor William R. O'Donovan. It now stands on the table in the entrance hall of the Academy. A bust of the late Dr. Lee Hurd was also accepted.

At the close of 1942, the Council ordered the appointment of a committee

> to be informed on the nature, quality and direction of the economic and social changes that are taking place now and that are clearly forecast for the immediate future; to define in particular how these changes are likely to affect medicine in its various aspects; to determine how the best elements in the science of medicine and its services to the public may be preserved and embodied in whatever changed social order may ultimately develop.

That was a big order. Dr. Goodridge, who was very active in urging establishment of the Committee, was later made its chairman, and its name was changed to the Committee on "Medicine and the Changing Order." It is interesting to note that in 1925 the title of Dr. George E. Vincent's Anniversary Address was "The Doctor and the Changing Order."

In 1942 the Academy lost a devoted friend and worker in the death of Dr. Walter L. Niles. Elected a Fellow in 1908, he had served long and faithfully, having been at various times a member of all the Standing Committees except Library. He had been on the Committee on Problems of Medical Practice for seven years, during four of which he was chairman, on Professional Standards for six years, and on Gifts and Bequests for four years. He was an elected Trustee 1928–1932, and a member of the Board's House

Committee for four years. Elected Vice-President in 1934, he therefore served on it as an ex-officio member for three years and was then elected for five more years, during which he was Chairman of the Board.

A born organizer, he had been made Dean of Cornell Medical College in 1919 and served for nine years. Owing to the illness of Dean Ladd, Dr. Niles was Acting Dean at the time of his death. Offered the Presidency of the Academy, he had declined, as his other duties would not allow time to do the office full justice.

A delightful personality, he justly won the confidence and friendship of a host of patients. He was only sixty-four at the time of his death.

The Council adopted these resolutions:

Few Fellows have rendered so much service and in so many capacities as did Dr. Walter L. Niles during his thirty-eight years of Academy Fellowship.

His devotion to Academy interests, added as it was to a life already over full of the responsibilities of a dean, a teacher of and practitioner of medicine, has always been of the sort that makes adequate expression of appreciation difficult.

He has contributed clearness of thought and soundness of decision to the proceedings of the Committees on Admissions, Public Health Relations, Problems of Medical Practice, Professional Standards, and Fund Raising, and as Chairman of the Board of Trustees and its Executive Committee, and a member of the Council.

Kindliness and gentleness of manner, patience and tolerance have colored every contact with his associates, and it is in this light that the memory of his accomplishments will live.

Dr. Samuel W. Lambert also died in 1942. The Library Committee adopted these resolutions:

By the death of Dr. Samuel W. Lambert the Library of the Academy of Medicine has lost one of its most devoted friends and staunchest supporters. The assembling of the collections in the Rare Book Room is to a great extent due to his interest and enthusiasm. He had much to do with making possible the purchase of the Streeter Collection, and later accessions.

His interest in the Anatomical Works of Vesalius led to a further search in Munich for the original wood-blocks and the discovery of many which had been lost up to that time. He originated the idea of the Library Publication Fund and from friends collected the necessary money to issue in our History of Medicine Series a beautiful Atlas containing all the Vesalian woodcuts which had been struck off nearly 400 years ago. He was a generous contributor up to his death and in 1941 he was made a Benefactor of the Academy.

Himself a Bibliophile of no mean attainments, among the rare books he was on his own ground. After his retirement from active practice, in 1932, it was rare for him not to drop in several times a week.

A member of the Library Committee from 1932 until his last illness, he was a regular, interesting and interested attendant at its meetings. The members who served with him will never forget his stimulating and often humorous remarks. His presence will be sadly missed.

The Library Committee wishes to record this appreciation of Dr. Samuel W. Lambert as a friend of the Library and a beloved associate.

The Council thus expressed for the Academy its appreciation of his services:

Since 1891, when Dr. Samuel W. Lambert first associated himself with its activities, the New York Academy of Medicine has profited greatly by his guidance and advice. During his Presidency, from 1927 to 1929 and for the following ten years as a Trustee, his influence was felt to advantage in all Academy procedures.

As a member of the Committee on Public Health Relations from 1929 to 1936, he contributed a keen perception of the delicate problems relating to the many questions of civic government constantly arising.

It was, however, in his ten years of service on the Committee on Library and to an even greater extent independently of that Committee, that his signal contribution was made. The Rare Book Collection will always connote a memory of Dr. Samuel W. Lambert and indeed every phase of the library work has benefited through support gained by his efforts.

Through it all, the burden of administration duties has been always lightened for his associates by his ready wit and humor.

The Trustees and Council wish to record their loss in the death of this good friend to the Academy and to them as fellow workers for its best interests.

Dr. Goodridge was urged to accept nomination for a third term, but he absolutely refused, feeling it was time for somebody else to take the Presidency. At the last meeting of the Council in 1942, Dr. Miller offered his congratulations to Dr. Goodridge for his service as President, and on his being able to resist the pressure to serve for a third term. Dr. Wilcox expressed his appreciation of his cooperation in everything connected with Academy management.

Dr. Arthur F. Chace was elected President.

1943–1944

Arthur F. Chace

DR. CHACE, thirty-eighth President of the Academy, was sixty-four years old when he took office. A Fellow since 1908, he had served on the Committee on Medical Education from 1924 to 1941, being its Chairman the last year, was Vice President 1937–1939, and a Trustee 1941–1942. He had also served in 1938 on the Committee on Academy Activities. He had been connected with the Post-Graduate Hospital and Medical School for many years.

In retiring, Dr. Goodridge spoke of the Academy's past with pride, and of its future with confidence, and he promised never to lose his interest in its activities and its ideals. Elected a Trustee, and as Chairman of the Committee on Medicine and the Changing Order, he kept his word.

Dr. Chace's address, "The Academy Meets the Challenge," promised support to the ever-increasing demands upon the Academy to blaze a trail for progress in solving the difficulties of the fast changing world in relation to medicine.

Early in 1943 a Moreland Act Commissioner reported on the administration of the Workmen's Compensation Law. The report showed that disgraceful practices were going on. Rebates from a commercial laboratory, amounting to some 40 percent and charged to carrier companies, were paid to physicians who referred diagnostic work to the laboratory. Loans were shown to have been made by physicians to an auditor of the State Insurance Fund, supposedly in the hope of securing approval of bills for services rendered to the claimant in compensation cases. Twenty Fellows of the Academy were accused of improper actions before the Moreland Commissioner. The charges were referred to the Committee on Professional Standards, which interviewed sixteen Fellows, the other four being in military service. Of the sixteen interviewed, the Committee was convinced seven were innocent of the charges and recommended that they be so informed, with a warning that, as Fellows of the Academy, they must avoid any *appearance* of participation in practices that might reflect unfavorably upon the standing of the Academy and the profession.

The Committee was "not convinced of the innocence" of seven others, but in some cases legally competent proof of guilt was not available. In two cases there was satisfactory evidence of guilt, one having confessed to receiving a small rebate. The Committee recommended that these seven should receive a reprimand from the Council, to the effect that their explanations, while perhaps *legally* satisfactory, were not *ethically* satisfactory.

The Council, after consulting legal Counsel, took immediate action, and sent a letter of clearance to those considered innocent, with warning against *appearance* of participation, and to the other nine, including the two considered guilty, a letter requesting their immediate resignation. Two promptly resigned and three asked for a reconsideration, which was refused.

To the pledge signed by applicants for Fellowship was added: "The undersigned agrees to accept the Council of the Academy as the sole and only judge of his qualifications to remain a Fellow."

The Constitution was amended in regard to discipline for *fee-splitting or receiving rebates* by adding:

By "fee-splitting" is meant the giving or receiving by a consultant or a referring physician, one to or from the other, of any portion of the remuneration paid to either by a patient for medical or surgical services rendered.

By "receiving a rebate" is meant the receipt by a physician of any moneys or gifts, or special privileges, from a laboratory, manufacturer or dispensing dealer to whom the physician has referred a patient or by whom service or material has been supplied to the physician's patient.

Both fee-splitting and receiving a rebate are to be considered unethical and a violation of the Constitutional regulations of the Academy.

During these two years the programs of the scientific meetings were harder to arrange, but they were carefully planned and were mostly well attended. In 1943 that dealing with the "Status of

Penicillin" attracted an audience of 674, and "The Present Status of the Treatment of Pneumonias" 325.

Many meetings were held at the Academy by outside organizations. The "Physicians' Forum" held a symposium on "Problems of Civilian Care in Wartime."

In February, 1943, at the suggestion of the Committee on Medical Information, the Academy cooperated with six health and relief organizations and the State and City Departments of Health in an all-day meeting commemorating the 100th anniversary of the publication of Oliver Wendell Holmes' paper on the Contagiousness of Puerperal Fever. Incidentally, it was also the tenth anniversary of the publication of the Academy's Report on Maternal Mortality. The day sessions were devoted to conferences on Maternal Health and Child Welfare, and the evening session was held at the Academy. Dr. Reginald Fitz of Boston spoke on "My Doctor Oliver Wendell Holmes" and Dr. B. P. Watson on "Oliver Wendell Holmes—a Century's Vindication of His Work on Puerperal Fever." An exhibition of the works of Holmes was prepared by the Library Staff.

In 1944 the attendance fell off, but 255 heard the papers on the use of plasma and plasma substitutes, and the treatment of burns, and 250 those on virus diseases; in only two instances the audience numbered less than 100.

Section meetings were also harder to arrange. In 1943 six of the eleven Sections had an average attendance of under 100; and the highest—Neurology and Psychiatry—was 168. In 1944 things were a little better, only two Sections having an average attendance of less than 100.

The Biggs Lectures were on "Malaria and Its Influence on World Health" by Lt. Col. Russell, and "International Health," by Dr. Wilbur A. Sawyer, Director, International Health Division of the Rockefeller Foundation.

For the first time in four years, in 1944, the May Stated Meeting of the Academy was resumed.

The attendance at the Library fell in 1943 to 37,458 and to 34,168 in 1944. That was a total decrease of 17,434, over 35 percent, since 1942.

The stack rooms had now become so crowded, even with the wooden shelves put up to meet the emergency, that in 1944 the Library was forced to box and move 40,000 duplicate volumes of periodicals to 10 East 103d Street, to join the boxes of "museum" material that were collecting dust and dirt there. These buildings are of course not fire-proof.

At the request of the Medical Consultant to the Eighth Service Command of the Army, a list of about 100 books, useful for an army hospital, was prepared, and all medical officers of the Army or Navy stationed near New York were invited to use the resources of the Library.

A legacy of $2,000 was received from Dr. Leo H. Shenier as a book fund, and Mrs. Hartwell added $1,000 to the principal of the Rare Book fund.

The Library staff was too busy to spare the time necessary to arrange many exhibitions. In 1943 a small collection of the works of Vesalius was exhibited to commemorate the 400th anniversary of the publication of *De Humani Corporis Fabrica.*

In 1944 a large shipment of 1942 issues of 220 periodicals, German, Italian and French, were received, and Swiss journals of 1942 and 1943.

During the first fourteen weeks of 1944 only thirteen Fellows used the Library on Saturday evenings. Keeping it open required the presence of five staff members, increasingly difficult to secure. It was voted, during the present emergency, to close the Library at 5 P.M. on Saturdays.

Among the important activities of the Committee on Public Health Relations were the working out of a program of medical selection for industrial education, to meet the demands for war manpower, which was adopted in full by local authorities; a revision of the medical standards of the Municipal Civil Service Commission, for positions calling for strenuous exertion; and support of the movement for recruiting practical nurses, which resulted in an increase the next year of 75 percent in the number of enrolled students in approved schools for practical nurses.

The Committee as usual, printed a leaflet on its activities in 1943. This called forth the following in the *Journal* of the A.M.A.:

BOOK NOTICES

This report reviews the active program in public health relations which should be studied by medical societies across the nation. It is a real program of public health relations, not merely a program of publicity. The committee of public health relations of the academy has actually gone to work and made studies, held conferences with interested groups and made contributions to a long list of problems and topics. The index alone gives an idea of the range of this committee's activities. Alphabetically the committee has had under consideration in 1943 abortions, adolescent delinquency, barbiturates, the Beveridge plan, malaria and world health, butter substitutes, pasteurization of certified milk, medical examinations by the Civil Service Commission, qualifications for a director of health education in schools, eye clinics, training the handicapped for war work, industrial medicine, inhalational therapy, qualifications of an ophthalmologist in the labor department, margarine, maternal mortality, qualifications of a commissioner for the mental hygiene department, payment of physicians in municipal hospitals, practical nurses, optical plans, the opticians' bill, optometrists in eye clinics, central file of psychiatric histories, the Public Health Research Institute of the City of New York, rebates, ringworm of the scalp, the compulsory examination of school teachers, social hygiene, speech rehabilitation, tuberculin tests, venereal disease instruction and youth correction authority. A real program of public health relations involves service, not mere publicity. This report exemplifies and summarizes such a program. It is recommended to the secretaries, medical or lay, of medical societies and to public health officials everywhere.

In 1944, the war having emphasized the need of rapid return of the sick and wounded to maximum efficiency, another conference, supported by the Josiah Macy, Jr., Foundation, was held on Convalescent Care. Its valuable findings were published. The whole subject of job placement of the disabled and crippled, as well as those discovered by the Selective Service Boards, occupied much of the Committee's time and effort.

The first edition of *Preventive Medicine in Modern Practice*, published by the Committee in 1942, had been out of print for over a year, but the shortage of paper had prevented a second edition to meet the constant demand for it. This appeared in 1944, and was well received.

The Committee studied intensively the status of Workmen's Compensation and made recommendations as to amending the law, which the Commissioner intimated were the most important received, and most, if not all, would be incorporated into the law.

In view of the Moreland Commissioner's investigation of unethical practices, the Committee was recommending strongly that the question of fee-splitting be reviewed. Recommendations were therefore made relating not only to Workmen's Compensation but to amendments to the general education law, in which fee-splitting, when proved, would constitute a cause for debarring a physician from the practice of medicine, with the penal law amended to make it a misdemeanor.

In 1943 the Committee on Medical Education inaugurated a new feature. The war had caused the suspension of meetings of special societies, at which reports of clinical research were usually presented. A "Clinical Research Meeting" was held at the Academy in three different halls, and some twenty-seven presentations were made. It was attended by research workers in the Metropolitan area, and brief abstracts of the papers were published later in the *Bulletin*. This meeting was held again, successfully, in 1944.

The Graduate Fortnights were held, the subject in 1943 being "Disorders of the Digestive Tract." The paid registration was 395. In 1944 "Infections and Their Treatment" was the subject, and 296 registered. When it is remembered how many younger physicians, those usually attending the Fortnights, were away in service, and that all medical officers in uniform were admitted without registration or fee, the numbers were surprisingly good.

In 1944 a permanent drug exhibit was established in the Academy for the double purpose of educating physicians in the use of the newer pharmaceuticals, and in recognition of the contribution of the great pharmaceutical houses to medical research and therapy.

It was opened at the time of the Graduate Fortnight; the total attendance during that period was over 2,000. After the close of the Fortnight, there was a daily average attendance of 62. The exhibit was under the control of a special subcommittee of the Committee on Medical Education.

At the request of Dr. Charles L. Mayer this committee awarded four fellowships of $2,000 each for research.

The Friday afternoon lectures were given as usual, with an average attendance of about 150.

Beside its regular work of issuing press releases, answering inquiries, reviewing manuscripts and supervising radio talks, the Committee on Medical Information was active and helpful in other ways. In 1943 it undertook, at the request of the Commissioner of Health, Dr. E. L. Stebbins, a study of the formation of a Bureau of Information in the Health Department. The Commissioner adopted the plan suggested.

In 1943 it held its Fourth Annual Health Education Conference, devoted to the subject of Radio in Health Education. This was well attended, with 170 participants representing thirty-six organizations. As a result of the conference, the "critical study" made with a grant from the Rockefeller Foundation, in 1942, and the papers presented at the Conference by the representatives of the radio industry, and official voluntary health organizations, were assembled, and in 1945 were published by the Columbia University Press, under the title *Radio in Health Education.*

The Laity Lectures were continued, and were well attended. In spite of the shortage of paper, the Columbia University Press continued to publish them, and those of 1943–44 caused many favorable comments in the medical press, including the *British Medical Journal.*

In 1944 an innovation was tried. The lectures, six in number, were given at intervals of two weeks, and were all on Psychiatry in Clinical Medicine. The average attendance was 650.

The Annual Press dinner, omitted since 1940, was resumed in 1944. Dr. Wightman, the steady supporter of this committee, again presided. Four representatives of the radio and eleven of the press attended, and all hoped the dinners would be continued.

It was a particularly active and constructive year for the Committee on Medical Information.

In 1944 the Academy Medal was awarded to Dr. Oswald T. Avery of the Rockefeller Institute for his work in Bacteriology.

In 1942 Dr. Miller had refused renomination as an elective Trustee.

The Trustees and Council passed this resolution:

The Trustees and Council are mindful that today they convene for the first time since 1925 without the official presence of Dr. Miller as a member of both governing bodies of the Academy in the capacity of a Trustee. This statement does not complete the story of the service rendered by Dr. Miller during the past many years, for the benefits of his advice have come to us through various channels.

A Fellow since 1904, there are few committees—be they Standing, annually appointed or subcommittees—on which Dr. Miller has not served greatly to the advantage of each.

He has been a member of the Committee on Public Health Relations since its inception in 1911, its Chairman from 1929 until he became President of the Academy for the years 1937 and 1938 and again has occupied this position of Chairman since 1942.

The recently published Thirty Year Report of this Committee is perhaps the best index of Dr. Miller's influence on the extent of important services rendered to the city, state, and nation. Too numerous to list in their entirety, many of these pronouncements are outstanding. Among the early studies those in connection with the Standard Nomenclature, the control of proprietary hospitals and the administration of Veterans' Relief, form a background for the important consideration of the Medical Aspects of the Workmen's Compensation Law—just finished and to Dr. Miller's valuable assistance in the activities of the Committee on Medicine and the Changing Order.

Not only are the Trustees and Council mindful today of these services but they are convinced that all those interested in the Academy activities will for a long time to come remain equally mindful and appreciative.

Finances were, of course, a tremendous problem during these years of war. The budget adopted for 1943 had estimated expenditures of $264,451 and income of $255,730. This meant an anticipated deficit of $8,721 even with "contributions" expected of $30,000. To meet the increased cost of living and to make replacements of absolutely necessary personnel—twenty-five had left for war service or defense work, which paid enormous wages and salaries—the adopted budget expenditures had to be exceeded by some $19,000. Salaries up to a certain point were raised 10 percent. The returns from investments were some $6,000 less, dues $1,600, and room assessments over $4,000 below expected income from these sources. On the other hand, contributions were over $22,500 more than expected and the *Bulletin* earned nearly $3,000 more than was estimated. All Standing Committee budgets were lived up to, or very nearly so. Several mortgages had to be foreclosed and "Foreclosed Property Expense" totaled over $10,000; because of this the Academy closed the year with a deficit of $11,840.91.

By the will of Mrs. R. T. Wilson, a legacy was received of $30,000, the interest to be used to pay the cost of lectures on medical subjects, the selection to be entirely in the hands of the Council, the only stipulation being that it be announced the lecture was given in memory of her first husband, George R. Siedenburg. The fund was accepted, thereby establishing a precedent in creating a lecture in memory of a layman.

Mr. R. T. Wilson also for three years gave annually $2,000 to support the Graduate Fortnight in memory of his wife.

Mrs. Stella L. Stone promised $5,000 annually to establish a fund to be known as the Dr. A. Richard Stone Memorial Fund, in income to pay expenses for medical lectures. This was accepted, and the final payment for the $25,000 promised was made in 1947.

In 1944, with an anticipated deficit of over $12,000, the Council appointed a committee to consider raising of dues or other means of increasing income from the Fellowship. Three hundred and fifty-five Fellows, of all classes, were exempt from dues owing to military service, the loss of income amounting to $13,500. The committee recommended there should be no permanent or temporary increase in dues; there should be no assessment, only justifiable in an emergency, which it felt did not exist; and it was opposed to a voluntary subscription to offset loss of dues.

The Comptroller reported that since 1931, there had been an increase of approximately $1,000,000 in the Academy portfolio, but the income was less than in 1931, owing to lower yield from investment.

The year turned out better than expected. Every source of income except room assessments turned in substantially more than estimated, and although expenditures were some $16,000 more than planned, income for the year was $12,470.55 more than expenditures. The returns from subscriptions and advertising made the *Bulletin* more than self-supporting.

The Steering Committee had been giving valiant service and contributions for the two years had amounted to $110,984. Large bequests from estates, and a few gifts, increased the endowment fund, general and for special purposes, by $343,650.

1945–1946

William Worthington Herrick
George Baehr

DR. HERRICK was in his sixty-sixth year when he became the thirty-ninth President of the Academy. He had long been connected with the College of Physicians and Surgeons and was much interested in the improvement of medical education. He had been a Fellow since 1910, but had not been intimately associated with Academy affairs, although he had presented several papers at Stated Meetings.

He brought to his duties a well-trained mind, an experience in organization, and a wide knowledge of present-day problems. His Inaugural Address, "Scientific Humanism in this Changing World," showed his appreciation of the Academy's position, responsibilities, and opportunities. He said, in closing, "The time calls for candid, honest and courageous leadership, a leadership based upon Truth. If we of the Academy continue to give such leadership in our proper field, we shall have done all that is possible in preserving for our calling that freedom of action that has given American Medicine its high standards and its efficient service to the public," and he suggested the adoption of "Scientific Humanism" as the goal.

It was a trying year for the Academy and its administration. The war came to an end in September, and in addition to the difficulties of war were added those of demobilization. There were the many problems of readjustment to face.

The Library probably had the most difficult time, and the Director in his report to the Council in December, gave an accurate account of some of its problems. During the previous twelve months, of the forty-one positions on the staff, forty had been filled. To keep those forty positions full, forty-five *new* persons had been employed, and five older employees had been transferred to more responsible positions. At the end of this period, of the eight stack assistants, on whose promptness and accuracy so much of the comfort of readers depended and whose efficiency required time to acquire, only *one* had been on duty for a year. Everyone had to "fill in" temporarily and it was no uncommon sight to see the Assistant Librarian, Miss Doe, at the reception desk.

The proper *replacement* of books is essential to finding them again. So unreliable were many of the stack assistants that a new system was adopted. All books replaced, instead of standing end up, were put back edge up, and subsequently checked by an experienced person and rightly placed. The number of readers fell in 1945 to 32,639, which was a help to the staff. In 1946 the shortage of help continued so acute that the replacing of books each day, which takes many hours, was impossible, and the Library was authorized to postpone opening to the public every day till 10.30, thus giving the staff a precious hour and a half to complete this essential work. It was open to Fellows, as usual, at 9 A.M.

In 1946 there were fifty-eight changes in the staff, mostly among the stack assistants. The long undelivered foreign periodicals, held by agents, began to arrive. During the year 576 packages of German and Dutch periodicals for 1941–46 arrived, and four large cases of French periodicals and other lots added to the work of the Library staff.

Readers increased nearly a thousand a month, and totaled 43,788 for the year.

Too much cannot be said of the spirit and patience of the staff during those years.

There was little chance to prepare exhibitions. An interesting collection of early feeding bottles was shown by Dr. L. H. Koplik in connection with a paper on "History of Methods of Feeding Infants," read at a joint session of the Sections on Pediatrics and on Historical and Cultural Medicine. Several other small exhibits were also arranged.

In the fall of 1945 a group of Fellows organized as the "Friends of the Rare Book Room of The New York Academy of Medicine, Inc." to "collect annually funds adequate for the purchase of such items as the Librarian deems desirable for the Rare Book Room. The 'Friends' also plan to stimulate gifts of money and books to the Rare Book Room from the general public." Several donations were received during 1946 from Fellows, through the "Friends," and early in 1947 three volumes were bought and presented.

In 1945, Mr. Frank Place, after forty years' service with the Library, retired. He had been Reference Librarian and also had had general supervision of the collection of portraits. An illuminated scroll, expressing the Academy's appreciation of his long and faithful service, was presented to him, and the Library Committee and a few friends presented, as a personal expression of esteem, several books which he had expressed a desire to own.

In 1945 the Committee on Public Health Relations, at the request of the Department of Health, studied the question of the promiscuous use of barbiturates and sulfonamids. Also on request, it studied, and reported on, health standards for teachers, periodic examination of hospital employees for tuberculosis, quarantine regulations, child adoption, medical care for the aged, Veterans' tuberculosis hospitals, and many other problems.

In cooperation with the State Society, letters of protest on the Chiropractic Bill were sent to the Legislature, and Dr. Aranow was delegated to represent the Academy at the hearing on the Bill.

Commissioner Stebbins resigned in 1946 to take a position at Johns Hopkins. The Mayor appointed Dr. Bernecker, Commissioner of Hospitals, as Commissioner of Health. The Public Health Relations Committee took exception to the appointment on the ground that the Charter, amended in 1936 at the Committee's insistence, required that the Commissioner of Health must have had at least eight years' experience in public health administration, or in teaching, or both; and that hospital administration could not be considered public health administration. These resolutions were sent to the Mayor by messenger and given to the press the next day. Two days later the Mayor reappointed Dr. Bernecker to his previous position as Commissioner of Hospitals and appointed Dr. Israel Weinstein Acting Commissioner of Health.

In 1946 the Committee, together with the Section on Historical and Cultural Medicine, cooperated with Commissioner Weinstein in celebrating the Eightieth Anniversary of the Health Department. The celebration was well attended.

The Committee undertook a study of rabies, its prevention, and control, which was accepted for publication in the *United States Public Health Reports.* Another extensive study was on the facilities for the care and treatment of alcoholism. This received a favorable write-up by the New York *Times* and was published in the *Quarterly Journal of Studies on Alcohol.* A conference was planned on the subject for 1947, with many groups to take part.

A study of the facilities and method of administration of birth control "Clinics" disclosed unsatisfactory conditions.

The Red Cross was anxious to continue its blood bank and blood plasma activity of the war and, failing to reach an agreement with the County Societies, appealed to the Academy for help. After long discussions, an arrangement was made by which Gamma Globulin was made available free of charge to all physicians for use in very young or delicate children exposed to measles. This is having surprising results.

Owing to the increased tendency in industry to eliminate physically handicapped persons, the United States Employment Service asked advice of the Committee; a conference was held, and it was decided to have the proceedings published by the United States Employment Office.

In 1945, with the cessation of hostilities, there was a great increase in requests for help in securing positions on hospital staffs, to round out training curtailed by the demands of the war, to secure qualification by one of the various Boards of Specialties. In the last three months of the year, 746 visits were made to the Committee on Medical Education as against 177 in 1944. In 1946 there were 1,971 visitors, looking for help or information; 1,578 were demobilized veterans and 232 were physicians from South America.

In 1946, the accumulated income from the Bowen Scholarships, unexpendable during the war, was allotted in "grants in aid" of $500 each, to nine young physicians who had been discharged from the Medical Departments of the Army and Navy, to allow them to complete their shortened interneships.

In both these years the Committee again arranged clinical research meetings, which drew good audiences. Twenty-seven reports were presented in 1945, but only nine in 1946, as the need for these meetings had become much less pressing.

The Fortnights were very successful. That of 1945, on "Contributions of the War Effort to Medicine," drew a paid registration of 282. In 1946, the subject of "Tumors" attracted wide attention; the expenses of the Fortnight were covered by a registration of 553, from twenty-five states and seven foreign countries. Ninety-seven percent of registrants came from New York State. In both years the lectures, demonstrations, and hospital clinics were well attended.

The Drug Exhibit, changed each year during the summer interval, was reopened in time for the Fortnight and drew a large number of physicians; the attendance was very good all through the year.

At the suggestion of the President, a subcommittee of the Committee on Medical Education studied the oft-recurring plan for a museum. It recommended the erection of a Hall for Exhibits, in order to display scientific material of current interest to the profession and the public and to furnish a live and changing exhibit rather than a static and cumulative collection such as a museum would provide.

The Stated Meetings were well planned and drew surprisingly good audiences in 1945. With the return of "peace" conditions, the attendance rose to between 400 and 600.

The Biggs Memorial Lectures were given and, although the fund did not pay expenses, excellent speakers were secured. In 1945 Dr. Laurence H. Snyder, Professor of Medical Genetics, Ohio State University, spoke on "Medical Genetics and Public Health," and in 1946 Dr. F. C. Bishopp, U.S. Department of Agriculture, discussed "The Medical and Public Health Importance of the Insecticide DDT."

In 1946, at the suggestion of the James Ewing Memorial Committee, the first "James Ewing Memorial Lecture" was given by

Dr. H. T. Karsner, Western Reserve University, on "Tumors of the Endocrine Glands." The Memorial Committee supplied the speaker.

The attendance at Section Meetings in 1946 increased markedly. The average was under 100 in only one Section, three had averages of over 200, and two over 300. The banner Section was Surgery, with an average of 337. The average for all Sections was 207.

In 1945 the New York Pathological Society submitted a series of questions as to whether certain procedures should be considered "fee-splitting." These were referred to the Committee on Professional Standards, which recommended, and the Council approved, that when a physician or a commercial laboratory submitted a pathological specimen to a pathologist, the latter must bill the patient directly; that when referred to a hospital pathologist, not receiving a salary from the hospital, the pathologist must bill the patient direct, but that if he did receive a salary, the hospital must bill the patient, and no part of the fee could be paid to the pathologist.

In October a five-day series of rather objectionable articles on Bellevue Hospital appeared in the press; five physicians on the staff were mentioned by name and quoted. The Committee on Professional Standards investigated, and the physicians mentioned by name appeared before it. When interviewed by the reporter they had thought he was writing a history of Bellevue. Two had no idea that what they said was for publication. The physicians were indignant that the Hospital authorities had not given them any chance to read what was to be printed. The Committee exonerated them and informed the Commissioner of Hospitals, the Medical Superintendent of Bellevue, and the Executive Committee of the Medical Board that the Committee on Medical Information was always ready to advise as to the character of material to be published in the press regarding hospitals, and suggested that in the future its services be made use of.

The Committee on Medical Information continued its busy career. Requests for opinions and advice were received in the usual large number.

The Laity Lectures in 1945–46 were devoted to the general topic of "Medicine Today" and gave a careful analysis of the various activities which were making medicine so complicated and so effective. They were rather more technical than heretofore and less devoted to practical matters. The attendance, though good, fell off somewhat. In 1946 the older plan of lectures on matters dealing with practical medical care of interest to the laity was resumed.

In both 1945 and 1946 Annual Health Conferences were again held and were well attended.

In 1945, the last year of the "five-year period," the Steering Committee, on its original plan to raise $250,000 for annual expenses during the five years, $300,000 for Library Extension, and an increased endowment, could show $313,886 received for current expenses, and $244,300 received for library extension. The Director in his report to the Council in December, 1945, stated the "Holdings" of the Academy at the end of 1940, were $3,135,462, with an income of $249,473, while for 1946 "Holdings" totaled $4,831,000, with an income of $342,000.

While the deficit for 1942 and 1943 was $32,000 and over, in the other three years the balance totaled $52,800, making $20,687 available for the "special reserve fund" during these five years.

The *Bulletin* of the Academy was paying for itself. It had a subscription list of around 800 and, when it is realized that Library exchanges were over 700, it is obvious that the Library saved many dollars thereby. Its total circulation was around 4,250.

In the budget for 1946, income was estimated at $318,000 and expenditures at $356,000. It was absolutely necessary to raise many salaries, "administration" expenses were $8,000 over the budget, and the Library's some $13,000. All other departments kept within the budget. Total income was $335,774, some $17,500 more than estimated, and expenses were only $7,000 more than expected. The year closed with a deficit of $27,950.

Effective January 1, 1947, dues were increased 25 percent for all classes of members and life membership fees were also increased according to actuarial methods.

Dr. Herrick died suddenly in June, 1945, in a heart attack. He had had warnings for a few months, but carried on as usual. He was the first President of the Academy in ninety-nine years to die in office. The Academy was, of course, inactive at the time. At the meeting of the Council and Trustees in October, the following resolutions were adopted:

> Dr. Herrick's choice of a title for his inaugural address, "Scientific Humanism," proved itself during the too short term of his service to be peculiarly descriptive of his own personality. His approach to every Academy duty was expressive of just this dominant personal characteristic, scientific humanism. He quoted a remark of another great physician, "I am too much in earnest for either humility or vanity," and he referred to an institution as being but the lengthening shadow of a man.
>
> We now have come to a full appreciation that he lengthened the Academy shadow to a degree all out of proportion to the five months period of his term of office. Indeed, as one reads that inaugural address in its entirety, the impression grows that the most suitable memorial has all unwittingly been written. The purposes to which the Academy's effort has been dedicated for nearly one hundred years have suffered a great loss in his untimely death.
>
> The trustees and Council would further emphasize their appreciation of the privilege of their personal contacts with Dr. Herrick.

A fine tribute to him was published in the *Bulletin.*

The Senior Vice President, Dr. Cornelius P. Rhoads, became President ad interim. The Constitution required a successor to be nominated and elected at a Stated or Special Meeting. The October meeting, coming so close to the Graduate Fortnight, had been omitted for several years. The first Stated Meeting was in November, and the Nominating Committee proposed Dr. George Baehr, who was elected in December, to serve till the end of 1946.

1946

Dr. George Baehr therefore became the fortieth President of the Academy, December 5, 1945. A Fellow since 1918, he was in his fifty-ninth year when elected. He had served long in many capacities. He had been a member of the Committee on Medical Education, 1924–27, and of the Committee on Public Health Relations, 1926–41, and its chairman from 1937 to 1941; away in service during the World War, he became a member again in 1944. He had also served on the Committee to Investigate Problems relating to Medical Practice from 1930 to 1941, and had been on the Editorial Board of the *Health Examiner* and its successor *Preventive Medicine* from 1934 till it was discontinued. He had been a Trustee from 1934 to 1939, and again in 1941–45, and a member of the Committee on Medicine and the Changing Order and of the Steering Committee from 1943.

At the May meeting of the Council, Dr. Miller asked for the floor and stated that he was deeply interested in the question of the Directorship of the Academy. Seven years ago Dr. Wilcox had come as Director. Now, though still a young man, in spite of being older in years, he felt that the time had come to resign. His place had been filled, but those seven years of close relationship with those around the table should not slip by without recognition of the extraordinary contributions Dr. Wilcox had made to the Academy. His service had been so well-rounded that one could not say what was most outstanding—his handling of finances, the staff, the Standing Committees, or the outside world. Dr. Wilcox had done a great deal not only to strengthen the Academy on the inside but had contributed tremendously to its prestige. This would be the last meeting he would attend officially and Dr. Miller thought it proper for the Council to put on record its heartfelt appreciation of his services, to wish him godspeed, a fine vacation, a long life and years of fun. All knew the Academy would always have his interest and support. Dr. Baehr echoed these sentiments and the Council then took a standing vote of thanks to Dr. Wilcox.

Dr. Howard R. Craig, on recommendation of the Council, and with the endorsement of Dr. Wilcox, was elected Director, to take office October 1, 1946. Dr. Craig had had much experience with Academy affairs. Elected a Fellow in 1927, he was for ten years Secretary and Chairman of the Section on Historical and Cultural Medicine and a member of its Advisory Committee. He had served on the Committee on Honorary Fellowships and Medal since 1935; the Library Committee since 1938, as chairman from 1942; the Committee on Academy History since 1942; and was also a member of the Steering Committee and the Committee on Medicine and the Changing Order. He was fifty-two years old when he took office.

At the December meeting Dr. George Baehr was reelected for a full term of two years.

In 1946 the Committee on Medicine and the Changing Order completed its work, and announced its report would be ready in the fall, or early in 1947.

In December, 1942, the Council had authorized the appointment of a committee "with unlimited latitude to study present trends in medicine." In January, 1943, the President was authorized to appoint a larger committee than originally intended, and its scope was made broader than a mere economic one. It was later given authority to solicit funds for its studies. The Committee met the first time February 25, 1943, "not sure what their objectives were." Its name, the Committee on Medicine and the Changing Order, was not adopted till later. In the June number of the *Bulletin* appeared the following announcement:

A COMMITTEE TO STUDY MEDICINE AND THE CHANGING ORDER has been organized by The New York Academy of Medicine. The objectives of this Committee are:

To be informed on the nature, quality and direction of the economic and social changes that are taking place now and that are clearly forecast for the immediate future; to define in particular how these changes are likely to affect medicine in its various aspects; to determine how the best elements in the science of medicine and its services to the public may be preserved and embodied in whatever changed social order may ultimately develop.

The Committee plans to survey the changes that are currently taking place in our economic and social organization and to consider also any changes which are likely to take place during the next decade.

In this survey the Committee will solicit information and opinion from a wide variety of groups, including sociologists, economists, representatives of organized labor, industrialists, bankers and politicians.

Also, in this connection, the Committee will solicit the cooperation of those intimately connected with medicine, hospital authorities, hospital clinicians, public health workers, those interested in graduate education, physicians in industrial medicine, medical social workers, and workers in voluntary health organizations.

We wish to emphasize the point that the Committee will devote itself primarily to the study of how, within the changing social order, the best qualities in medical service, in medical education and in medical research can be preserved and developed.

It is expected that the study will continue until sufficient evidence has been accumulated to make possible a considered report.

The members of the original Committee were:

Dr. Malcolm Goodridge, *Chairman*	Dr. Tracy J. Putnam
Dr. Arthur F. Chace	Dr. Wilson G. Smillie
Dr. James Alexander Miller	Dr. Jean A. Curran
Dr. Alan Gregg	Dr. Herbert B. Wilcox
Dr. George Baehr	Dr. Howard R. Craig
Dr. Harry Aranow	Dr. E. Tolstoi
Dr. I. Ogden Woodruff	Dr. E. H. Pool
Dr. Paul Reznikoff	Dr. Robert E. Pound
Dr. Henry W. Cave *	Dr. Iago Galdston, *Secretary*

Committee Associates

Mr. John W. Davis
Mr. W. S. Gifford

* Resigned at the first meeting

From time to time other members were added, until the Committee numbered fifty, of whom thirty-five were physicians, two clergymen, one a dentist, three registered nurses, nine of the laity, and two representatives of labor. The latter two resigned from the Committee during 1946.

The Committee formed a "Program and Planning Committee" composed of fifteen members, later called the "Reviewing Committee." This Committee and the whole Committee met 120 times, with a full attendance. Reliable information was sought on every possible angle of the wide field of study. Forty-eight experts were invited to give their individual experience and opinions on special phases—economics, sociology, industry, labor, insurance, public health services, the hospital, rural and urban medicine, nursing, dentistry, pre-medical and medical education, the problem of the Negro physician, and research. Thirty-eight of these individuals were nonmembers of the Committee. The two labor members did not personally appear but sent detailed reports, which were read. Special subcommittees studied all phases of the special problems involved. It should be noted that the Chairman presided at every meeting held except one, when he was prevented by illness.

The Committee had prepared for publication, before its official report appeared, ten valuable reports:

"American Medical Practice in the Perspectives of a Century," by Bernhard J. Stern, Ph.D.
"Government in Public Health," by Harry S. Mustard, M.D.
"A Future for Preventive Medicine," by Edward J. Stieglitz, M.D.
"Medicine in Industry," by Bernhard J. Stern, Ph.D.
"Nursing and Nursing Education," by Agnes Gelinas, R.N.
"Medical Services by Government—Local, State, and Federal," by Bernhard J. Stern, Ph.D.
"Medical Education and the Changing Order," by Raymond B. Allen, M.D., Ph.D.
"The American Hospital," by E. H. L. Corwin, Ph.D.
"Dentistry: an Agency of Health Service," by Malcolm W. Carr, D.D.S.
"Health Insurance in the United States," by Nathan Sinai, Dr. P. H., Odin W. Anderson and Melvin L. Dollar.

Two other monographs were in preparation: "Medical Research" and "Rural Medicine," and a further volume of "Essays" relating to Medicine and the Changing Order was planned.

The Commonwealth Fund, Milbank Memorial Fund, and the Josiah Macy, Jr., Foundation contributed $54,000 for the expenses of the study, and in addition, the Commonwealth Fund published the ten monographs and the final report, "Medicine in the Changing Order."

In May, 1946, Dr. Baehr, with Drs. Craig and Galdston, appeared before the Committee on Education and Labor of the United States Senate. Dr. Baehr made a fine statement of the Academy's stand on the whole subject of compulsory health insurance and its objections to Bill S. 1606, known as the Wagner-Murray-Dingell Bill, then before that Committee. His testimony in full was printed for the use of the Senate Committee.

Again in December, 1946, Drs. Baehr, Miller, Craig, and Galdston were invited by a group of Senators to discuss with them informally the subject of legislation in regard to Health Insurance. This was *not* before a Senate Committee, and there is no printed report.

The final report appeared in March, 1947, during the celebration of the Centenary. It attacked the problem: How could medical service be bettered? How did economic and social conditions and changes affect it? The report emphasized the futility of viewing medical care as an isolated phenomenon; it must be viewed as a part of present-day-living. Every phase of medical service is related to every other, and this must be understood to appreciate the entire picture.

Many far-reaching recommendations were made, concerning a multiplicity of problems of varying geographical, social, economic, and educational circumstances: Origins of Present Problems in American Medicine; Medicine and the Changing Order in recent Decades; The Health of the Nation; Medical Care in Urban Areas; Medical Care in Rural Areas; Extension of Public Health Services; The Quality of Medical Care; Preventive Medicine; The Hospital; Nursing; Medical Insurance: Voluntary and Compulsory; The Method and the Goal.

There was wide editorial comment and approval. The *Times* said, in part:

> Though not every possible solution of the problem presented by medical care has been or could be considered, this succinct, temperate document is well worth the money and the effort expended on its preparation. It comes from an eminent body of medical men, who have consulted representatives of the public as well as physicians and health officers. It should be required reading for legislators, county medical societies, private practitioners and the public.
>
> . . . The Committee concludes against "compulsory health insurance at the present time." But the corollary conclusion is "that everything should be done . . . to hasten the growth of voluntary medical insurance."

Those who see the Wagner-Murray-Dingell bill as the final answer may be tempted to dismiss this committee's findings as merely what was to be expected of any study under medical auspices. Any such dismissal would be a grave error. The study uses the historical approach to point the vast gap in experience which must be bridged before any final reorganization of medical practice is made. The only experience there is to draw on with compulsory insurance chiefly European indicates that "national compulsory medical insurance would not and could not realize the promises made for it and would inevitably create new and formidable evils of its own.". . .

The American tendency is to look for immediate action, usually in the form of cover-all legislation, to correct any such inadequacy as is now recognized in the field of health and medical care. In this case hasty legislation, the committee points out, is "a leap in the dark; the results are at best uncertain, may even be disastrous and, in any event, are irrevocable." No citizen who is sincerely interested in wider distribution of good medical care, either from an individual or from a social and humanitarian viewpoint, can afford to dismiss the academy committee's report.

The Academy had been planning for its Centennial, in a general way, for some months. With the retirement of the Director, things rather held back, and it was not until October that the work began with full vigor. A most detailed program was arranged, with an extensive exhibit illustrating its development, at the Academy, and other exhibitions relating to the Academy and to early medical history in New York were shown at the New York Public Library, New York Historical Society, Museum of the City of New York, and Metropolitan Museum of Art. Kennedy & Co. gave an interesting exhibit of prints, and the International Business Machine Corporation, Dry Dock Savings Bank, and the College of Physicians and Surgeons gave small ones. All this was in 1947 and details do not come within the scope of the "First One Hundred Years of the Academy."

Suffice it to say, the Academy celebrated its Centennial.

The Start of a Second Century

FROM A SMALL GROUP of 185 men, a number of whom were influenced by motives of self-advancement; without an official home and with little immediate prospect of obtaining one; torn by internal rivalries and jealousies; originally administered by ten officers, a President, four Vice-Presidents, a Recording Secretary, Domestic and Foreign Corresponding Secretaries, a Treasurer, a Librarian, and five Standing Committees, all elected for one year only; without paid assistance, except for a professional collector of dues; with a hoped-for annual income of only $555.00; but with a full measure of determination and boundless optimism—from these beginnings has developed the present New York Academy of Medicine. It now has a membership of 1,646 Resident, 516 Non-Resident, Associate and Research Fellows, all paying dues, 20 Honorary, and 81 Corresponding Fellows. More than 200 Fellows have paid dues for thirty years or more, and are now exempt. Total membership in all classes is over 2,400. Dues for 1947 were $88,750.

The Academy owns its own building, free of debt, occupying a plot 100 x 125 feet, and the adjacent lot, 75 x 100 feet, for the proposed and much needed extension. It has an endowment of $4,536,562, and had, in 1946, an income of $335,774.59.

Incorporated under the laws of the State of New York, its purposes as stated in the Constitution of 1940 are the advancement of the science and art of medicine, the maintenance of a public medical library, and the promotion of public health and medical education.

Its organization consists of a President, elected for two years, three Vice-Presidents, serving three years, one retiring each year, a Secretary and a Treasurer elected for three years.

According to the Charter, the Board of Trustees consists of "not less than ten, nor more than twenty-three." Ten are elected, to serve five years, two retiring each year. The President, Secretary, and Treasurer are also members, ex officio. The Trustees have charge of all the finances, vested funds, personal property, and real estate of the Academy; all expenditures must be authorized by them.

The Council transacts the general executive business and determines policies. It has general supervision of Academy activities, as well as of its Sections. It is composed of the six officers of the Academy, the ten elected Trustees, and the chairmen of the six Standing Committees, twenty-one members in all. (A Vice President is appointed Chairman of the Committee on Sections.) The Council passes on all recommendations of the various committees of the Academy. It has authority to discipline any Fellow, except by expulsion, which must be voted by the Academy. In a case of fee-splitting, however, of which a Fellow is found guilty, he may be expelled by a three-fourths vote of the Council.

The Council appoints the Director of the Academy, and the Executive Secretaries of Standing Committees.

The President is the titular head of the Academy. He presides over all meetings of the Academy and of the Council, and appoints all non-elective committees to serve during his administration. He is, ex officio, a member of all Standing and other Committees, except that on Nominations. He cannot commit the Academy to any course of action without the approval of the Council.

The entire administration is the responsibility of the Director, who sees that all orders of the Council are carried out, and that the building is properly run and kept in repair. (The maintenance personnel numbers twenty.) All orders of each department pass over his desk. He attends meetings of all committees. With him work the Comptroller, Mr. Arthur E. Eberle, and a staff of nine.

The Academy is always in need of increased income to meet its budget. That from Endowment and Fellows' dues is entirely inadequate. The raising of money is in the hands of the Steering Committee, composed of thirteen Fellows. The routine work is carried on by the Public Relations Counsel, Mr. Donald Price. It is advised by a Lay Council, consisting of fifteen gentlemen, whose chairman is Mr. Walter S. Gifford. This Lay Council renders most valuable service. The Academy is in desperate need of more endowment.

Legal Counsel is Mr. John W. Davis, of Davis, Polk, Wardwell, Sunderland and Kiendl. Deeply interested in the Academy, he has been an active and most valuable legal adviser.

The Library is the most important activity of the Academy. Its affairs and policies are watched over by the Library Committee, established in 1875. It consists of nine members, three being elected and three retiring each year. It meets each month, from October through May. It establishes the rules of the Library, the days and hours of opening and closing, subject to the approval of the Council, and recommends its budget for the year.

The Library contains 251,981 bound volumes, exclusive of duplicates, and 148,446 pamphlets. It is the largest medical library, public or private, in the United States, next to that of the Surgeon General, and serves more readers than any other medical library, 43,788 in 1946. It occupies all of one floor, almost all of a mezzanine floor, eight floors of stack room, and nearly half of the basement. For lack of space in the building, two adjoining tenements are used for storage of little used duplicates.

The detailed administration is carried out by a librarian, Dr. Archibald Malloch, and an Assistant Librarian, Miss Janet Doe, both members and past officers of the Medical Library Association. The Library consists of five Departments, each with a "Head" and a number of assistants.

The Reference and Circulation Department is in charge of Miss Louise D. C. King, and six library-trained assistants, one other assistant and seven stack assistants. They serve readers not only in obtaining and delivering books from the stacks, but in answering innumerable requests for advice and information; these requests are also received by telephone and by mail. The magnitude of the service can only be appreciated by seeing and hearing what is going on.

On the shelves of the main reading room are bound volumes of over 500 of the most used journals and transactions issued during approximately the last ten years. These are immediately accessible at all times. For all books taken from the stacks there must be an order slip made out and later filed. When the day's work is over all books from the stacks are checked against the order slips and then replaced in the stacks, together with those taken from the shelves of the reading room. Fellows, and certain others, are allowed to take a limited number of books out for a definite time. For these a separate record is kept, and when the time allowed has expired, a request for their return must be made out and sent, sometimes more than once.

The Periodicals Department, administered by Mrs. Sarah Wilson George with two assistants, all library trained, and three other assistants, is in charge of unbound current issues of journals from all over the world. In 1946 it received 1,652 journals. Before the war caused the discontinuance of many, it received 2,320, some of which are beginning to appear again. As soon as a "volume" is completed, it is assembled in this department and prepared for the binder; when bound, it passes to the care of the Reference and Circulation Department.

The Catalogue Department is perhaps the most driven branch of the Library. One or more cards must be made for every new book, journal, and pamphlet, and it must also be entered on the "Shelf-List." Constant changes are being made in the catalogue. It is all very technical work, and requires the time of a "Head," Miss Duvall, a first assistant and four others, all library trained, and three other assistants.

The Bibliographical Department is constantly occupied in providing bibliographies, preparing abstracts, translations, and references on a multitude of subjects. It requires the time of a "Head," Miss Helen Sayer, and an assistant, both library trained.

The Rare Book and History Department is in charge of Miss Gertrude L. Annan and one assistant, both library trained. It is quartered in the beautiful Rare Book Room on the mezzanine floor. It has so outgrown its quarters that four other rooms have had to be used for the overflow. Here are stored all Incunabula, valuable old books, books on the history of medicine, manuscripts, diplomas, and the collection of photographs of distinguished physicians and scientists numbering over 9,500. The department also has charge of all articles of historical interest, and maintains a separate catalogue of all items in its care. The staff are constantly occupied in giving information of all kinds on matters of historical character.

A valuable part of the Library Service is the Photostat and Photograph Section, which reproduces old records, photographs, articles in current and old journals, and anything desired. In 1946, it made 39,920 photostats, 706 photographs, and 267 lantern slides for Fellows, subscribers of the Library, and the public. It is well run by two skilled assistants. Every request is checked and confirmed by a member of the staff of the Reference and Circulation Department, which occupies practically her entire time.

One of the best pieces of educational work done by the Academy is in aiding other medical libraries to build up their collections through Academy Library duplicates. During the years 1936–46, inclusive, 14,792 bound volumes and 152,807 issues of unbound journals were given away. Most of these gifts were made through the Exchange of the Medical Library Association, but since the close of World War II hundreds of books and magazines have gone to European and Asiatic libraries also.

The Library Staff also includes an entrance-desk assistant, who sees that every reader signs the register, answers general questions, and tells readers where to find what they are looking for; three assistants constantly employed in mending and marking books; a messenger-shipping clerk who handles all miscellaneous donations, and a library-trained "order assistant." They, as well as many others, perform other duties as occasion demands.

The Library is open to the public from 9 to 5 (temporarily 10.30 to 5) and to Fellows from 9 A.M. to 10 P.M., except on Saturdays and, during the summer, except Wednesdays, when it closes to all at 5 P.M. It is also at present closed on Sundays and certain holidays.

The Committee on Admissions, the only other Standing Committee elected by the Academy, now consists of twelve members, four retiring and four being elected each year. Its duty is to investigate the ethical, personal, and professional qualifications of each candidate for election. It makes its own rules, subject to the approval of the Council. It can refuse to recommend any candidate. It has no paid staff.

The Committee on Public Health Relations was founded in 1911. Its personnel consists of an Executive Secretary, Dr. E. H. L. Corwin, who has served continuously since that time, and five assistants. The thirty-five Committee members are appointed by the President each year, with the approval of the Council. Each of five County Medical Societies, New York, Kings, Queens, Bronx and Westchester, is represented by a Fellow of the Academy whom the County Society designates as its delegate. The Committee meets once a month from October to May, inclusive, and the Executive Committee every week.

It is constantly engaged in studies on important matters relating to public health in the broadest sense: hospitals, education, and welfare; organization and administration of City and State Departments; and the budgets of the city Department of Health and of Hospitals, and the Medical Examiner's office. By the vote of three-fourths of its members, and with the approval of the President, it is authorized to speak for the Academy on matters of public health interest.

The Board of Health appeals to the Committee for expert advice on medical problems which may require changes in the Sanitary Code of the city or the public health laws of the state. It holds many conferences with heads of departments and is in constant contact with the National, State and City Administrations. In addition to official agencies, the Committee serves as adviser on matters of health and hospitals to hundreds of voluntary agencies, local and national. Members of the Committee are designated by the Council to represent the Academy on the Health Council, Hospital Council, and Welfare Council and other bodies concerned in public health.

It arranges an occasional Stated Meeting of the Academy and has charge of the annual Hermann M. Biggs and A. Walter Suiter Memorial Lectures. Its work is so widespread that it is forced to call upon Fellows outside of its own members, and even outside of the Academy Fellowship, to serve on various subcommittees. During its more than thirty-five years of existence it has presented over 700 reports, many of which have been published and have received widespread comment.

The Committee on Medical Education is the result of the fusion, in the fall of 1924, of the "Society for the Advancement of Clinical Study in New York" (formed in 1912) and the "New York Association for Medical Education" (founded in 1919). Both had offices in the Academy, and the former had published a daily bulletin of surgical operations. The Committee is now composed of thirty members, appointed each year by the President, subject to the approval of the Council. It meets each month from October to May. Dr. Mahlon Ashford is the Executive Secretary and his staff numbers seven.

The By Laws of 1926 state that this Committee shall "take cognizance of any or all matters relating to *graduate* medical education in New York City or elsewhere," maintain a Bureau to give information regarding facilities for clinical study and opportunities for postgraduate instruction here and abroad, and publish bulletins of facilities for such instruction as occasion arises. The By Laws of 1940 broaden the field by including *all* medical education; the Committee's activities have been confined primarily to postgraduate education, almost from the first.

The Bureau of Medical Education publishes a daily bulletin of surgical operations, hospital conferences, rounds and lectures, as well as a weekly bulletin of medical clinics and non-operative clinics in medical and surgical specialties, and a synopsis of courses in postgraduate education. It has been doing this almost since its organization. It is consulted by hundreds of physicians on where and how to obtain general and special postgraduate instruction. Since 1941 it has maintained an "Inter-America Division," at the request of the State Department, to advise physicians from Central and South America. Since cessation of hostilities it has rendered assistance to hundreds of medical officers relieved from duty, in securing opportunities to round out their education, interrupted by the war.

The Committee has other and varied functions. In 1925 it inaugurated, and continues to arrange, the Friday afternoon lectures, twenty each year, on important medical subjects, given by distinguished speakers from all over the country.

In 1928 it arranged the first "Graduate Fortnight," consisting of evening lectures and daily demonstrations, hospital clinics, and an exhibit on the subject chosen. Each year, hundreds of physicians are attracted from all over the country and from other lands.

Up until 1926, the By Laws required two Stated Meetings each month, on the first and third Thursdays, from October to May. In February, 1926, this was changed to "such dates and at such times as the Council may prescribe." Since 1927 the programs for Stated Meetings have been planned by this Committee, and since October, 1928, the second Stated Meeting each month has been arranged and conducted by the Harvey Society "in affiliation with the New York Academy of Medicine," the Harvey Society retaining its complete autonomy.

Since 1930 the selection of recipients of the Bowen and Harlow Brooks Scholarships has been made by the Committee on Medical Education. The Committee also has charge of the annual exhibit illustrating "Progress in Therapy," to acquaint physicians with the "uses, limitations and dangers of new remedies" and with the "contributions of leading pharmaceutical companies in the development of these remedies." The annual exhibit opens with the Graduate Fortnight each year and is continued until spring. It is entirely revised during the summer. At the request of the United Hospital Fund, the Committee has advised on grants for experimental work by members of the Fund.

During the war, owing to the discontinuance of meetings of many of the special societies, the Committee also arranged a Research Symposium at which workers in the Metropolitan Area described their work. This was continued through 1946. Abstracts of the papers were published in the *Bulletin.* In addition to all these activities, this Committee publishes the folder of coming meetings at the Academy and edits the *Bulletin* of the Academy.

The Committee on Medical Information was established as a Standing Committee in 1939. Its purposes are:

1) to serve agents of public education as an interpreter of the mean-

ing, purposes and advances in medical and allied sciences;

2) to assist agencies of communication,—the press, radio, popular magazines and publishers—concerning medical and pharmaceutical matters, the reliability of statements thereon and in obtaining further authoritative information;
3) to furnish agencies of public information with reports of important actions or events at the Academy.
4) to answer requests for information from professional, public health, and social groups, industry, business, advertising, federal, local and foreign governments on matters relating to medicine and allied subjects;
5) to assist and guide physicians in their contacts with the press, radio and other publicity agencies;
6) to arrange and direct an annual series of lectures to the laity on medical subjects and matters of interest to them, and the publication of the same;
7) to conduct conferences on problems of interest to the professional health educator and public health worker;
8) to make from time to time, as needed, studies on subjects related to health education and the instruction of the public, cooperating with public and private organizations in so doing, and to publish important reports on such subjects.

The work of this extremely busy Committee requires the full time of its Executive Secretary, Dr. Iago Galdston, and three assistants. A group of over 200 special consultants is also available for opinions on special subjects.

The last Standing Committee, that on Sections, was established in 1930. It is composed of twenty-three members, a Vice-President appointed by the Council to serve as chairman, and the chairmen and secretaries of the eleven Sections. It meets at least three times a year, and takes "cognizance of all matters relating to the scientific work of the Academy, and shall consider ways and means of advancing the efficiency of the Sections." It does not have much to do, for each Section has an Advisory Committee of five who consult with officers of each Section in planning its program.

In addition to these six Standing Committees, a number of others (ten in 1946) are appointed annually by the President. For special purposes and only called upon occasionally, these committees are: Nominating, Revision of the By Laws, Honorary Fellowship and Medals, Gibbs Prize, Salmon Memorial, Louis Livingston Seaman Fund, Academy History, Professional Standards, and an Editorial Board of the Bulletin.

The only other Committee which really worked hard through 1946 was that on Medicine and the Changing Order; its work is terminated, but it will be reorganized and continue its activities.

Altogether on all committees there are 255 positions which are filled by 179 Fellows. Thus is organized The New York Academy of Medicine on completion of its first hundred years.

Index

THE HISTORY OF MEDICINE SERIES

ISSUED UNDER THE AUSPICES OF

THE LIBRARY OF THE NEW YORK ACADEMY OF MEDICINE

---

1. Incunabula scientifica et medica. By Arnold C. Klebs. A short title-list appeared in *Osiris,* IV (1938), 1–359.

2. De contagione, libri III. By Hieronymus Fracastorius. Venice, 1546. With translation and notes by Wilmer Cave Wright. New York & London: G. P. Putnam's Sons, 1930. Pp. 356.

3. Icones anatomicae. By Andreas Vesalius. New York: New York Academy of Medicine and the Library of the University of Munich, 1934. Ninety-five folio pages containing over two hundred woodcuts from the original blocks, together with one hundred and thirty pages of text.

4. A Bibliography of the Works of Ambroise Paré. By Janet Doe. Chicago: University of Chicago Press, 1937. Pp. 266.

5. How the President, Thomas Jefferson, and Doctor Benjamin Waterhouse Established Vaccination as a Public Health Procedure. By Robert H. Halsey. New York: The Author, 1936. Pp. 58. OUT OF PRINT.

6. The Role of Scientific Societies in the Seventeenth Century. By Martha Ornstein. Revised edition. Chicago: University of Chicago Press, 1938. Pp. 308.

7. De morbis artificum diatriba. By Bernardino Ramazzini. Latin text of 1713, revised, with translation and notes by Wilmer Cave Wright. Chicago: University of Chicago Press, 1940. Pp. 549. OUT OF PRINT.

8. The New York Academy of Medicine: Its First Hundred Years. By Philip Van Ingen. New York: Columbia University Press. 1949.